WORDS OF PRAISE FOR THE WORDS OF WISDOM IN
FEMININE HEALING

"Elias and Ketcham have gathered a harvest of ways to perceive, ways to center, ways to dance the dance of women's health. It is an offering cleverly crafted, modern in application, yet grandmotherly in wisdom."
—Dianne M. Connelly, Ph.D., author of *Traditional Acupuncture: The Law of the Five Elements* and *All Sickness Is Homesickness*

"Increasingly mainstream medicine is traveling the road paved by generations of natural healers. . . . FEMININE HEALING not only helps in paving that road, but in taking readers on a journey of self-awareness."
—Niels H. Lauresen, M.D., Ph.D., author of *Getting Pregnant: What Couples Need to Know* and *It's Your Body*

"A work of art . . . with practical recommendations."
—Wayne B. Jonas, M.D., co-editor of *Alternative Therapies in Health & Medicine*

"Blending tradition and current thinking, general advice and precise prescriptions, softness and strength, FEMININE HEALING is essential reading for the modern woman who seeks a wholesome, integrated understanding of her own biology."
—Valentin Fuster, M.D., Ph.D., director, Cardiovascular Institute, and dean for academic affairs, Mount Sinai Medical Center

"The essence of his book is centered on respect of human life forces brought together by [Elias's] impressive multiple healing experiences the world over. The book is a miraculous synthesis of his universal experience and the universality of his wonderful soul."
—Serafina Corsello, M.D., The Corsello Centers for Nutritional-Complementary Medicine

more . . .

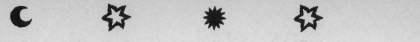

"Elias and Ketcham have written a book that is full of practical information, in a very tender and warm style . . . clearly a book that will prove to have value for women all their cycles, and all their 'seasons.'"
—Kenneth A. Bock, M.D., founder and director, Rhinebeck Health Center, Rhinebeck, New York, and Center for Progressive Medicine, Albany, New York

"A welcome voyage into the feminine healing spirit."
—Simon Y. Mills, author of *The Essential Book of Herbal Medicine* and director, Center for Complementary Health Studies, University of Exeter, UK

"The authors have done a remarkable job in illuminating both the soulful and practical paths that lead to this state of health and wholeness. FEMININE HEALING sets a new standard of integrity toward which all future health guides would do well to aspire."
—Joseph Jastrab, author of *Sacred Manhood, Sacred Earth*

"FEMININE HEALING is an inspirational journey toward self-awareness and complete health. By including a directory of twenty-one herbs and a description of the major acupuncture points, the reader has the foundations for personal holistic health awareness."
—*Horoscope* magazine

"Autobiographical and scholarly at the same time, this is a profound and many-layered volume with treasures for women and men, consumers and healthcare professionals alike."
—*Health Inform*

"Elias illustrates how acupuncture, herbs, diet, and, importantly, understanding underlying emotional issues can correct imbalances, release vital energy, and remedy problems with menopause, osteoporosis, and PMS."
—*Publishers Weekly*

"Both comprehensive and practical for today's woman. I highly recommend it as an indispensable companion on our collective journey toward wholeness. Rarely have I encountered so many pearls of women's wisdom in one volume! This book is a must for everyone interested in women, the feminine, and healing."
—Christiane Northrup, M.D., author of *Women's Bodies, Women's Wisdom*

JASON ELIAS *and*
KATHERINE KETCHAM

FEMININE HEALING

A

Woman's Guide

to a

Healthy

Body, Mind,

and Spirit

WARNER BOOKS

A Time Warner Company

Grateful acknowledgment is made to reprint from the following:

Jacob the Baker by Noah Benshea, © 1989 by Noah Benshea, reprinted by permission of Villard Books, a Division of Random House, Inc.

Daughters of Copper Woman by Anne Cameron, © 1981 by Anne Cameron, reprinted by permission of Press Gang Publishers, Vancouver, Canada.

Tao Te Ching by Stephen Mitchell, translation © 1988 by Stephen Mitchell, reprinted by permission of HarperCollins Publishers, Inc.

"The Tale of the Sands" from *Tales of the Dervishes* by Idries Shah, © 1967 by Idries Shah, used by permission of Dutton Signet, a division of Penguin Books USA, Inc.

Originally published as *In the House of the Moon*

Warner Books, Inc., 1271 Avenue of the Americas, New York, NY 10020

Visit our Web site at
http://warnerbooks.com

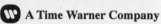 A Time Warner Company

Printed in the United States of America
First Trade Printing: September 1997
10 9 8 7 6 5 4 3 2 1

Library of Congress Cataloging-in-Publication Data
Elias, Jason.
 [In the house of the moon]
 Feminine healing: a woman's guide to a healthy body, mind, and spirit / Jason Elias and Katherine Ketcham.
  p.   cm.
 Previously published in 1995 by Warner Books under the title: In the house of the moon.
 Includes bibliographical references and index.
 ISBN 0-446-67271-8
 1. Women—Health and hygiene. 2. Alternative medicine. 3. Healing 4. Mind and body. I. Ketcham, Katherine, 1949—. II. Title.
RA778.E394   1997
613'.04244—dc21
                                        97-20474
                                         CIP

Cover design and illustration by John Martinez
Book design, moon phase art, and acupuncture point illustrations by Giorgetta Bell McRee
Illustrations of the five elements by Jeanne McMenemy

ACKNOWLEDGMENTS

"All wisdom is plagiarism; only stupidity is original."
—*Hugh Kerr*

Whatever wisdom we can claim in this book comes to us as a gift from ancient sages and modern-day wise women and men who have shaped our search for meaning with their intelligence and grace. Because this work is co-authored, we offer separate acknowledgments.

To my teachers who have gently shaped my mind and spirit, I offer my deepest respect and gratitude. I first learned that the answers to life's most basic questions must come from within while working at a psychiatric hospital and reading Fritz Perls's autobiography, *In and Out of the Garbage Pail*; Perls's vision reframed my own and initiated my odyssey to Esalen in the summer of 1969. At Esalen and later in New York, Ilana Rubenfeld took me in, sharing her vision of the continuity of mind, body, and spirit.

Moshe Feldenkrais and Ida Rolf helped me to understand the wisdom of the body and showed me how to approach the body as a doorway to the mind and spirit. Judy Leibowitz, Debbie Caplan, Aileen Crow, Rachel Zahn, and Sarnie Ogus, friends and teachers of the Alexander technique, helped me find a softer way to access the body's innate wisdom. David Elizalde and Helen Morgante accepted me into their hearts and homes and taught me the power of psychic surgery, initiating a nice Jewish boy from Brooklyn into the Church of the Black Nazarene in the Philippines. Bhagwan Rajneesh opened my eyes to the light of ancient wisdom. Mark Seem, director of the Tri-State Institute of Traditional Chinese Medicine, always encouraged me to develop my own style of acupuncture. Bob Duggan, founder of the Traditional Acupuncture Institute, continues to teach me to trust the metaphoric gifts inherent in acupuncture; his genuine warmth and compassion are the signs of a true healer. My dear friend and mentor Simon Mills introduced me to the fine art of herbal medicine; in our summer sojourns into the English moors, I learned a deep and abiding reverence for Mother Earth. Ted Kaptchuk shared his vision of the essence of Chinese herbal medicine, offering invaluable insights into the "spirit" of the herbs. Leon Hammer, beloved friend and teacher, took me into his heart, showed me how to integrate Chinese medicine and Western psychology, and always emphasized that "the kingdom of heaven lies within."

Numerous friends have offered encouragement, love, trust, and support. Rupa Cousins enriched my life and catalyzed my encounter with Rolling Thunder. I am deeply grateful to Nancy Hutchins for her friendship and for introducing me to my literary agent, Janis Vallely. On faith alone Janis agreed to represent me, and her spirit and grace guided the book from its inception to its publication. Kathy Ketcham came into my life as a writer and co-author; through the process of researching and writing this book together, she became my spiritual soul mate. Both Kathy and I are equally indebted to the publishing pros at Warner Books, and especially to our editor, Colleen Kapklein.

My clients allowed me to share in their transformative experiences and gave me permission to include their stories in this book; for their trust and faith, I am deeply grateful. Inanna Champagne introduced me to the work of Brooke Medicine Eagle, Carol Pepper-Cooper gifted me with her "clipping" skills, and Martha Frankl generously offered friendly literary advice.

I am deeply indebted to the following friends and colleagues for their consulting skills and advice on the manuscript: Arya Nielson, M.A., L.Ac., for her support and counsel on the Chinese medical aspects; Susun Weed, wise woman herbalist, for her advice on gynecological herbs; Carol Robbins, D.C., for sharing her knowledge of women's health issues; Jennifer Houston, midwife and educator, for her insights into the emotional and psychological aspects of women's health; Larry Perl, gynecologist and obstetrician, for his advice and suggestions for improvements; Serafina Corsello, physician, healer, and supreme nurturer, for invaluable assistance and counsel; Marc Grossman and David Lester, friends and co-founders of Integral Health Associates, for their support and constant encouragement; Berkana Gervais for her organizational skills and sense of humor; and especially Sil Reynolds, R.N., nurse practitioner, for so generously sharing her wisdom and opening her heart to me and to the book.

My family gave me many precious memories of the past, which support me firmly in the present and give me hope for the future. My father, brothers, and sister gifted me with a sense of home and the security of knowing I could always count on them. Uncle Pincus and Aunt Sulica offered me their precious memories of my great-grandmother, my father's childhood, and the Holocaust. My mother's constant love and acceptance allowed me to be true to myself. To my wife, Birgit, and my son, Adam, I owe the largest debt of thanks, for my consuming relationship with "the book" took many hours away from our time together; I am forever grateful for their unquestioning love and support.

—JASON ELIAS

I am profoundly grateful to my father, Frank Ketcham, for his passion, sense of humor, and the lessons he taught me about life and death. Joan Davidson Ketcham's kind heart and gentle spirit continue to influence my life in subtle and mysterious ways. Dick Nagle, my first cousin, showed me that the moon rises; in that moment and many others, he has been the guiding spirit of my life. Mike, John, Billy, and Debbie, my brothers and sisters, teach me still about the meaning of home and the power of love to transcend disagreement. Melinda, Marilyn, Sharon and Julie, friends for a lifetime, continually remind me about the depth and breadth of love women can offer to each other. Jane Dystel, my literary agent, gently but firmly guides my career and shelters me from the more mundane aspects of the publishing world. Ernest Kurtz introduced me to the power of storytelling and continues to send me precious stories to feed my soul. Sarah Blattler, interlibrary loan assistant at Whitman College, offered invaluable assistance in completing the endnotes. Kevin Scribner loaned me many books from his eclectic lending library and reminded me that "what goes around comes around."

Jason Elias, one of the most compassionate human beings I have ever been privileged to meet, brings a new dimension to the term "co-author"; I cherish his friendship and his gentle, illuminating wisdom.

Patrick Spencer, my husband and best friend, embodies all that is good and gentle and kind in male and female alike. And Robyn, Alison, and Benjamin Spencer, the most precious gifts of my life, forgive me for all my imperfections and remind me every day about the real meaning of life.

—KATHERINE KETCHAM

DISCLAIMER

The information herein is not intended to replace the services of trained health professionals. You are advised to consult with your health care professional with regard to matters relating to your health, and in particular regarding matters that may require diagnosis or medical attention.

CONTENTS

PRELUDE

The day my father died, my uncle Pincus and his family arrived to "sit shiva," the Jewish family tradition of celebrating and honoring the spirit of the dead. Night after night, long after everyone else had gone to sleep, Pincus and I stayed up crying, laughing, and telling stories about the past. Pincus told me about his family's decision to smuggle my father, just thirteen years old but young and fearless, aboard a Greek cargo ship sailing to Manhattan, where, it was hoped, he would make his fortune and send for the rest of the family to join him. But World War II intervened, and eight members of my father's family died in the ovens at Auschwitz. Only my grandmother Nona and her son Pincus, who lost his wife and three children at Auschwitz, survived. After the war, my father sent for Nona, Pincus, his new wife, Sulica, and their two young children, and for years we lived together as one family—broken but whole.

In those first days after my father's death, Pincus gave me the gift of his memories of his older brother, my father; as the nights wore on into the early-morning hours, he inevitably wandered farther back in time, sharing his recollections of childhood on the Greek island of Kastoria. My great-grandmother loomed large in these remembrances, for she was the much-loved island healer, a tiny woman with astonishing resources of energy whom the islanders called "the little doctor." Brewing her complicated herbal potions in a cast-iron pot suspended above an open-hearth fire, ministering to the sick and the dying with her healing herbs, gentle hands, and rich collection of prayers and incantations, my great-grandmother allegedly performed many miracles. One time, as legend has it, she secluded herself in a one-room hut with a young man who was dying of a dread disease. When they emerged three days later, the dying man was completely restored to health and lived to tell his grandchildren about his experiences of death and rebirth at the hands of "the little doctor."

My great-grandmother's healing powers were passed down to her daughter, my grandmother, who lived with our family in Brooklyn until she died of pneumonia at age seventy-six. Whenever one of her grandchildren caught a cold or the flu, Nona would toss a handful of strange-smelling herbs into a special pot simmering on the kitchen stove and after much tasting and clucking over her treasured recipes, she would offer the vile-tasting brew to her reluctant *"bubbas,"* encouraging us with a mixture of Yiddish, Greek, and Spanish phrases intended to make the medicine more palatable. When a sickness was particularly tenacious, Nona would cover our naked bodies with healing balms and strategically place the glass *bonka* cups on our backs to draw up the "bad" energy and release it through the pores of the skin. Onions were just the thing for abrasions; cucumbers worked wonders for bruises and black eyes; and if everything else failed, there was always chicken soup, the all-purpose remedy for injuries to body, mind, or spirit.

As I talked with Uncle Pincus in the days after my father died, listening to his stories of my great-grandmother and sharing my cherished memories of Nona, I began to understand the power of the blood that coursed through me. I was my father's son, but it was his mother's and grandmother's blood mixed with my mother's loving support that directed my destiny, for like my female ancestors, I was fascinated by the art of healing and the complex interconnections between body, mind, and spirit. In college, I majored in psychology and was immediately drawn to the humanistic psychology of Maslow and Perls and the writings of Carl Jung, who was heavily influenced by Eastern philosophy, noting in his foreword to the Chinese classic *The I Ching* that "the thoughts of the old masters are of greater value to me than the philosophical prejudices of the Western mind."

But my father had always disapproved of my interest in psychology and healing. "That stuff is for women, not for men," he used to chide me, clearly hoping that I would toughen up and show an interest in the family wholesale clothing business. My brother, Butch, who during his high school years led the teenage street gang called the Garrisons (so named because they wore studded Garrison belts that doubled as weapons), agreed with my father that I was at risk of becoming "a yellow-bellied sissy"—certainly the worst thing that could happen to a Jewish boy in the Brooklyn ghetto known as Hell's Kitchen. And so I acted tough, excelled at the rough-and-tumble sports, swaggered and whistled at the girls like Butch taught me, but I always felt like a fraud. I grew up knowing that somehow I didn't fit, for my behavior was perpetually at odds with the softer, more empathic and intuitive side of my nature, which was fascinated by the intricate relationships between human beings and haunted by the ghosts of female relatives who devoted their lives to caring for others.

The summer after my father's death I traveled to Big Sur, California, to study Gestalt therapy at the Esalen Institute, where I met and trained with such luminaries as Ilana and Frank Rubenfeld, Ida Rolf, Alan Watts, Al Huang, and Joseph Campbell. At Esalen, I began to understand that the gentler side of my nature, which was so powerfully drawn to the world of psychology and connected so strongly to the sufferings of others, was in fact my strength rather than my weakness. With that dawning awareness, I began the process of accepting back into myself the complicated emotions and spiritual yearnings that I had spent so much of my youth trying to disown.

When I returned to New York after that summer at Esalen and began studying for my master's degree in psychology, I felt strengthened and renewed; for the first time in my life, I knew that I had nothing to hide. My friends looked at me sideways, commenting that I seemed different— more "together," even more masculine. I was deeply affected by the irony, for I knew that what they were witnessing on the outside was precisely what I had been experiencing on the inside: a sense of the torn and broken pieces being stitched back together again, mending, healing, becoming a whole. Because the male and female aspects of my nature were finally learning how to complement and complete each other, I was no longer at war with myself.

After several years of private practice in New York City as a psychotherapist, I decided to use the small inheritance my father left me to travel around the world and study various healing traditions. I was particularly interested in the age-old concept of energy healing, for every major world culture (except ours) practices a variation of the ancient art of laying on of hands, using invisible sources of spiritual energy to guide and invigorate the healing process. In my own practice I had witnessed the astonishing effects of the mind and the spirit on the body's ability to fight illness and disease, but because the Western medical world remained stubbornly skeptical about healing methods that involved the spirit, I knew I had to look elsewhere for answers to my questions.

In Japan, I continued my studies of Aikido, the art of using your opponent's energy *(ki)* to defeat him. Like the Chinese martial art Tai Chi, Aikido taps into the quintessentially "female" power of receptivity and yielding. The Aikido master feels the negative energy approaching him, moves out of its way before it can harm him, and then uses his inner strength to turn the energy back against his attacker, rendering him powerless. Aikido and Tai Chi seek to emulate the power of water, which is fluid and yielding but over time is capable of wearing down even the highest mountains. The ancient Chinese philosopher Lao-tzu described the nature of water's soft power in his beautiful collection of poems titled *Tao te Ching:*

> *Nothing in the world*
> *is as soft and yielding as water.*
> *Yet for dissolving the hard and inflexible,*
> *nothing can surpass it.*
>
> *The soft overcomes the hard;*
> *the gentle overcomes the rigid.*
> *Everyone knows this is true,*
> *but few can put it into practice.*

In the Philippines, I studied psychic surgery, a bizarre healing art that finds its roots in the unlikely mixture of fervent Catholicism and tribal superstition. I watched psychic surgeons reach into patients' bodies, using their hands as instruments to remove blood clots and tumors. Although no anesthetic was used, the patients appeared to feel no pain whatsoever and, after the procedure, would pronounce themselves cured, walking home in their blood-stained clothing with rapturous looks on their faces. While psychic surgery is unmistakably aggressive and invasive, the healers believe that they are merely the receptacles for the healing powers of Jesus, the Virgin Mary, and ancient tribal spirits. Their faith guides them into the spirit world, where they claim to tap into a powerful healing energy capable of restoring health and vitality to the sick and wounded.

After six months in the Philippines, I traveled to Hong Kong, where I apprenticed with a Chinese acupuncturist and herbalist and witnessed firsthand the dramatic effects of these ancient healing arts on disorders ranging from ovarian cysts to arthritis to migraines. The Chinese believe that the human body is covered with a matrix of energy channels flowing along specific meridians; by intervening in the energy system through the use of acupuncture needles, massage, herbs, and various lifestyle changes, imbalances in the *chi*[1] (energy) are corrected, and health is restored.

My final stop was India, where I lived in a spiritual community known as an ashram, and studied Ayurveda, the ancient art of Indian medicine in which the energy of the mind and spirit is thought to balance the life force *(prana)*, which flows through numerous invisible channels in the body. Ayurveda employs diagnostic techniques similar to those used by the Chinese, such as pulse and tongue analyses, and relies on the healing actions of herbs, yoga, breathing exercises, various ritual purgings, diet, meditation, and prayer to keep the *prana* in balance and harmony.

In all these cultures and healing traditions, the underlying themes are the same. The body, mind, and spirit are considered essential parts of the whole, and thus an imbalance in one area necessarily affects the entire system. If the disharmony is not corrected, pain and discomfort result, and if these symptoms are not adequately addressed, illness and disease may occur. Balance is created by living in harmony with nature and with other human beings, remaining flexible and adaptable, and opening the mind and the spirit to the healing energies that flow in, through, and around our being. All the healers with whom I studied and trained approached their patients with humility, openly acknowledging that they were merely a vehicle to assist the body, mind, and spirit in the healing process and using as their primary interventions the archetypally feminine traits of tender care, gentle touch, or massage, close attention to behavior and temperament, sensitivity to the individual's emotional needs and spiritual longings, and the deep-rooted belief that health and happiness cannot be sustained without a reverence for nature and a willingness to live in harmony with her eternal laws.

When I returned to the United States in 1974, I established a private

[1] We choose to use the phonetic spelling of *qi*.

practice using a combination of psychotherapy, acupressure, massage, and the basic philosophical tenets of energy healing. As time went on, I was increasingly drawn to the philosophy and practice of Traditional Chinese Medicine, which I believed captured most eloquently and effectively the wisdom of the ancient healing arts. In 1980, I enrolled in a three-year training program in the techniques of traditional acupuncture; after I was certified and licensed as an acupuncturist, I spent three summers in England with herbalist Simon Mills and later completed a two-year certification program in Chinese herbal medicine.

My practice gradually evolved to the point where acupuncture and herbal medicine became my mainstays, for Traditional Chinese Medicine offered the unifying metaphor that helped to bring the body, mind, and spirit into a dynamic whole. Approximately 75 percent of my clients were women, with problems ranging from recurrent acne to infertility and from fibroids to osteoporosis. No matter what their age, medical history, or background happened to be, my female clients seemed to intuitively understand the connections between body, mind, and spirit and the need to look beyond the physical symptoms of pain and discomfort to the deeper emotional and spiritual issues that underlie all illness and disease.

As I worked with them, I kept recalling Lao-tzu's famous dictum "The more you know, the less you understand." Indeed, the more experience I had, the more humble I became, for I realized that my task was to use insights, metaphors, stories, and reassurances to open the door to healing, and then step out of the way to give the seeds of change space to germinate and grow. My role as a participant in the healing process was to guide without interfering, helping my patients to become whole by locating, reclaiming, and reintegrating the lost and broken parts of the self. I even began to mistrust the word *healer*, because it implied that I was responsible for restoring health when I was, in fact, only contributing to the powerful process of self-healing. In truth my patients guided me, for they intuitively understood where they were most deeply wounded. If I asked the right questions, they invariably led me, with great courage and resolve, to the root of the problem.

As I continued to witness the astonishing impact of Traditional Chinese Medicine on my patients' innate powers of self-healing, I began to think about writing a book on "complementary medicine." So many of my patients talked about their feelings of hopelessness and powerlessness after encounters with Western medicine; they all told me similar stories about seeking out alternative therapies in the hope that they would be treated like a whole human being with a mind and a soul rather than just a physical body with a specific diagnosed illness. But if Western medicine fails in terms of its ability to relate to the whole human being, it is enormously successful in diagnosing and treating acute, life-threatening illnesses. Traditional Chinese Medicine and other ancient healing arts, which emphasize prevention and gentle healing techniques, cannot provide all the answers to the problems and plagues of the modern world—even the Chinese are quick to look for a Western doctor when a situation is life-threatening and a dramatic intervention is required. It seemed to me that we needed to create a partnership in which East and West could merge their separate strengths to create a system of healing that transcends the limitations of both. Western medicine would provide the advanced technology and life-saving interventions, while Eastern medicine would be used to prevent disease and reconnect the patient to the emotional and spiritual ramifications of illness.

I took my idea to literary agent Janis Vallely, and when she expressed interest in the book, I suggested that she come to my office for a treatment, hoping to assure her that my work was deeply grounded in age-old wisdom. Janis and I talked for two hours, I took her pulses and examined her tongue, needled six points on the Liver meridian to get the energy flowing through the "stuck" channels, told her several teaching stories, and prescribed a healing tonic of Native American and Chinese herbs. Janis pronounced herself "amazed" by the energy she felt coursing through her after just one treatment, and with mounting enthusiasm, we sat down to discuss the book.

"You keep talking about your female patients and how much they teach you about the healing process," Janis commented at one point. "Why not focus your book on the problems affecting so many women in our modern-day culture, offering your perspective as an acupuncturist and herbalist and interspersing the narrative with case histories and teaching stories?"

I was intrigued with the idea, but I knew that I couldn't presume to speak or write for women. I needed a female guide who could take me into the soul of the female experience and help me communicate the lyricism and poetry of Chinese energetics. Janis contacted veteran literary agent Jane Dystel, and Jane immediately recommended Katherine Ketcham for the project. From my very first conversation with Kathy, I knew that I had discovered a soul mate, for ours was a spontaneous, heartfelt connection. As we discussed our dreams for the book, we realized that they were the same dreams, which led us to the awareness that the feminine spirit of healing was guiding even the writing of this book—the book, it seemed, was creating itself, gently encouraging us to follow its lead.

As the weeks of researching, organizing, and writing stretched into months and then years, *In the House of the Moon* took on a spirit of its own. We understood that we needed to go backward before we could move forward; we had to go deeper than the practical information, deeper even than the philosophy and poetry, and travel back into the distant past to the time when the words *feminine* and *healing* were synonymous. Thus, the first part of the book evolved into a quest for "the lost keys," the bits and pieces of wisdom that were systematically destroyed as Western civilization became increasingly driven by the need to dominate and control, and the art of healing gradually metamorphosed into the science of medicine with its precise delineations of body and mind.

But the feminine spirit of healing was never wholly lost. While the Western world was becoming increasingly enamored of heroic treatments and chemical cures, doggedly pursuing the analytical, linear pathway to knowledge, the Eastern world remained firmly rooted in the vital connections between health, healing, and wholeness. In part II, we explore the lyrical pragmatism of ancient Chinese thought, offering a detailed look at the diagnostic framework of the "Five Transforming Powers." Every human being has a distinct constitutional attraction to one of these powers, and this "affinity" influences her body, mind, and spirit in profound ways. When she understands the nature of the powers that flow through her, she can learn how to recognize when they are out of balance and initiate the process of self-healing that lies at the heart of all traditional healing methods.

In part III, we celebrate the seasons of a woman's life, reframing the transitional stages of puberty, motherhood, menopause, and advancing age (the wisdom-gathering years) as the quintessential stages for tapping into the innate power of the female spirit. Female blood is life giving and life sustaining; through her monthly cycles a woman is given the opportunity to strengthen and revitalize her connections to the natural world. When she gives her blood away every month, she participates in the mysterious, ongoing cycle of life, death, and rebirth; when her cycles begin to wane and eventually cease during the menopausal years, she gives the gift of the blood back to herself, fortifying her body while cleansing and renewing her spirit for the challenges and adventures that await her in the final decades of her life.

In many Native American cultures the power of menstrual blood has been revered as the sacred source of life, and women have been held in awe and respect as the vitalizing force capable of generating and sustaining life. During the time of their bleeding, women have retreated to the Moon Lodge to rest, reflect, dream, and gather wisdom. In the House of the Moon, they learn how to live in harmony with the moon's cycles, nurturing their bodies, concentrating their mental energies, and refining their spirits. With each lunar cycle, women feel the moon pull on their inner tides, drawing them deeper into the shadows and dark mysteries. Just as the moon sheds her shadow to be born again, so do women shed their blood in an ongoing process of renewal and regeneration. Filling with light and emptying into darkness, the moon has come to symbolize the dynamic, eternal nature of life, and women, because their bodies are privileged to follow these natural cycles, carry within their hearts and souls the moon's gentle wisdom.

In the House of the Moon seeks to honor the cyclic, sacred nature of the female experience, offering insights and suggestions for strengthening our connections with the world of mind and soul. These lessons are culled from female experience, but they are not for women alone; men can also learn how to reclaim the healing wisdom of the female spirit and use it to create wholeness in their lives. "When male and female combine," counsels *The I Ching*, "all things achieve harmony."

PART I

THE
LOST
KEYS

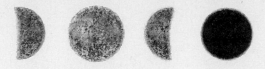

CHAPTER 1

A SENSE OF BALANCE

What can we gain by sailing to the moon
if we are not able to cross the abyss
that separates us from ourselves?
——*Thomas Merton*

If you want to become whole,
let yourself be partial.
If you want to become straight,
let yourself be crooked.
If you want to become full,
let yourself be empty.
If you want to be reborn,
let yourself die.
If you want to be given everything,
give everything up.
——Tao te Ching

The ability to yield and to flow—to merge, melt, and unite—carries within its heart the understanding that all of life is a circle with no beginning and no end. What modern American culture has come to imagine as two rigid parallel lines—male and female, dark and light, night and day, sun and moon, heaven and earth, life and death—are, in truth, two gentle arcs bending toward each other, curving until they join forces and continue on as one, unbroken, whole, complete. We are all, male and female alike, part of the circle of life, what the Native Americans call the sacred hoop, and the Chinese call tao.

When illness threatens, when we are wounded in body, mind, or spirit, when we are separated from the whole of which we were once part, we feel pain, grief, and fragmentation, that feeling of coming apart at the seams that William James, translating from the German *zerissenheit*, called "torn-to-pieces-hood." At these times, we experience a craving for wholeness, a yearning for serenity, a healing for our torn-to-pieces-hood.

How can we begin to heal our wounded nature and become whole once again? The feminine spirit of healing teaches that the first essential step to wholeness requires coming out of ourselves and reaching out toward others. For only when we operate at "the level of the heart," as Joseph Campbell explains in *The Power of Myth*, are we able to "move out of the field of animal action into a field that is properly human and spiritual." This awakening to the heart is made possible by the wholly human ability to feel compassion—to participate in another person's suffering so fully that their pain and anguish become our own. Compassion involves the recognition that we are all wounded, and that only by joining together can we heal the injuries to body, mind, and spirit and become whole again.

This ancient insight continues to be honored by many modern-day healers. One of my favorite modern healing stories is told by Dr. Rachel Remen, who relates her experiences with a twenty-four-year-old cancer patient whose leg had been surgically removed at the hip. Recovery was slow and painful, for the young man could not imagine himself as anything other than a shattered replica of his former self. In one therapy session he drew a picture of a vase with a jagged crack running through it and insisted that his body, like the vase, was broken and therefore useless.

As time passed, however, he began to emerge from his isolation and self-pity and open up to others who were also wounded and despairing. Through his very vulnerability—his woundedness—he achieved a heightened sensibility to the sufferings of others. One day, while looking at his early drawings, he announced that the picture of the cracked vase wasn't finished. Pointing to the black line running through the vase, he explained that it was there—in the broken places—that the light shines through. Then he drew streams of light radiating outward from the crack.

Like so many stories, this is actually a story within a story within a story, a wondrous unfolding of questions within answers within questions. As the young man journeyed through his pain and loss to discover the healing power of compassion and other-centeredness, he was privileged to participate in the feminine spirit of healing as it has been practiced throughout the ages. His physician, certainly a wise woman healer in the ancient sense, understood that even though his disease was cured, he was not yet whole. With compassion and great patience, she relied on the healing power of metaphors, images, and cleansing soul-talk to take the healing process deep into the heart and soul. Over time, the patient realized that he was not alone in his suffering, and he began to come out of himself and reach out toward others. Fractured and broken, he became whole again with help from others who were also wounded and who needed his assistance with their healing journey. The "cracks" in his body, mind, and spirit did not diminish his strength but, instead, created the space and thus the potential for the light of compassion and concern to shine through and illuminate the darkness. When he accepted himself—*I am what I am, wounds and all*—he created himself anew.

All healing is concerned with balance and harmony, for healing is the act and art of restoring to wholeness that which has been broken apart. From the very beginning of human time, healing has been considered a feminine art, embodied in the loving, nurturing relationship between a mother and her child. Women are life-givers, but they are also life-sustainers who understand that the healer's most powerful ally is simple human contact—the willingness to listen, to guide without interfering, to touch with tenderness, to respect the body's inherent capacity for self-healing. Healers have always sought to imitate the mother/child relationship, offering tender compassion, intuitive wisdom, images, metaphors, myths, and stories to soothe the wounds of body, mind, and spirit.

Illness and disease are considered symptoms of a deeper disorder, guiding the healer to look beyond the superficial aches and pains for potential disruptions or disharmonies in the relationships between the individual and her family, community, and Mother Earth. While the physical wounds are tended, careful attention is paid to the broken connections, discordant relationships, and unfulfilled longings that continue to divide and do injury to the whole.

Healers from time immemorial have understood the wisdom of the spirit and the ways in which a sick spirit can make itself known through various physical and mental symptoms. With sensitivity and compassion, they have sought to restore the severed connections, knowing that the health and integrity of the whole depends on the balance and harmony of each individual part.

In the last several hundred years, however, the ancient art of attending to body, mind, and spirit as equal, essential elements to health and wholeness has been systematically dismantled. The body and mind have been separated into distinct, disconnected realities, while the spirit has been relegated to a minor role, considered of interest only to the philosophically inclined. As healing has evolved into a scientific discipline consumed with solutions, and as the science of medicine has come to dominate and overshadow the ancient art of healing, we have lost our sense of balance and essential harmony. The classically feminine virtues of spiritual nurturance, love of peace and harmony, and sensitivity to the needs of others have been subordinated and suppressed in a world increasingly enamored of the archetypally masculine ideals of competition, confrontation, and conquest.

As cooperation has given way to competition, synthesis to analysis, and intuitive wisdom to rational knowledge, the dynamic balance between the male and female aspects of the human experience and their complementary modes of knowledge (what the Chinese call yin and yang) has been disturbed. In this last decade of the twentieth century, we feel the long-term effects of this imbalance. We are dangerously off-kilter, swinging precariously on the bent axis of a fractured consciousness. Every one of our relationships is affected, for as sages and saints from all cultures and traditions teach, everything in life is connected. Our sense of kinship and connection to our families, our communities, our own bodies, minds, and spirits, and the earth itself suffer from the loss of the nurturing and regenerative powers of feminine wisdom and experience. Favoring mind over body, we have lost our soul—the compassionate, healing center of the human experience.

How do we begin the process of restoring balance and putting the broken pieces back together again? Healing necessarily begins with recognition of our woundedness and the need for relationships—male *and* female, logic *and* intuition, analysis *and* synthesis, mind *and* body *and* spirit—to mend the wounds and create the balance that underlies wholeness. In its most basic form, healing is awareness—the art of being awake and aware of the moment as it is happening, not in spite of our wounds but because of our wounds, which remind us that only by reaching out to each other can we find the self. Our symptoms of pain, fear, and dislocation are the means of our salvation, for they remind us that something is wrong and that it needs to be put right again.

As we grope in the dark for the answers to our questions, we discover that we are not alone, and this insight guides us slowly but surely toward the light of healing and wholeness. In one of my favorite collections of modern stories, a simple man known as Jacob the Baker affirms the need to unite together in order to overcome our fear and confusion.

> *A neighbor of Jacob's needed to start on a journey, but it was the middle of the night.*
> *Afraid to begin, afraid not to begin . . . he came to Jacob.*
> *"There is no light on the path," he complained.*
> *"Take someone with you," counseled Jacob.*
> *"Jacob, what do you mean? If I do that, there will be two blind men."*
> *"You are wrong," said Jacob. "If two people discover each other's blindness, it is already growing light."*

Healing, as Jacob the Baker understands, is a matter of meaning, a deeply moral response that affirms the inherent integrity of the human body, mind, and spirit. Healing looks beyond the self to others who are in pain, requiring a kind heart, a listening ear, and an open mind. The other-centeredness of healing is crucial, for isolation intensifies our suffering, while community—that sense of knowing that our lives matter to someone beyond ourselves—is the wellspring, the very source of our humanity.

Healing begins with questions—*Where did I come from? Who am I? How am I to live my life?*—but it can proceed only if we are willing to acknowledge that with each answer we discover, we sink deeper into the question. John Updike once said that a problem with a solution is not a problem. Gertrude Stein was even more forceful. "There ain't no answer. There ain't going to be any answer. There never has been an answer. That's the answer."

As we begin the journey to rediscover the ancient art of healing, we will dance with the question of what it means to be *wholly* human. *In the House of the Moon* will not provide the one, final answer to this question, for even the presumption that one answer will suffice diverts us from the mysteries we seek to explore. Rather than follow the analytical straight line away from the territory of heart and soul, this book expands the boundaries of both questions and answers by telling stories, myths, parables, and legends, which circumnavigate the globe of human consciousness and inevitably, miraculously, bring us back home to ourselves.

> *There once was a child made all of salt who yearned to know who she was and where she had come from. One day she embarked on a long journey, traveling to many foreign lands to seek the answers to her questions. Eventually she came to the coastline of a vast ocean.*
>
> *"How wonderful!" she exclaimed, putting one foot in the water.*
>
> *"Don't be afraid," the ocean whispered to her, "for if you continue, you will find what you seek."*
>
> *The salt child put her other foot in the water and waded deeper and deeper, her body dissolving with each step. When she was fully immersed, she cried out in a voice filled with wonder, "Ah, now I know who I am."*

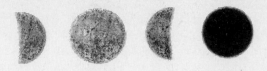

CHAPTER 2

THE WISDOM OF THE WHOLE

All know that the drop merges into the ocean but few know that the ocean merges into the drop.

—*Kabir*

Your vision will become clear only when you can look into your own heart. Who looks outside, dreams; who looks inside, awakes.

—*Carl Jung*

In the point of rest at the center of our being, we encounter a world where all things are at rest in the same way. Then a tree becomes a mystery, a cloud a revelation, each man a cosmos of whose riches we can only catch glimpses. The life of simplicity is simple, but it opens to us a book in which we never get beyond the first syllable.

—*Dag Hammarskjöld*

In the far distant past our ancestors imagined the world as a circle, with every location along its arcing curve at once the beginning and the end, the original and the final point. All of life was contained within the circle, and human beings assumed the responsibility of maintaining balance and harmony by strengthening the spiritual connections between the creatures of the earth and the forces of the universe. But as the centuries passed, the harmony of the whole began to matter less than the value of each individual part, and the spirit of kinship and unity gave way to the pursuit of self-interest. Holes and tears appeared in the delicate fabric of the sacred hoop, and the structure began to break apart into separate, disjointed pieces. The wisdom of the old ways was scattered to the four winds, and even the stories were lost, for storytelling and listening require an appreciation of the balance and harmony of life.

As humans severed their connections with the spirit world and its dark mysteries, our hands came unclasped, and we drifted off to confront the seemingly hostile universe alone and without the aid or comfort of others. Dazed by the seething intensity of the unfamiliar, we wandered far off track, experiencing the deep, haunting emptiness that all children feel when they are separated from their families and long for the welcoming nearness of home. Straying farther and farther from the center, we became disconnected from each other and from the whole of which we were once part. In our fear and confusion, we began to break the world into smaller, more manageable pieces, hoping that in the fragments, we might discover the wisdom that would help us to reclaim what we had lost.

A well-known story centers on this sense of dislocation and the yearning to reconnect the pieces in order to recreate the whole. I remember my mother reading a version of this story to me when I was five or six years old. Listening to her voice, with its old-world lilting charm, I would shut my eyes and stroke her arm, feeling the skin and soft muscles moving like clay underneath my fingers. Then I'd traverse the knobby ridges of her knuckles and glide along her fingernails, smooth as glass, and I would wonder: Is this what the blind men felt? Are these mountains and plains, hidden valleys and channeled rivers the whole of my mother?

Many hundreds of years ago a King and his army traveled across the high mountains of India to impress the common people with his wealth and omnipotence. Most impressive of all was the King's mighty elephant, whose size and strength awed the populace.

One day the King's entourage set up camp outside a small village in which every inhabitant was blind. At night several blind men stole into the camp, hoping to discover the truth about this extraordinary creature so that they could share this knowledge with their blind neighbors. When they returned to the village, they related with great excitement the facts that they had gathered.

"It is large and rough," said the blind man who had touched the elephant's ear, "and it moves in the breeze like a heavy canvas tapestry."

"No, no, that is not at all the case," interrupted the blind man who had felt the elephant's trunk. "It is, in fact, like a powerful, rough-skinned snake that coils and uncoils but does not strike."

"I beg to differ," said the blind man who had touched the creature's legs, "for it is solid and firm like a tree with rough, furrowed bark."

Each of the blind men had felt only a part, but each believed that he understood the whole. Because they shaped reality to their limited perception, the truth remained obscured.

The story took my breath away, for I understood that the world was much more complicated than the simple mathematical formula that insisted that one plus one equals two. As I grew up and continued to reflect on the meaning of the story, I knew that my reality was only one version of the whole story, and as my reality changed—and it seemed to change every day—the story itself became more difficult to grasp. I began to understand the ancient truth that when we look only with our eyes, we see only what our eyes can see. When we touch only with our hands, we feel only what our hands can feel. When we seek out the truth, blindly hoping to discover "the real facts," we shape reality to our expectations. Possessing knowledge of the broken parts, we mistakenly assume that we understand the wisdom of the whole.

The ancient Hindu fable of the blind men and the elephant illuminates the enduring human propensity to sever the whole and seek answers in the disjointed parts. For thousands of years, human beings have attempted to understand the world by breaking it apart and sifting through the scattered pieces for bits of truth. But not until the seventeenth century was this systematic fact-finding tendency called "science" and instituted as the real and only way to knowledge and understanding. When seventeenth-century philosopher and mathematician René Descartes developed the scientific method, which consists of breaking problems into pieces that can then be arranged in logical order, he took the interlooping arcs and curves of the world and flattened them into straight, parallel lines. As the web of interconnections between human beings, the earth, and the cosmos was systematically leveled and planed, the sacred hoop of the world evolved into a square with rigid, straight-line boundaries.

Descartes insisted that mind and body were two independent, fundamentally distinct realms, arguing that "there is nothing included in the concept of body that belongs to the mind; and nothing in that of mind that belongs to the body." With the mind separated out and set aside, the body could be understood as a precision instrument governed by specific mathematical laws. Comparing animals to a clock "composed . . . of wheels and springs," Descartes extended the metaphor to humans. "I consider the human being as a machine," Descartes pronounced. "My thought . . . compares a sick man and an ill-made clock with my idea of a healthy man and a well-made clock."

What of soul and spirit, the intuitive, metaphorical, and synthesizing aspects of the human being? Descartes offered these nonscientific intangibles to the Church in exchange for the right to study the flesh-and-blood body machine. The Church agreed, accepting the Cartesian argument that dissection of bodies wouldn't harm the soul, and the deal was done. Human beings were effectively split apart, with scientists taking what could be analyzed, weighed and measured, and religious leaders accepting as their primary domain the ethers of consciousness wherein drifted the soul.

The body as machine was a mind-capturing metaphor for a new age in which scientists searched for specific causes of disease, relying on anatomy and structure as their guides. The metaphor found its way into human consciousness, as metaphors tend to do, and there it remains to this day. "Think of your body as a superautomobile," exhorts the self-help book *How to Live Cheap but Good.* "If you don't drive it too fast for too long, and if you feed it the right fuel, give it periodic checkups, and maybe wash it occasionally, you'll prevent rumblings."

If the "superautomobile" body does send up rumbles of disease or dissatisfaction, the owner is advised to call a specialist and request a tune-up. And sure enough, when the battery gets low and our energy sputters, we feel an unmistakable urge to kick the stubborn old jalopy into action. Feeling helpless, out of control, and disconnected from "it"—that carnal shell housing the heart and soul—we look outside for answers to our questions. We ingest potent chemicals, agree to high-tech invasions, and even submit to the excision or replacement of essential parts in the hope that we can resume our journey as quickly and efficiently as possible.

From the Cartesian split between mind and matter, we have come to imagine our bodies as separate from our minds and spirits. Thus, when the body breaks down, we are more than willing to hand over this fragmented part of ourselves to the expert mechanic—the medical doctor or, as some wryly translate the acronym M.D., the Medical Deity. We are so out of touch with our bodies that we don't know we're out of balance (or even out of order) until someone else pronounces the verdict.

When artificial heart recipient Murray Haydon wondered about his condition, he quipped, "Would you please turn on the television? I'd like to see if I'm still alive and how I'm doing." Although Mr. Haydon may have been reacting to the excessive media attention he was receiving, I like to think that having a man-made, mechanical instrument imbedded in his otherwise human chest gifted him with sudden insight. Perhaps he understood with special poignancy the modern truth that the mind and body have become so separated and cut off from each other that one does not know how the other is doing without seeking the priestly opinion of high technology.

We have all had the experience of visiting a doctor for some vague complaint, answering a few questions, and then waiting patiently for the verdict to be handed down from on high. We know something is wrong, but we're not sure what it is, and we have no idea how to fix it. If the laboratory tests and various diagnostic workups place us in the normal range, we are informed that nothing is wrong—an analysis that does not correspond with an internal sense of imbalance and disharmony. If we are told we have a disease or a disorder requiring medical attention, we continue to wait patiently for additional information, but rarely receive the attention we deserve. Here's a joke doctors like to tell on themselves:

"Hi," the caller said to the nurse. "You have a patient on your floor—a Mr. Hipp. Can you tell me how he is?"

"He's doing fine," she said. "The doctor expects to remove the stitches tomorrow and he'll be up and about within a week."

"Thanks," said the caller.

"Would you like me to tell Mr. Hipp who phoned?"

"This *is* Mr. Hipp," the caller said. "My doctor won't tell me anything!"

The more awkward, anguished side of the problem comes into focus when we listen to the long-term impact of such a disastrous breakdown in communication. In my practice, I see many people whose illnesses and disorders have been treated with great skill and efficiency by their doctors, but who continue to feel sick in heart and spirit. They have been cured, but because they have been treated like bodies without souls, they have not been healed. As one woman, who was in remission from cancer, told me, "When my doctors touch my body, it's as if they forgot that there is a human being inside."

In his autobiography, *At the Will of the Body*, Arthur Frank tells his story about suffering a heart attack at age thirty-nine; he survived but eighteen months later was diagnosed with testicular cancer. *"What is happening to me?"* was the question he was literally dying to ask.

> My physician provided the medical answer, but it has taken me years to understand why it was not *my* answer. We talked about my heart as if we were consulting about some computer that was producing errors in the output. "It" had a problem. Our talk was classier than most of the conversations I have with the mechanic who fixes my car, but only because my doctor and I were being vague. He was not as specific as my mechanic usually is.

What Frank's body, mind, and soul craved was an opportunity to make sense of his suffering, to talk about the changes illness was creating in his life, to communicate to another human being the intense drama of his personal experience. He needed to know *how to live with illness*. "The help I want is not a matter of answering questions but of witnessing attempts to live in certain ways," Frank explains, centering his discussion in the present tense even though his disease is in remission. "I do not want my questions answered; I want my experiences shared."

This intense need to share our life dramas with others does not fade away with time. Perhaps the most effective healing act I can perform for my elderly patients is to listen to their stories and through the simple act of paying attention, acknowledge that their life and experience have value and meaning. In our culture, we look at the elderly and see the ravages of time on the body and mind; we pay no attention to the deep and abiding wisdom of the soul. In Ram Dass's book *How Can We Help?* a resident of a nursing home describes her need to tell her story—the story of her life—and to have someone listen, understand, and appreciate the gift inherent in the story. But listening, she has discovered, is a lost art.

Heard . . . if they only understood how important it is that we be heard! I can take being in a nursing home. It's really all right, with a positive attitude. My daughter has her hands full, three kids and a job. She visits regularly. I understand.

But most people here . . . they just want to tell their story. That's what they have to give, don't you see? And it's a precious thing to them. It's their life they want to give. You'd think people would understand what it means to us . . . to give our lives in a story.

So we listen to each other. Most of what goes on here is people listening to each other's stories. People who work here consider that to be . . . filling time. If they only knew. If they'd just take a minute to listen.

In our narrow focus on the body as separate from the mind, we have lost touch with the feminine spirit of healing, which seeks to reconnect the body, mind, and spirit into a functioning whole. We have, in truth, lost the *art* of healing: the *art* of listening without offering answers or solutions; the *art* of taking a moment to stop and participate in another person's life experience; the *art* of recognizing the profound changes that illness creates and marking their significance; the *art* of understanding that whatever affects the body also touches the mind and the spirit—the life—of the human being.

The body has become a thing, detached and distant, a space we happen to inhabit, an *it* to measure, weigh, and objectify. How we live in that body, how we experience life within its chemical folds and atomic corners, is a question few are willing to ask, for we are uncomfortable with questions that harbor no easy answers. We have lost patience with paradox. Because our minds have been carefully trained to break apart the whole and analyze the parts, we have difficulty conceiving of the *whole* as anything other than an entity waiting to be dismantled, like a jigsaw puzzle or a building-block toy that is less satisfying in its intact state than in its disarray of jumbled parts.

But when human beings are seen as collections of parts that can be ranked according to prestige, power, or influence, something irrevocably precious is lost. Disconnected pieces can't interact; cut off from their source, they blindly seek but cannot find the place where they fit. Disorder and dislocation replace a sense of harmony and balance, and we suffer the effects of fragmentation in every aspect of our lives.

Out of touch with our own bodies, we have lost touch with the basic truth that what happens to the self also happens to the concentric circles of family, community, earth, and cosmos that sustain and ensure the continuation of life. Having lost sight of the basic truth that all life is interconnected and interdependent, a vast, textured web of relationships, we have lost our footing and drift without direction or purpose in a world that no longer makes sense.

What we have spent so many years breaking apart we must now find a way to put back together again. For thousands of years human beings have turned to metaphors and images to reframe reality. Myths and stories create a subtle shift, gently guiding us to expand our boundaries, pushing out the edges of reality and helping us to create a "home"—a place where we fit within the larger whole. When we listen to stories, the full impact may not be felt for days or even years, for stories work like time-release capsules in which the wisdom seeps out in small doses, giving us time to adjust and adapt. Story "medicine" is powerful and long lasting. "It can be a fatal error to underestimate the power of myth," writes Riane Eisler in *The Chalice and the Blade*. "The human psyche seems to have a built-in need for a system of stories and symbols that 'reveal' to us the order of the universe and tell us what our place within it is. It is a hunger for meaning and purpose seemingly beyond the power of any rationalistic or logical system to provide."

Because the stories and symbols we embrace as meaningful will function as our guides, shaping our perceptions and our thoughts, defining what is right and wrong, just and unjust, morally acceptable or morally condemnable, we have a responsibility to select those stories that celebrate life rather than death, cooperation rather than competition, peace rather than war, and harmony with, rather than conquest of, nature. Happily, we do not need to spin these stories out of new cloth, for they are interwoven in the wisdom traditions handed down to us from the ancients.

One of my favorite myths centers on the story of the ancient Egyptian goddess Isis, whose name literally means "the giver of life." When Joseph Campbell discusses the remarkable powers of Isis in *The Power of Myth*, he focuses on a particular scene in which Isis lies upon the dead body of her husband, Osiris, and conceives a child, thus reenacting the transcendent power of the female to create life from death. My favorite version of the myth was retold by Dr. Gerald Epstein in a lecture on mind/body medicine presented to the Acupuncture College in New York City. I have adapted Dr. Epstein's version of the story from my notes of his lecture.

Deeply in love with her husband, Osiris, Isis conceived and gave birth to a son, Horus. As Horus grew into manhood, he became envious of his parents' devotion to each other and arranged to have his father murdered. Fearing the strength of his mother's life-giving powers, Horus took his father's corpse many hundreds of miles away to a foreign land.

When Isis learned of her husband's death and her son's betrayal, she sent out expeditions to recover the body, and from the deep reservoir of her love and passion, she breathed life back into the corpse. Enraged by his mother's death-defying powers, Horus was determined to remove his chief rival for eternity. Once again he arranged to have his father murdered, but this time Osiris's body was dismembered into fourteen pieces, which were scattered throughout Egypt.

Isis commanded her people to search for the pieces of her husband's body and return them to her. When all fourteen pieces were re-collected, she breathed life back into Osiris by re-membering him and restoring his body to wholeness.

In this ancient myth, a powerful woman is assigned the role of the compassionate healer who is responsible for the renewal and regeneration of life. After collecting the lost and scattered pieces of her beloved, Isis was able to restore wholeness through the process of remembering and reconnection. Through her love and passion, she was able to heal the wounds and recreate the miracle of life.

The ancients believed in the power of miracles. But our modern minds, assiduously trained in the logic of rational thought, have difficulty accepting the fact that a sense of the sacred underlies all life. A popular cartoon illustrates our refusal to entertain the notion that some mysteries cannot be explained:

Two men stand at the blackboard, staring at a complicated mathematical equation consisting of three steps. In the second step of the equation, between two complex jumbles of symbols, are the words *"Then a miracle occurs."*

The older man, stoop-shouldered and balding, frowns and offers his advice to his colleague: "I think you should be more explicit here in Step Two."

Then a miracle occurs. The ancients understood the dark wisdom of those words, while moderns see only an incomplete equation and sloppy inattention to detail. But the cartoon also points out the annoying paradox of modern life, for as smart as we may be, we don't have all the answers. Sometimes the only answer is "Then a miracle occurs." Faced with that conundrum, we can worry the problem to death, ignoring the admonitions of Oscar Wilde, who insisted that "thinking is the most unhealthy thing in the world, and people die of it just as they die of any other disease." Or we can learn to speak more like the poets, recognizing the mysteries as yet unexplained and celebrating the limitless potential for miracle.

Acknowledging our ignorance may be the route to our salvation. All wisdom traditions teach that the more we learn, the less we know, a paradox that became disturbingly clear to twentieth-century physicists struggling to understand the complexities of the atomic and subatomic world. The dilemma faced by such eminent physicists as Albert Einstein, Max Planck, Niels Bohr, and Werner Heisenberg is described by physicist Fritjof Capra in his brilliant book *The Turning Point*:

> Every time they asked nature a question in an atomic experiment, nature answered with a paradox, and the more they tried to clarify the situation, the sharper the paradoxes became. In their struggle to grasp this new reality, scientists became painfully aware that their basic concepts, their language, and their whole way of thinking were inadequate to describe atomic phenomena. Their problem was not only intellectual but involved an intense emotional and existential experience.

Capra suggests that the inability to make sense of the universe reflects the inadequacy of the scientific method, which seeks to accumulate knowledge by breaking the whole into its constituent parts. When physicists attempted to disassemble the atomic world in order to better understand it, they realized that at this most basic level the world could not be broken apart. Capra tells a story about Werner Heisenberg, whose late-night discussions with Niels Bohr frequently ended in confusion and despair. Afterward, Heisenberg would walk alone in the park, asking himself one question over and over again: "Can nature possibly be so absurd as it seemed to us in these atomic experiments?"

Perhaps it was the fact that their questions never called forth a complete answer, but eventually these brilliant scientists let go of their struggle and gave in to wonder, an embrace of paradox, and an acceptance of the underlying unity of life. "As we penetrate into matter, nature does not show us any isolated basic building blocks," Capra writes, "but rather appears as a complicated web of relations between the various parts of a unified whole."

Physicist James Jeans expresses a similar belief, arguing that the mechanical conception of the universe is breaking down and giving way to a new reality, a vigorous and dynamic brainstorm of activity. "Today there is a wide measure of agreement," he writes, "that the stream of knowledge is heading towards a nonmechanical reality . . . the universe begins to look more like a great thought than like a great machine."

Imagine a distinguished scientist chasing a thought around his laboratory, trying to pin it down in order to analyze its constituent parts! The idea of a dynamic, coherent, continually evolving universe echoes the ancient conception of the cosmos as a vast musical symphony, what the sixth-century B.C. Greek philosopher and mathematician Pythagoras called the "harmony of the spheres." While observers may not be able to make sense of each individual note or even decipher the minor motifs, there can be no doubt that the *whole* is magnificent, awe inspiring, filled with wonder.

Capra invokes the musical metaphor when he speaks of matter being in "a continuous dancing and vibrating motion whose rhythmic patterns are determined by the molecular, atomic and nuclear configurations." As the science of physics was infused with art (if not poetry), matter could no longer be conceived of as sleepy stuff, immobile sludge waiting passively for something to bump into it and set it in motion. Rather it was reimagined as all aquiver and alive, skipping to a beat just beyond human comprehension. This dancing subatomic motion was not viewed as random, disconnected convulsions of activity (a quark standing in a cosmic corner, headphones secured, shuddering to some unfathomable beat), but rather as an elegant waltz in which each individual movement and response functions as an integral part of a single, undivided whole.

The universe, delicate and complex beyond imagining, was being newly conceived (or more accurately, newly discovered) as a whole underlaid by a symmetrical web of relationships in which each subatomic strand contributed to balance and integrity. Some of the most brilliant minds of the twentieth century were confirming the ancient view of the universe as a sacred hoop: "The world thus appears as a complicated tissue of events," Heisenberg lyrically articulated, "in which connections of different kinds alternate or overlap or combine and thereby determine the texture of the whole."

Theoretical scientists were using the spirit-soaked words of poetry to bridge the gaps in their knowledge. What William Wordsworth called "a sense sublime" seems to have slipped through the straight-edged seams of their senses:

> *And I have felt . . . a sense sublime*
> *Of something far more deeply interfused,*
> *Whose dwelling is the light of setting suns,*
> *And the round ocean and the living air,*
> *And the blue sky, and in the mind of man:*
> *A motion and a spirit, that impels*
> *All thinking things, all objects of all thought,*
> *And rolls through all things.*

If physicists, who study matter, motion, and energy, can speak of dances, rhythms, tissues, and textures, what do scientists who study human beings have to say about the unanswerable problems they face in their work? While mainstream science remains focused on observable and verifiable facts, growing numbers of neurologists, immunologists, psychiatrists, and psychologists are stripping off their shrouds of scientific invincibility and embracing the everyday mysteries—indeed, the miracles—that confront them. Their minds and souls also have been touched by Wordsworth's "something far more deeply interfused." They, too, hear the voices of the ancients calling to them.

Bill Moyers's groundbreaking book *Healing and the Mind* is filled with interviews with highly educated, powerfully intelligent men and women who are not afraid to open their minds to the motion and spirit that in Wordsworth's words "rolls through all things." These brilliant iconoclasts do not talk with the arrogant assurance or scientific precision of scholars obsessed with concepts and certainty. They falter for words, confess their shortcomings, and willingly permit the gentle persuasions of soul and spirit to nestle in with the hard body of scientific facts. The new science of mind/body medicine, with its wealth of unanswered questions, fascinates and intrigues them.

"We know more about the body than the mind, or we think we do," Thomas Delbanco, associate professor of medicine at Harvard Medical School, hesitatingly explains. "Actually, we know incredibly little about the body, either—but it's staggering how much we have to learn about the mind."

Is Delbanco itching to get his hands around the mystery in order to fill in the holes of his gaping ignorance? Astonishingly, no.

"In a sense, I don't even want to learn about the mind because the mind is part of the mystery of you, and I like that sense of mystery," he says, adding that he feels the need to enfold the science of medicine into the art of understanding soul and spirit. "I've got to go beyond the technical aspects of this test and that part of your body. I've got to somehow try to understand your spirit and maybe even touch it at times."

The idea of a physician struggling to touch the human spirit is analogous to the image of the physicist chasing the great thought that is the universe around his four-walled laboratory. Something playful and astonishing is happening in the waning years of the millennium. Centuries-old distinctions between the mind and body are breaking down, and scientists are giving themselves permission to think and talk like mystics. When Moyers asks neuroscientist Candace Pert to describe the mind, she excitedly discusses the activities of neuropeptides, strings of amino acids that function as information molecules allowing cells in different parts of the body to talk to each other.

"Intelligence is in every cell of your body," Pert explains. "The mind is not confined to the space above the neck. The mind is throughout the brain and body."

But what exactly is the mind, Moyers wants to know.

Pert tackles the question with mischievous intensity: "What is the mind? Gosh, how frightening! I'm a basic scientist, and I'm having to answer, 'What is the mind?' " But then she offers a definition that is infused less with science than poetry: "The mind is some kind of enlivening energy in the information realm throughout the brain and body that enables the cells to talk to each other, and the outside to talk to the whole organism."

Enlivening energy? Information realm?

Immunologist David Felten, professor of neurobiology and anatomy at the University of Rochester School of Medicine, was looking through a microscope at blood vessels in the spleen when he noticed a snag of nerve fibers. *Now what are nerve fibers doing in the spleen all tangled up with immune system cells?* he wondered. He kept cutting up tissue sections, and there they were again, those pesky nerve cells setting up house where they didn't belong. As he continued slicing away and subjecting the tissue samples to painstaking analysis, he eventually came to a reasonable and yet wholly illogical conclusion: Mind is *in* the body, Felten realized with sudden insight; the mind is literally talking to the cells, coaxing them along, influencing hormonal output, signaling distress and—*just as astonishing*—the body talks back.

But what about the old Cartesian concept that the mind and body are separate and never the twain shall meet? That notion, Dr. Felten insists, is "down the drain," which means that people who study the brain and people who study the body are going to have to start talking to each other. "And in the past, heaven forbid that immunologists and neuroscientists would ever use each other's language," Felten says. "They'd rather use each other's toothbrushes. But that's no longer a viable approach. We have to learn how to talk to each other and to educate each other."

Once again we come back to the need to admit our ignorance, for learning how to talk to and educate each other necessarily entails giving up the claim to have all the answers. The willingness to communicate with each other involves the admission that there may not be answers, at least not the logical, rational answers we have been taught to seek.

In the eighties, Dr. David Spiegel, professor of psychiatry and behavioral sciences at Stanford University School of Medicine, conducted a study involving eighty-six women with advanced breast cancer. The women were randomly assigned to two groups: one group received routine cancer care (radiation and chemotherapy), and the other group received experimental group support in addition to the routine care. "The group therapy," Spiegel explains in his recent book *Living beyond Limits*, "consisted of sharing their fears, planning means of coping with the threat of death, grieving the losses of members, teaching the women self-hypnosis to control their pain, and learning to savor the preciousness of life."

Three years later, after evaluating his subjects' moods, pain levels, coping styles, and family interactions, Dr. Spiegel concluded that the women in the experimental group were less anxious and depressed and experienced only half as much pain as the women who received standard care. These positive but expected results were dutifully published in psychiatric journals. Several years later, with the idea of disproving alternative medicine claims that the mind can control the progression of a bodily disease, Spiegel decided to find out what had happened to the women in his study. When he received the computer printouts analyzing the "survival curves," which show the number of women still alive at a given time after the study began, he was literally knocked off his feet.

I had to sit down when I got the first (of what would prove to be hundreds) of printouts. The two survival curves overlapped initially, but diverged markedly at twenty months. By four years after the point at which the women were enrolled in the initial study, it turned out that all of the patients in the control group had died, but fully one third of the patients who had received group therapy was still alive. . . . In other words, on average, patients who had been in the experimental treatment program had lived *twice as long* from the time they entered the study as did the control patients. This was a difference so significant that statistical analysis was almost unnecessary—all you had to do was look at the curves. And I had been expecting no difference at all!

It seems wonderfully appropriate that Dr. Spiegel was studying the female disease of breast cancer and that the group therapy sessions employed the basic tools of the feminine spirit of healing—listening with compassion, guiding without interfering, nurturing, protecting, comforting, and caring. But how exactly did these ancient healing arts help the women live longer? How did the mind have such an astonishing effect on the body? The wise doctor acknowledges both the miracle and his inability to analyze it. "Something in the group appears to have helped these women live longer," Spiegel concluded. "But what that is, I don't know."

Once again the eminent scientist stands at the blackboard, chin in hand, trying to figure out what to do with that perplexing phrase, "Then a miracle occurs." Will our most capable, energetic minds ever be able to analyze the *miracle* of human contact? Can a kind word be synthesized, a loving touch be dissected, a moment spent in quiet reflection be weighed, measured, or objectified? While we can witness the effects of caring and compassion, can we ever hope to explain these intangibles in terms of atoms and molecules or break them down into a mathematical formula or chemical equation? Can we say anything more profound than the words "Then a miracle occurs"?

Even if we had the language or the intellectual constructs to explain the miracle of human contact, the analysis would not necessarily reduce our sense of wonder. In the 1970s, a group of investigators at Ohio State University designed a study to test the effects of a high-fat, high-cholesterol diet on rabbits. They expected their findings to replicate numerous other studies showing that such a diet causes obstructions and ulcerations in the rabbits' arteries (a process known as atherosclerosis that causes heart attacks and strokes in humans). At the end of a specified time period, the rabbits were killed, and their arteries were microscopically examined for evidence of cholesterol deposition. While most of the animals demonstrated the predicted atherosclerotic changes, one group was wildly out of line, showing 60 percent less evidence of disease.

The investigators were dumbfounded. What was it about these rabbits that defied logic, allowing them to resist the proven toxic effects of a high-cholesterol diet? Sifting through the possibilities, they eventually isolated an unexpected variable. During the course of the experiment, a student in charge of feeding this particular group of rabbits regularly took the animals out of their cages to hold and pet them.

But was it really possible that a loving relationship between caged rabbits and their human caretaker would have such a marked effect on the animals' immunity to physical disease? The original experiment was replicated, and once again the group of rabbits given tender loving care demonstrated a 60 percent lower incidence of atherosclerosis. Wary of coincidence (and unaccustomed to miracle), the researchers again repeated the experiment, again with the same results: the rabbits who received loving attention and affection were obviously and significantly healthier than their neglected cohorts.

Scientists investigating the new frontier of mind/body medicine seem most impressed with their own ignorance. "We're just in the infancy of our explorations," they say. "We know very little." "We don't know how the relationship works." "We don't have the right language." "There are big holes all over the place." "Perhaps someday we will understand." And then, wistfully, inevitably, "I wish I knew. . . ."

But the "big holes" seem to concern them less than the misguided attempts to jump over the holes and concentrate only on what can be held, touched, measured, or quantified. In fact, many scientists are beginning to wonder if the holes in our knowledge may be precisely those places where true wisdom resides. In an epilogue to a recent book, Dr. David Felten writes:

> Just as the physical world of rainbows, lightning, and stars was not understood in the centuries before modern physics and astronomy, so also the more elusive and complex aspects of the human mind are not understood at present, even with the impressive technology we have at our command. Can we afford

to ignore the role of emotions, hope, the will to live, the power of human warmth and contact just because they are so difficult to investigate scientifically and our ignorance is so overwhelming?

Sages and scholars have always taught that when the soil of our consciousness is seeded with the knowledge of our own ignorance, wisdom can take root. Awareness of our ignorance is the necessary precondition for comprehending that which we do not know and perhaps can never fully understand. This is the "beginner's mind" that was described by the ancient Chinese philosopher Lao-tzu as the *knowing of not knowing*: "To know yet to think that one does not know is best; Not to know yet to think that one knows will lead to difficulty."

McDonald's founder, Ray Kroc, translated Lao-tzu's ancient insight into pithy Americanese: "When you're green, you're growing; when you're ripe, you rot."

Only by immersing ourselves in the depth of our own ignorance—that dark, impenetrable place where we acknowledge and accept what we do not know—can we begin to move into the light of knowledge and understanding. This is a deceptively simple beginning, however, for plunging into the darkness in an attempt to discover the light is a paradox too difficult for most of us to grasp. Rather than admit our shortcomings and accept our limitations, we search in the light for the answers to our questions . . . even if we know there is no hope of finding what we seek.

One of my favorite teaching stories employs a loving sense of humor to approach this human tendency to avoid the shadow places:

> *Mulla Nasrudin was outside his house, down on his hands and knees desperately searching through the dirt. A neighbor walked by and asked if he might be of some help.*
>
> *"What are you looking for, Mulla?" the neighbor asked.*
>
> *"I lost my key," said Nasrudin.*
>
> *The neighbor got down on his hands and knees to help Nasrudin and for quite some time they searched for the lost key. When it appeared that their search was futile, the neighbor turned to Nasrudin and said, "Think carefully, Mulla. Where exactly did you lose the key?" he asked.*
>
> *"Why, I lost it in the house," Nasrudin replied.*

"Good heavens!" exclaimed the exasperated neighbor. "Then why are you searching for it outside?"

"Because the light is better here," said Nasrudin.

Mulla Nasrudin, the wise fool of many Sufi stories, holds up a mirror and allows us to see the folly of our ways. We search in the light—the well-traveled, brightly illuminated pathways—for what can only be discovered in the depths of our own souls, busying ourselves with doing in order to avoid being. Like the blind men trying to describe the elephant, we touch a part and immediately assume that we understand the whole. When our efforts fail, we ignore our inner wisdom and intuition, hoping that someone will come along and help us out of our predicament. Facts and truths obsess us; enigmas and unknowns make our hair stand up on end.

"When we must deal with problems, we instinctively resist trying the way that leads through obscurity and darkness," wrote psychoanalyst Carl Jung, who understood the nature of human resistance to the darkness of our own ignorance. "We wish to hear only of unequivocal results, and completely forget that these results can only be brought about when we have ventured into, and emerged again from, darkness." We resist the plunge into darkness because we know that there we will encounter ambiguity and paradox, those muddy, murky obstacles that slow us down in our efforts to discover the light of wisdom. Unaccustomed to inactivity, uncomfortable with isolation, and unwilling to walk when we can just as easily fly, we seek shortcuts to enlightenment.

One of the devotees in the temple was much admired for his faith and discipline. All day and all night he would sit in meditation, refusing to eat, refusing even to sleep. As the days and weeks passed, he became emaciated and appeared near collapse.

"You must slow down and take better care of yourself," advised the master of the temple. But the devotee continued with his prayers, refusing to heed the master's advice.

A few days later the master again approached his disciple. "Tell me," he said kindly. "Why are you so zealous? What's your rush?"

"I am seeking enlightenment," replied the disciple, "and I cannot afford to waste my time."

"But how do you know that enlightenment is running on ahead of

you, so that you have to hurry to catch up with it?" asked the master. "Perhaps it is behind you and in order to encounter it, you need only stand still. And yet all this time you have been running away from it!"

The master knows that the light of wisdom and truth does not shine from some elevated, external source, illuminating a pathway that only the swift and nimble can travel. Enlightenment radiates from within. The winds of change and circumstance may cause the flame to flicker and fade, but in those who understand that "the meaning is in the search," it can never be extinguished.

> *An old man was bitter and challenged Jacob with a complaint.*
> *"All my life I have searched for meaning," he said.*
> *"The meaning is in the search," said Jacob, waving off the man's distress.*
> *"Then I will never find the meaning?"*
> *"No," said Jacob. "You will never stop looking."*
> *Jacob held his voice for a moment, unsure if he had been too harsh.*
> *"My friend," Jacob began again, "know that you are a man with a lantern who goes in search of a light."*

In the darkness, we seek the light and discover that we have possessed it all along. We arrive at the point of understanding that only by slowing down and *being*—*being* awake, *being* aware, *being* patient, *being* truthful— can we also be open and receptive to the mysteries that promise not answers but insights, not an end to our journey but a new beginning.

Where is enlightenment to be found? A Zen parable speaks of the finger pointing to the moon, an image with two clear focal points—the finger, which symbolizes the wise teacher, or guide, who points the way to wisdom and truth; and the moon, which signifies the goal, the endpoint, the mystery revealed. But in this simple metaphor, we may miss the most significant space waiting to be explored: the expanse between the finger and the moon, which represents the experience of life itself.

In that mysterious space that contains both the fear of emptiness and the promise of fullness, each of us must begin the journey toward wholeness, guided only by the light of our intuitive wisdom. When we let go of fear and the desire for control and release ourselves into the wonder of being alive, we understand that the answers to our existence have been waiting for us all along. Leaping into darkness, we discover what we cannot hold between our hands, what we cannot touch and cannot speak: the lost keys to the shadowlands of heart and soul.

> *"COME TO THE EDGE."*
> *"No, we will fall."*
> *"COME TO THE EDGE."*
> *"No, we will fall."*
> *They came to the edge.*
> *He pushed them, and they flew.*
> *—Guillaume Apollinaire*

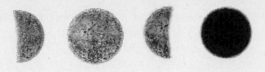

CHAPTER 3

THE GODDESS
AND THE WITCH

When you have a Goddess as the creator, it's her own body that is the universe. She is identical with the universe. . . . She is the whole sphere of the life-enclosing heavens.

—*Joseph Campbell*

This is a story we like to tell ourselves in the night when the fire seems nothing but dying embers winking out and the labor is too hard and goes on too long . . . When we are afraid, when it hurts too much, we like to tell ourselves stories of power. How we lost it, how we can reclaim it. We tell ourselves the cries we hear may be those of labor; the pain we feel may yet be that of birth."

—*Starhawk, poet, teacher, wise woman*

The journey toward wholeness—toward a balance of yin and yang, female and male, intuition and logic in ourselves and in our society's healing practices—necessarily begins with an understanding of what we have lost. For once upon a time the world was gently but firmly guided by the feminine spirit of healing. A sense of awe and wonder at the magnificent harmony and delicate balance of the universe permeated all of life, and women, who embodied the nurturing and regenerative powers necessary for the ongoing cycles of life, were invested with great powers of healing and renewal. Females were revered as the spinners of the web, the guardians of the invisible threads linking human beings to the cosmos. Passionate, fiercely protective, and highly intuitive, women kept human beings in touch with the healing energies of the natural world, appealing to the wild and untamed powers of nature in daily rites and seasonal celebrations.

When disease threatened the body, women used their knowledge of healing herbs, soothing ointments, and cleansing rituals to restore the body to health and wholeness. When the mind was troubled or the spirit unsettled, women healers relied on myths, symbols, and dream imagery to restore balance. Any disorder in the individual, family, or community was viewed as a symptom of disharmony with the natural order, and the healer assumed the responsibility of guiding the torn and broken pieces into their rightful places, creating a dynamic, self-healing social structure with deep ties to Mother Earth and the world of soul and spirit. This was the time, in Merlin Stone's famous phrase, when God was a woman, and when women were revered as the earthly representatives of the Great Goddess's gentle wisdom.

Whenever I think back to the peace and harmony of these ancient societies, I am filled with a sense of loss. But my grief is balanced with hope, for all of life is characterized by change, and even the forward march of history can be imagined as a gentle arc in which the end and the beginning are inevitably joined. The circle completes itself over and over again. While it may seem that we have wandered far off course, many signs indicate a return to ancient values and healing traditions.

In the waning years of the twentieth century, we are witnessing a renewed respect for the earth, which is once again honored with the name "Mother"; a resurgence of interest in the wisdom and healing arts of the Native American peoples; a fascination with earth- and mother-centered cultures; a revival of interest in holistic medicine and healing techniques that honor the deep connections between body, mind, and spirit; and a growing recognition that the linear, analytical approach to problem solving has contributed to the alienation of male from female, individual from family, and the human community from the cosmos. Women and men alike are looking to the past for guidance about how to live and survive in the modern, technological age. But what exactly are we hoping to recapture and reclaim?

To understand the roots of the feminine spirit of healing, we must journey back in time to the historical periods archaeologists call the Paleolithic (the "Old Stone Age," from 30,000 to 7500 B.C.). and the Neolithic (the "New Stone Age," from 7500 to approximately 3500 B.C.). Numerous scholarly works, most notably Marija Gimbutas's masterwork *The Goddesses and Gods of Old Europe* and Joseph Campbell's four-volume series *The Masks of God*, reveal the existence of ancient societies that were stable, culturally advanced, and deeply committed to the feminine spirit of healing. Paleolithic art offers a visual testament to our early ancestors' awe at the miracle of birth, their reverence for nature, and the association of women with the powers that govern fertility, birth, life, and death. Burial chambers reveal an abundance of female symbols commonly called Venus figurines, arranged in a centrally located position. Vagina-shaped cowrie shells were carefully arranged around the corpse, and red ochre pigment, which symbolized the life-giving powers of female blood, was used to coat both the body and shells. Scenes of ritual dances featuring priestesses and prominent female symbols suggest the existence of an early form of religion in which the life-giving and life-sustaining powers of the female were considered divine.

In the Neolithic, family and communal life centered around the figure of the Great Goddess, who represented values aspired to by both women and men—love of truth and beauty, passion for justice, commitment to healing, cultivation of wisdom, and above all, deep and abiding respect for Mother Earth. Indeed, the Goddess was synonymous with Nature Herself, the ultimate source of all healing and harmony. Second-century A.D. writer Apuleius gave the Great Goddess a voice with which to speak of her powers in his novel *The Golden Ass*:

> I am Nature, the universal Mother, mistress of all elements, primordial child of time, sovereign of all things spiritual, queen of the dead, queen also of the immortals, the single manifestation of all gods and goddesses that are. My nod governs the shining heights of Heaven, the wholesome sea breezes, the lamentable silences of the world below. Though I am worshipped in many aspects, known by countless names, and propitiated with all

manner of different rites, yet the whole round earth venerates me.

In numerous archaeological excavations ranging from India to England and as far south as the Mediterranean island of Malta, Goddess shrines and figurines appear in abundance. In southeastern Europe alone, a total of three thousand sites has yielded thirty thousand miniature sculptures made of clay, marble, bone, and copper; evidence of temples, pictorial paintings, charms, amulets, surgical tools, and various herbal prescriptions confirm that these primarily agrarian societies were sexually egalitarian, sophisticated in the healing arts, and permeated with a deep spiritual reverence for the Great Goddess, who personified the unity of all living creatures and their life-giving connections to Mother Earth.

For four thousand years, the Great Goddess served as the compassionate, healing center of Neolithic society. She was both nurse and mother, human and divine, protecting the weak, tending the sick, enfolding the dying in her loving embrace, and at all times affirming the beauty, harmony, and integrity of life. Mistress of Life, Giver of All, Guardian of the Dead, the Lady of Nature, Queen of the Ghosts, Opener of the Womb, Life-Giver and Life-Taker, she was, in Joseph Campbell's words, "the whole sphere of the life-enclosing heavens." Filled with the powers of both heaven and earth, she affirmed the divine in humans while celebrating the wholly human ability to love and care for each other.

Tender compassion for the weak and feeble was her trademark, but erotic love was also part of her domain, for the Great Godess served to honor through her own sexuality the vital, pleasure-loving link between males and females. In the book *Inanna: The Queen of Heaven and Earth*, the Sumerian goddess relates her passion for her lover, the shepherd Dumuzi:

> He shaped my loins with his fair hands,
> The shepherd Dumuzi filled my lap with cream and milk,
> He stroked my pubic hair,
> He watered my womb.
> He laid his hands on my holy vulva,
> He smoothed my black boat with cream,
> He quickened my narrow boat with milk,
> He caressed me on the bed.
> Now I will caress my high priest on the bed,
> I will caress the faithful shephered Dumuzi,

I will caress his loins, the shepherdship of the land,
I will decree a sweet fate for him.

When God was a woman, the relationship between females and males was distinguished by respect, affection, and a joyous, uncensored passion. Neolithic societies worshiped the vital, life-giving connections between the sexes, making no attempt to rank men and women according to superiority, dominance, or power. While the Great Goddess was the divine authority and supreme moral force governing these peaceful societies, there is no evidence of a hierarchical system in which men were subjugated or suppressed; in fact, Neolithic imagery frequently portrayed male gods in important partnership roles. "The male divinity in the shape of a young man or male animal appears to affirm and strengthen the forces of the creative and active female," writes archaeologist Gimbutas. "Neither is subordinate to the other: by complementing one another, their power is doubled."

Images of male domination, female submissiveness, battle scenes, noble warriors, conquering heroes, or enchained slaves simply do not appear in the art of the Neolithic, for with the Great Goddess as a reigning deity, power was wielded with love and respect for life. Men and women lived in peaceful cooperation, as equal partners working together for the common good. "The whole of life was pervaded by an ardent faith in the goddess Nature, the source of all creation and harmony," writes archaeologist Nicholas Platon, who spent fifty years of his life excavating the island of Crete. "This led to a love of peace, a horror of tyranny, and a respect for the law. Even among the ruling classes personal ambition seems to have been unknown; nowhere do we find the name of an author attached to a work of art nor a record of the deeds of a ruler." Among both men and women, Platon writes, "the fear of death was almost obliterated by the ubiquitous joy of living."

For many thousands of years, the peaceful Goddess-centered civilizations of the Neolithic flourished. But beginning around the fifth millennium B.C., the archaeological remains reflect a growing state of chaos and disruption. Armed invaders from the Asiatic and European north swept down in three separate waves, overpowering the peaceful agrarian societies and violently altering their way of life. These invaders—semi-nomadic peoples later called the Kurgans or Indo-Europeans—worshiped a vengeful male God, glorified war rather than peace, and invested their growing resources in technologies of destruction and domination.

With her love of peace and harmony and her dedication to the healing arts of caring and compassion, the Great Goddess was powerless to protect her people from the invading hordes with their oppressive male gods. In an ancient myth that presaged the destruction of the feminine spirit of healing, the Sumerian goddess Inanna wandered into the lower regions of the world. As she passed through the gates of the netherworld, her divine powers were taken from her, and she was held prisoner, never again permitted to ascend to the world of the living. When word of Inanna's fate reached Enki, the god of wisdom, he understood the terrible curse that had befallen the human world. For without the healing presence of the goddess Inanna, Enki foretold that the world would lose its center of balance, peace and harmony would be destroyed, and life itself would be at risk.

The myth was prophetic, for civilization suffered grievously as the Goddess Societies crumbled under continual, brutal assault. As male gods of war replaced the female goddesses of healing and compassion, the respectful alliance between men and women disintegrated. The partnership societies of the Goddess-worshiping peoples were gradually replaced with a patriarchal system in which males assumed positions of dominance, and females were relegated to a subordinate, subservient status. Women were no longer allowed to work as doctors, priestesses, or scribes and were forbidden to pursue formal education in the healing arts. As education and training were denied to them, their independence and authority were severely restricted.

In her book *Woman as Healer*, Jeanne Achterberg tells a story about the Athenian physician Agnodice, a skillfull, compassionate healer who defied the customs of her male-dominated society in order to minister to the women of Athens.

One of the better known woman physicians of all time was named Agnodice, a great favorite among the women she treated. She wore men's clothing, probably trying to disguise her sex. By then (the third or fourth centuries B.C.), women were in disrepute as healers, and her disguise may have allowed her to practice with less scrutiny. Agnodice was forced to stand trial when her ruse was discovered. The women of Athens rushed to the tribunal with vociferous declarations of loyalty. According to legend, they threatened to condemn their husbands and with-hold certain favors if she were not released immediately. The strategy was effective. Agnodice was released and allowed to continue to practice, and to dress in whatever way she chose. . . . It is said that after her release, she lifted her skirts to proudly display her womanhood.

The Great Goddess would have smiled on such an act of moral courage, but the spiteful male gods would have been sorely displeased by such brazen, disrespectful behavior. Resourceful and courageous women such as Agnodice were greatly feared by the ruling elite, for they reminded the citizenry of the peaceful past, when a divine mother instilled in her people a love of nature, joy in living, and equality between the sexes.

The feminine spirit of healing nurtured the unquenchable human desire for peace and harmony; such yearnings threatened the stability of a society that increasingly emphasized the brutal domination of the weak by the strong. And so it was inevitable that efforts would be made to destroy the feminine spirit itself. Priestesses were stripped of their powers, goddess temples and shrines were demolished, and women were banned from positions of importance in the healing arts. To consolidate the power of the male gods, scribes (who were all men, for by 700 B.C. women were no longer permitted to pursue the occupation) were assigned the duty of revising the laws and rewriting the ancient myths with the express purpose of humiliating and defiling the Great Goddess. New myths and legends were created in which goddesses were portrayed as minor deities or companions to the all-powerful male God. In many stories and legends, the Great Goddess was captured, brutally raped, and then murdered.

In the most famous myth ever created, we learn that man was made first in the image of God, and woman was produced later from man's (presumably spare) rib. God presented woman to man as a gift to keep him from being lonely and as "a helper fit for him." All was well in paradise until the villainous serpent slithered along (in Goddess societies, snakes were venerated as the symbol of nature's mysterious, immortal powers), and Eve foolishly decided to listen to the serpent's counsel. After tasting the forbidden fruit from the tree of knowledge of good and evil, Eve became aware of her own sexuality and was immediately possessed of the need to tempt man to join her in sinful sexual pleasures.

The vengeful male God was swift and cruel with his punishment: "I will greatly multiply your pain in childbearing; in pain you shall bring forth children, yet your desire shall be for your husband and he shall rule over you." By divine proclamation Eve and all her female descendants were destined to suffer grievously in childbirth and to desire only their husbands, who were assigned the privilege of ruling over them.

The myth of Adam, Eve, and the serpent reveals the emerging view of the female as inherently carnal and corrupt. Sex, sin, and the female were intimately linked in the very first pages of the Bible, and throughout this sacred text the message was repeated in endless permutations. Fearing woman's power, which was rooted in her passionate, intuitive nature, the Hebrew priests created the myths and drafted the laws that would attempt to destroy her, making her a possession of man and subjecting her to swift and cruel punishment if she dared defy the male God's commands.

The Bible is filled with punishments and humiliations meted out to women in an attempt to curb their strong, sensual nature and force them into submission. In the books of Leviticus and Deuteronomy, written between 1000 and 600 B.C., the cruel laws and severe punishments for infraction are carefully explicated:

- All women must remain virgins until marriage. While husbands can possess numerous wives or concubines, a legally married woman can have sexual relations only with her husband.
- If a woman commits adultery, both she and her lover will be condemned to death.
- If a man rapes a virgin, he "owns" her and will be forced to marry her; the rape victim automatically loses all rights as a free and independent woman.
- If a married or betrothed woman is raped, she and the rapist will be stoned to death.
- If a husband discovers some "uncleanness" in his wife, he can write a note announcing his divorce and send her out of his house.
- If daughters of priests "play the whore," the punishment is death by fire.

The New Testament continues the tradition of putting woman in her place. In his letter to the Ephesians (5:22–24), Paul wrote:

> Wives, submit yourselves unto your own husbands as unto the Lord. For the husband is the head of the wife even as Christ is the head of the Church and he is the savior of the body. Therefore as the Church is subject unto Christ, so let the wives be to their own husbands in everything.

In I Timothy 2:11–14, the Garden of Eden myth is invoked to make the point that because the first woman was so easily deceived, all her descendants should be forced into silence:

> Let the woman learn in silence with all subjection. But I suffer not a woman to teach, nor to usurp authority over the man, but to be in silence. For Adam was first formed and then Eve and Adam was not deceived, but the woman being deceived was in the transgression.

In I Corinthians 11:7–9, the same story is repeated in yet another version:

> But the woman is the glory of the man. For the man is not of the woman but the woman of the man. Neither was man created for the woman but the woman for the man.

Throughout the centuries, the saints reiterated the basic message. Saint Clement, considered the father of the Roman church, quoted the Bible as justification for urging women to avoid physical sports and to content themselves with spinning, weaving, and cooking. Saint John Chrysostom, a fifth-century Christian teacher, declared that "woman taught once and ruined everything. On this account . . . let her not teach." Saint Augustine relied on the Bible's authority in his insistence that man is complete alone, for he is made in God's image, but woman is not complete without man.

In the fifteenth century two Dominican monks used the creation myth to explain the carnal nature of witchcraft, emphasizing throughout their treatise the imperfections and deceptions of the female sex:

> For as regards intellect, or the understanding of spiritual things, they seem to be of a different nature from men. . . . The natural reason is that [a woman] is more carnal than a man, as is clear from her many carnal abominations. And it should be noted that there was a defect in the formation of the first woman, since she was formed from a bent rib. . . . And since through this defect she is an imperfect animal, she always deceives. . . . Therefore a wicked woman is by her nature quicker to waver in her faith, and consequently quicker to abjure the faith, which is the root of witchcraft.

The metaphor had become the reality. Woman was defective; therefore she was carnal; therefore she was deceptive; therefore she wavered in her faith and was susceptible to the devil's charms. Woman was feared because woman was powerful, and her sexual powers were feared most of all. Indeed, her unforgivable sin was her inherent sensuality. Like nature herself, the female sex was viewed as receptive—warm, moist, enfolding— and like the earth, she could be violently unpredictable, her "storms" of intuition, compassion, and maternal protectiveness clashing with the reasoned calculations of those who insisted that good and evil were abso- lutes, with God occupying heaven and Lucifer banished to hell.

That morality might be relative, an ebbing and flowing that depends on values, relationships, and circumstance, was akin to heresy in a world ruled by the supreme authority of an intolerant and imperious male God. That knowledge of sexuality and delight in sensual pleasures might be a privilege, even a right of the human species, was an affront to the male God's code of morality, in which sensuality was considered the devil's doorway. That females could think independently, live alone, own property, and use their healing powers in the service of others directly defied God's command that woman be submissive and defer to the greater wisdom of man.

The entire female sex had evolved from the ancient image of the compas- sionate mother to the church-inspired conception of the deceiving tempt- ress, who by her very presence could endanger the souls of decent men. This view of the inherently depraved nature of the female captured the imagination of the Indo-Europeans, was institutionalized in the Bible's teachings and the Christian religion, and found its most grotesque expres- sion in the European witchcraze, a tale of such profound and unfathomable evil that the mind cringes from its horror.

In sixteenth- and seventeenth-century Europe, tens of thousands of "witches"—some scholars place the number in the millions—were hanged, tortured to death, strangled, boiled in oil, or burned at the stake during the church-sanctioned reign of terror. Lawyers, priests, and scholars penned the monstrous witch-hunting manuals that painstakingly described how the pious could identify, torture, and destroy the devil's earthly representa- tives. In thousands of witch trials, professional male doctors (for by that time the tradition of forbidding women from education and training in the healing arts was formalized by law) provided the testimony that stripped women of their possessions, subjected them to barbarous methods of torture, and sealed their doom. Kindhearted observers who requested leniency and skeptics who questioned the barbarous methods of the Inquisition were accused of heresy and, in many cases, joined the witches at the stake.

Eighty-five percent of the victims were women, for in this time of plague, war, and religious oppression, women had become the scapegoats for every possible misfortune. If a baby was stillborn, the midwife was blamed (midwifery, once honored as a noble profession, was now considered beneath the dignity of the university-trained male doctor). If a cow's milk ran dry, the female neighbor (or any woman who happened to have been in the vicinity) was condemned. If a man was impotent, Saint Thomas Aquinas himself proposed that the wife or mother-in-law should be held accountable. Any oddity or nonconformity turned a woman into a potential suspect. Old women, young women, outspoken women, painfully shy women, homely women, beautiful women, unmarried women, widowed women, rich women, poor women, and women with moles, warts, or birthmarks were all potential suspects.

If a woman practiced the art of herbal healing, ignoring priestly pronouncements that sickness and suffering were God's chosen punishments for sin, she risked being called a witch. If she met in secret with other women to worship female goddesses and ancient "pagan" religions, she was pronounced a heretic. If she was young and fetching, wore her hair long and unrestrained, slept naked, or in one way or another inflamed the passions of those who equated sensuality with the devil, she was in jeopardy of being tortured and burned at the stake.

But in truth it didn't matter whether a woman was rich or poor, young or old, attractive or unattractive, married, spinstered, or widowed. What mattered was that she was a woman. In the notorious *Malleus Maleficarum*, the most famous of all the witch-hunting manuals (available in English, German, French, and Italian, with at least thirty editions appearing before 1669), the authors, both Dominican priests, explain why women were susceptible to the devil's seductions:

> All witchcraft comes from carnal lust, which is in women insatiable. . . . Wherefore for the sake of fulfilling their lusts they consort with devils. . . . It is sufficiently clear that it is no matter for wonder that there are more women than men found infected with the heresy of witchcraft. . . . And blessed be the Highest Who has so far preserved the male sex from so great a crime.

The ability to think and reason independently—traits that could be said to characterize any woman who called herself healer—was evidence enough for suspicion. "When a woman thinks alone," the *Malleus* declared, "she thinks evil." In the *Compendium Maleficarum*, a lesser-known but equally malignant witch-hunting manual, the author (also a monk) warns witch-hunters to view the entire female sex with suspicion, for it is in a woman's nature to be foolish, impetuous, and unwise:

> For other things being equal, greater faith is to be placed in the revelations of men. The feminine sex is more foolish, and more apt to mistake natural or demoniacal suggestions for ones of Divine origin. Women, too, are of a more humid and viscous nature, more easily influenced to perceive various phantoms, and slower and more loath to resist such impulses. Therefore women are quicker to imagine, but men are less obstinate in holding to their imaginings; and since women have less power of reasoning and less wisdom, it is easier for the devil to delude them with false and deceptive apparitions.

The *Compendium Maleficarum* denounces any woman "whose fervour is too eager, captious and unbridled, and therefore suspect." Be on the lookout, the author warns all prospective witch-hunters, for specific female traits that indicate a haglike temperament; such vigilance is essential not only to bring the sorceress to justice but also to protect the purity and integrity of the unlucky male who unwittingly crosses her path.

> Further, since women are lascivious, luxurious and avaricious in their manner of life (as Apollonius has remarked), it must be noted whether such prophetesses are particularly garrulous, of a roaming disposition, evildoers, greedy of praise, passionate, and whether in their teaching or in their attitude towards the Sacraments of the Church they show themselves in any way opposed to the Apostolic doctrine. For women of this sort not only deceive themselves, but drag even learned men to destruction.

Through their exhaustive descriptions, biblical anecdotes, and saintly proscriptions, the witch-hunters left no doubt that the entire female sex was to be feared and reviled. Women were feared because women had great sexual and intuitive powers, and no woman was more powerful or more greatly feared than the wise woman healer, who, it was believed, procured her prodigious healing powers not from God but from the devil. The following story about a wise woman witch is related by Jeanne Achterberg in her book *Woman as Healer*:

> Gilly Duncan was a young servant woman in the employ of David Seaton, deputy bailiff of a small town near Edinburgh. Gilly had established a reputation as a healer and cured those who were troubled or grieved with any kind of sickness or infirmity. Seaton felt her exceptional skill was unnatural. He also claimed to have seen her going to unexplained places at night. He obtained torture devices and began to question her. He jerked her head around with a rope, applied the thumbscrews, and examined her for the devil's mark. She finally confessed to the wicked allurements and enticements of the devil. Satisfied with his work, Seaton turned her over to the authorities. They forced her, with their own means, to name her accomplices. Those accused, the so-called witches of North Berwick, were tried and hanged in about 1592.

In the *Compendium Maleficarum* a sad and bizarre tale is related about another wise woman healer. The long story begins with a description of her astonishing healing powers, which the author insists she used for evil purposes:

> At Dammartin [France], December 1587, Nicole Stephanie of Saint-Pol was induced by a reward to purge the castle from the plague which was afflicting it, since she had a reputation for skill in such matters. She performed this task with great care: but after a sufficient period to prevent any fear of further contagion, and when she had been paid her reward and was allowed to depart, she was angry at being dismissed earlier than she expected and at the thought of losing the good rich living she had been enjoying, and thought that she could provide an excuse for delaying her departure by casting some spell of sickness on the Chatelain's wife, who had been very prompt and eager to dismiss her. So without any hesitation she decided to afflict that lady with a disease, so that she might again be asked for her services in removing it.

Nicole Stephanie's mistress was suddenly tormented by a terrible trembling and "such pain in her feet that they were horribly curled up so that the toes were twisted round to the heels." Terrified servants reported conversations in which Nicole Stephanie allegedly boasted that she had learned her healing skills from a famous he-witch who impregnated her and was later condemned to die for his necromantic crimes. The fear of witchcraft spread throughout the castle with the speed and virulence of the plague itself. After her son was tortured and forced to confess that his mother had inflicted a spell on the castle's inhabitants, the "witch" was kicked, beaten with sticks, and dragged to the fire by two lusty peasants. She eventually confessed to her crimes and was burned at the stake along with her son.

In small towns and rural villages throughout Europe, wise women healers like Gilly Duncan and Nicole Stephanie were accused of witchcraft, tortured unmercifully, and put to death for their godless crimes. Their problems typically began with a strange, unexpected, or inexplicable circumstance; soon enough, rumors and gossip began to spread, sexual impropriety was suggested, torture was used to extract the confessions, corroboration was sought in the deeds (good or bad) the alleged witch performed or in the actions she refused to undertake, and proof was painstakingly alchemized from the bubbling fear and hysteria of peasant superstitions and religious fervor.

Good deeds were as suspect as evil-doing, for healing itself was considered a nefarious art. When plagues and epidemics swept through rural villages, priests attempted to comfort the peasantry with the knowledge that their afflictions were sent by God as punishment for their sins. But after offering their confessions, the villagers appealed to the local wise women for help with their suffering. Herbs were gathered, poultices applied, potions brewed, and throughout Christendom the sick and the dying were "miraculously" restored to health by the ancient arts of feminine healing.

Such flamboyant ministrations inflamed the passions of the priests, who insisted that the wise women healers (and any male doctors who were brave or foolish enough to rely on the simple curative power of herbs) were dabbling with magic and interfering with the will of God. With religious leaders providing the necessary spiritual impetus, laws were written proclaiming that all women who practiced the healing arts without having attended a university were witches and must die for their crimes. Because older, well-established laws strictly forbade women from attending universities, the only officially sanctioned healers were men. And since only the rich could afford the services of the university-trained male physicians, the peasantry was doomed to suffer in silence or risk their lives by consulting the healing witch. Just asking a witch for help (even if that help derived from her healing powers) was enough to seal your doom in some localities; a Scottish law of 1563, for example, decreed that not only witches be condemned to death but any and all who consulted them.

Herbs and ointments, the witch-hunters argued, were useless vegetative matter that could only "heal" when invested with powers derived from the devil. Thus, any healing through simple, natural means generated automatic suspicion of witchcraft. The *Compendium Maleficarum* expressly states that herbs and ointments are a "cover" for witchcraft:

> There is no curative virtue in any of the external remedies used by witches for the sicknesses they have caused, such as herbs, unguents, baths and such things; but these are merely a cover for their witchcraft which, through fear of the severity of the law, they dare not show openly.

"For this must always be remembered, as a conclusion," a well-respected and influential English witch-hunter intoned, "that by witches we understand not only those which kill and torment, but all Diviners, Charmers, Jugglers, all Wizards, commonly called wise men and wise women . . . and in the same number we reckon all good Witches, which do no hurt but good, which do not spoil and destroy, but save and deliver. . . . It were a thousand times better for the land if all Witches, but especially the blessing Witch, might suffer death."

The blessing witch—the wise woman healer who did no harm but only good, easing the pain of women in labor, ministering to the sick with gentle herbs and natural, time-proven remedies—was considered even more dangerous than the witch who poisoned cattle, conjured murderous lightning storms, or flew to the orgiastic sabbats on her bread paddle, for by using her powers to help her fellow human beings, she placed herself above God. Catholic doctrine taught that only God had the power to decide who would live and who would die. By using their considerable powers to heal others—powers that according to the witch-hunters' twisted logic could only have been acquired with the devil's help—the wise women healers attempted to mimic God's power and usurp His will, crimes punishable by swift judgment and excruciating torture and death.

Midwives were particularly despised and feared, for the miracle of birth was now contaminated with the shame and degradation associated with the sexual act. Midwives who sought to ease the pain or intensity of labor directly defied the biblical pronouncements that women should suffer in childbirth as penance for their original sin. When a baby was stillborn or died soon after birth, superstition and fear pointed to the midwife, for the witch-hunters insisted that these compassionate healers were actually witches in disguise who murdered scores of newborn babies and used the boiled and cooled fat to cover their bodies with "devil's grease." Thus anointed, they were able to fly through keyholes or up chimneys to join friends and neighbors at the sabbat, where revelers joined in frenzied dances, engaged in sexual intercourse with attending demons and witches, and topped off the festivities with feasting on such delicacies as boiled children, exhumed corpses, or fricassees of bats.

Nothing was beyond the evil of the wise woman witch. In a crazed section of the *Malleus*, the authors describe how witches collected male genitals, stored them in boxes or birds' nests, and fed them grain to keep them "alive":

> And what, then, is to be thought of those witches who in this way sometimes collect male organs in great numbers, as many as twenty or thirty members together, and put them in a bird's nest, or shut them up in a box, where they move themselves like living members, and eat oats and corn, as has been seen by many and is a matter of common report? It is to be said that it is all done by devil's work and illusion, for the senses of those who see them are deluded in the way we have said. For a certain man tells that, when he had lost his member, he approached a known witch to ask her to restore it to him. She told the afflicted man to climb a certain tree, and that he might take which he liked out of a nest in which there were several members. And when he tried to take a big one, the witch said: You must not take that one; adding, because it belonged to a parish priest.

For such imagined misdeeds, the witches burned, but their tortured confessions did not ease the anguished fears and thinly disguised longings of the witch-hunters. In censuring the witch, the witch-hunters exalted her innate female powers, particularly her power to heal, comfort, nurture, and protect; in condemning her, they betrayed the desires of their own souls. When a Basque judge in 1609 branded witches as "usually lascivious and wanton wenches, living only for the flesh," his words revealed the depth of his own passionate nature. Tortured and inflamed, his lust for beauty, for love, for life itself is transparent in its intensity:

> When you see them with their hair on their shoulders flying in the wind, then in this gorgeous ornament of their hair they appear so beautiful that when the sun shines through it as if through a cloud, the radiance is indescribable and gives off blazing lightning; this is how enchantment comes from their eyes which are just as dangerous in love as in witchcraft.

The madness ended in England in 1684, when the last witch was officially hanged, in America in 1692, and in Germany in 1775. When the metaphysical battle between God and Satan was replaced with a new cosmology in which science was deified, the devil of the underworld and his dastardly human incubi and succubi gradually loosened their hold on the human imagination.

In the sixteenth century, Copernicus initiated the cosmological shift by redefining the earth as a minor star on the fringes of the galazy; this was such a heretical view that the scientist waited until 1543, the year of his death, to publish his theories. Galileo (1564–1642), who was condemned by the Roman Inquisition, confirmed and extended Copernicus's heliocentric theory, encouraging the use of mathematical language to decipher and express the laws of nature and insisting that scientists restrict themselves to that which can be objectively measured and quantified. From the seventeenth century onward, soul, consciousness, and spirit were banished from the domain of science, and the devil became an anachronism, an old-fashioned myth that had outlived its usefulness. Man's energies were gradually redirected from torturing and enslaving women to the grander, more challenging task of torturing and enslaving Nature Herself.

In his position as attorney general for King James I, Francis Bacon presided over numerous witchtrials in seventeenth-century England, and his courtroom work had an obvious impact on his scientific musings. Bacon proposed that nature, like the witch, should be hounded, subdued, constrained, and "bound into service." Arguing that the domination and control of nature should be the goal of the new scientific method, Bacon

encouraged his fellow scientists to "torture nature's secrets from her."
Nature and the female, intimately linked since the beginning of human
time, were tormented first in the name of God and later in the service of
science. The enduring wisdom of the Great Goddess, who represented the
joyful, sensual, life-affirming aspects of being human, was defiled, woman
herself was humiliated and disgraced, and man, as the degrader, debased
himself.

When we ravage the earth, raping and plundering her resources, we
sever our own lifeline to the future and cut ourselves off from the ultimate
source of healing and wholeness. When we divide humanity into two
unequal halves, disparaging one-half as less trustworthy, intelligent, and
spiritually advanced, we cleave our own souls in two. For what we do to
each other, we do to ourselves; what we do to the earth, we do to our
own souls. Everything in life is connected, and when any part is cut off
or broken apart, the whole feels the insult and must struggle to maintain
balance and harmony.

A modern story adds a deeper level to the biblical creation story to
demonstrate how men and women are each the source of the other:

> There was a man who was married to a very wise woman. In time,
> the man became jealous of his wife's wisdom.
> Insecure inside and angry outside, the man argued to himself that,
> since man was created before woman, man was clearly superior.
> Seeking support for his insecurity, he sought Jacob at the bakery.
> "Woman was created from the rib of man," said the husband,
> beginning to build a case for himself.
> "Yes," said Jacob, barely looking up. "Woman was made from the
> rib of a man. But, from what was man created?"
> "Well, from the ground, the earth, of course."
> "And," said Jacob, "isn't a woman the earth which receives your
> seed?"
> "Yes," said the man, feeling foolish.
> Jacob stopped what he was doing and spoke with the ease of truth.
> "Each of us is the source of the other. And our only strength is in
> knowing this."

From the very beginning of human time, the feminine spirit of healing
has guided the wounded to the insight that we are each the source of the

other. Only when we accept the basic truth that we are interconnected and interdependent will our wounds be healed. Only when we embrace our sensuality and enfold what is wild, passionate, and intuitive into the rational and reasonable world, will we become whole once again. The healing power of the female spirit leads us to search for the lost and broken pieces and, with patience and faith, begin the process of restoring them to the whole. Healing is synonymous with reintegration, and the most healing act of all is the ability to reach out to others in the spirit of love and forgiveness, knowing that whatever has happened before is in the past and it is to the present that we must direct our attentions. Resentment opens up old wounds and refuses healing; forgiveness, which is at the heart of healing, eases our pain and soothes our troubled spirits.

"The memory of things past is indeed a worm that does not die," wrote Dominic Maruca. "Whether it continues to grow by gnawing away at our hearts or is metamorphosed into a brightly colored winged creature depends . . . on whether we can find a forgiveness we cannot bestow on ourselves."

Perhaps we can learn how to forgive (and, more important, learn how to *be* forgiven) from an innkeeper who knew how to keep his "accounts."

> *"How should one pray for forgiveness?"* the disciple asked Rabbi Elimelech of Linzensk. After considering the question for a moment, the rabbi suggested that the disciple spend his time in the days before Yom Kippur observing the behavior of a certain innkeeper. The disciple took a room at the inn and for several days kept careful watch over the innkeeper. To his great disappointment, nothing he observed seemed to illuminate the nature of forgiveness.
>
> Then, on the night before Yom Kippur, the disciple watched as the innkeeper sat alone in his room, his desk illuminated by a candle and two large ledgers spread out before him. Reading from the first book the innkeeper recited all the sins he had committed during the past year. Then he turned to the second book and proceeded to describe all the pains and woes that had been visited upon him in the previous year.
>
> Finished with his recitations, the innkeeper looked up toward Heaven and said, "Dear G-d,[1] it is true I have sinned against you, but it is also true that you have done many upsetting things to me. Now it is time to start a new year, so let us take this opportunity to wipe the slate clean. I will forgive you, and You will forgive me."

[1]Traditional Orthodox practice refrains from writing out the divine name.

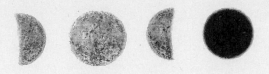

CHAPTER 4

SPEAK TO THE EARTH

Speak to the earth and it shall teach thee.

—The Book of Job 12:8

The purpose of good medicine is to make it simple.

—Mad Bear, Native American medicine man

The earth forgives all. She is the unchanging center, the tranquil core around which all life and movement revolves. She grounds our being, feeds our bodies, and nourishes our souls. Even when we deeply wound her, she heals herself and continues to provide. Polluted rivers and streams are pulled deep within her breast, where minerals remove the contaminated ions, and underground channels return the newly purified waters to the surface. In compost heaps and garbage dumps, the earth sends forth its armies of bacteria to break down wastes into fertile soil, providing the essential nutrients for the vegetables and plants that sustain human life.

From the muck at the bottom of the stream the lotus takes root, driving upward with strength and purpose to open its finely petaled face to the life-giving energy of the sun.

For thousands of years, wise women healers, medicine men, and shamans have honored the earth as mother, gratefully accepting her healing plants and herbs as gifts of renewal and regeneration. Even today more than 80 percent of the world's population rely on simple herbs and crude plant extracts for health and healing. Of all the diverse earth-centered societies, none is more passionately connected to the earth than the Native Americans, whose vast knowledge of healing plants impressed early settlers like Albert Isaiah Coffin (who eventually became an ardent advocate of herbal therapy). Deathly ill with tuberculosis, Coffin was cured by a Seneca wise woman, who gathered an apronful of herbs and nursed him back to health in exchange for a gallon of cider.

The ancient art of herbal medicine is still practiced by certain wise women and men who wander the hills and valleys looking for herbs, which they call "helpers." One of the most famous is the Shoshone medicine man Rolling Thunder, whose wisdom has been sought by numerous individuals and organizations committed to rediscovering the healing powers of Mother Earth. In 1974, a series of events led me to Rolling Thunder, an encounter that would have a profound impact on my life. I was studying the Japanese martial art of Aikido in New York City when I ruptured the meniscus—the cushion separating the upper and lower legs—in my knee. Because the meniscus does not have a blood supply of its own, it cannot spontaneously heal itself, and two orthopedic specialists informed me that surgery was my only option.

Having just returned from a year traveling around the world to study Chinese, Japanese, Philippine, and Indian healing methods, all of which emphasize the innate self-healing powers of the mind and body, I chose to ignore the advice of the specialists and for two months worked hard to heal myself, using massage, gentle exercises, acupuncture, and Chinese herbs. Although my knee gradually improved, it remained swollen and painful, and I continued to look for new techniques that would help stimulate the healing process.

One day a friend loaned me the recently published book *Rolling Thunder*, in which journalist Doug Boyd describes his experiences with Native American wisdom-seeker Rolling Thunder. I was immediately struck by the similarity between Rolling Thunder's vision of the human being as a microcosm of nature ("Every person is a model of life, so the true nature of a person is the nature of life") and the Taoist philosophy in which human beings are regarded as exemplars of the natural world and encouraged to live in harmony with nature's immutable laws.

In one of those serendipitous events that seem to guide our individual destinies in life, I told another friend about the book, and she mentioned a seminar Rolling Thunder was scheduled to lead on an Indian reservation in Georgia. Hoping to learn more about Rolling Thunder's healing techniques (and continuing to search for a nonsurgical alternative for healing my knee), I flew down to Georgia for the conference. I arrived several hours before the first session and decided to take a walk along the river bordering the Indian reservation. At first I walked slowly, for I was accustomed to extreme discomfort whenever I exercised; but to my surprise, my knee didn't bother me at all. After a few minutes I broke into a run and jogged for perhaps ten minutes, experiencing no pain whatsoever. When I recall the events of that morning, I like to think that just being near the great medicine man healed my knee; or perhaps my knee was simply the vehicle for putting me in touch with Rolling Thunder and, having performed that function, it spontaneously healed itself.

I spent four days with Rolling Thunder, who spoke eloquently and passionately about his function in life and the specific talents and insights of the Native Americans—"the red people," as he called them. "The red people are the custodians of Mother Earth," Rolling Thunder explained, "and our wisdom is essential now because the Mother is in a state of crisis. The other three colors—the black, yellow, and white peoples—need to actively seek their visions and learn of their purpose so that we can all unite together to heal our many wounds and become whole once again." As Rolling Thunder talked about healing the wounds of body, mind, and spirit, he often discussed the invaluable assistance of herbs, or helpers. Because herbs are divine gifts of the earth spirit, we must learn to use them with knowledge and reverence. All plants, like all living things, have a value and a purpose—what Rolling Thunder called "a reason for being"—and when we find the power plant that we are seeking, we must speak to it, pay our respects to the chief, and carefully explain why we are taking the plant's roots, leaves, berries, or flowers. After speaking to the earth, asking for her help, and receiving her permission, we must take only those parts of the plant that are needed and never more, and we must always use what we have taken for a good purpose—to heal and make whole.

When Rolling Thunder spoke to Mother Earth, he did not say, "I feel sick, fix me," but instead he sought to communicate this message: "My body, mind, and spirit are out of balance, and I need your help to get better." Entering into a partnership with the herb, he gratefully accepted its help while acknowledging his own responsibility to take an active role in "getting better," which, he insisted, is more than just feeling better but includes thinking better, acting better, and becoming a better human being. The highest goal of living, Rolling Thunder believes, is to treat every living thing including yourself with respect, for everything in life has a reason for being.

In the book *Rolling Thunder*, the great medicine man described his philosophy of life, which, not coincidentally, is synonymous with his philosophy of healing:

> The most basic principle of all is that of not harming others, and that includes all people and all life and all things . . . Every being has the right to live his own life in his own way. Every being has an identity and a purpose. To live up to his purpose, every being has the power of self-control, and that's where spiritual power begins.

The power of self-control can be understood as the power to assume responsibility and heal ourselves. The underlying theme of all ancient and traditional forms of healing is contained in those simple words, which emphasize the fact that all human beings have the innate ability to take charge of their own destinies. Healing is not something that is done to us only when we are sick, but an ongoing process that we initiate and maintain ourselves even when we are feeling energetic and healthy. Traditional Chinese and Japanese medicine, Indian Ayurvedic medicine, early European and Middle Eastern healing arts, Native American medicine, and other traditional healing methods teach that health is not just the absence of disease but a state of well-being that results from a "dynamic balance" of harmony and centeredness.

"Find your center," a Taoist proverb teaches, "and you will be healed." Rolling Thunder phrases the same basic message in a slightly different way, urging the red, black, yellow, and white people to actively seek out their identity and purpose, a process that will put them in touch with their spiritual power. The Chinese philosophy of finding your center and the Native American concept of tapping into your spiritual power emphasize a continuing process of healing, growth, and renewal. Because life is dynamic and ever-changing, every human being will cycle in and out of balance many times. When we are out of balance, we feel sick, disoriented, irritable, anxious, and out of sorts. When we are in balance, we feel centered, at *home* with self, family, and community, at *one* with the world.

The gradual process of cycling in and out of balance occurs over a period of time and can be traced to a multiplicity of causes—lack of sleep, inadequate exercise, poor diet, environmental pollution, unrelieved stress, or a general state of disharmony with family, community, and especially self. The experience of disharmony, or off-centeredness, was described by Siddhartha Gautama (the Buddha) as *"dukkha,"* which literally means a bone torn from its socket and connotes a state of being broken or torn apart from oneself. Because illness is thought to result from a complex pattern of causes leading to disharmony and imbalance, feeling sick or out of sorts is considered much more significant than a mere symptom of disease or disorder. Illness is imagined as a message emanating deep from our center that we do not fit comfortably into the whole of which we are part. Our symptoms of distress call out for a creative response, which requires the commitment to move inward, toward our core self. For only when we go deep into the center, where the heart and soul reside, will we learn how to right the imbalance, fix the brokenness, heal the wounds, and become whole again.

All traditional cultures view illness as both natural and meaningful, for the experience of being out of balance offers an opportunity to adapt to crisis and in the process grow stronger physically, mentally, and spiritually. Traditional medicine reveres the inherent wisdom and integrity of the human body, for as flexible and adaptable creatures, we have the power to stabilize ourselves and put ourselves *right* again. The medicine man, shaman, wise woman, and traditional healer know that their job is to assist and support nature, honoring at all times the sacred connections between the individual, the community, and the environment.

The only healing method that deviates dramatically from these concepts of balance, centeredness, self-control, and natural healing is modern techno-logical medicine. While ancient healing traditions think in terms of circles and cycles, spirals, and continuums, modern scientific medicine focuses on margins and perimeters, vertical ascensions, and horizontal declines. The natural world is perceived by the analytical mind as a bounded region of straight lines, abrupt turns, and sharp corners; human beings are imagined as machinelike creatures of stimulus and response; and the human experience of illness is reduced to the symptoms and signs of disease.

A humorous story illustrates how deeply this philosophy of cause and effect has permeated our thinking about illness and disease:

> "I hate it, I hate it, I *hate* it!" Feldman wailed. "I can't *stand* having a cold."
>
> "You'll just have to be patient," the doctor told him. "People get colds in the winter, and there's no cure—"
>
> "But it's making me crazy. You've *got* to do something."
>
> "Tell you what you can do," the doctor said. "Take a cold shower, wrap a towel around your waist, and run around outside the house for an hour."
>
> "But Doctor," said Feldman, "then I'll get pneumonia."
>
> "Yes, but *that* we have a cure for!"

The doctor, of course, is responding to his patient's demands for a cure. "You've *got* to do something," the patient whines, abrogating his responsibility to help his body heal itself while expressing impatience at the time and energy needed to restore balance, and the inconvenience of having to wait while nature does its job. By reducing his illness to the status of disease and turning to the outside expert for a quick and effective cure, he denies himself the power of self-healing.

The doctor's response to his patient's demands reveals both the limitations of modern medicine and its significant potential, for while conventional M.D.s can't do anything to cure the common cold, all sorts of amazing remedies are available if the patient happens to get *really* sick. But if we expand the definition of healing to include caring as well as curing, the potential remains, while the limitations become less restrictive. When faced with illnesses for which there is no quick fix, modern-day healers can listen to the words being spoken—"I hate it," "I can't stand it," "It's making me crazy"—and look for the source of the patient's problem in those clear expressions of impatience and futility. A good doctor (and there are many patient and perceptive physicians operating within the modern technological model of medicine) listens to his patients and enlarges the symptoms and signs of disease to include the illness— the *human experience* of living through the disease. By focusing on the patient's subjective feelings, thoughts, and emotions, as well as the objective symptoms and signs of disease, the doctor treats the patient as a whole person with interdependent spiritual, psychological, and physiological needs.

In an interview with Bill Moyers in *Healing and the Mind*, internist Thomas Delbanco describes an incident that brought home to him this idea of the "whole person" for whom illness can be a meaningful and life-changing experience. When a friend became seriously ill with a strange assortment of symptoms, a much-admired professor agreed to diagnose her problem and suggest a course of treatment:

> When she came out, we were all waiting with our fingers crossed. "Well, what's the prescription?" And she said, "He tells me I've got to get a washing machine. I'm working too hard at home." That was the diagnosis. . . . You don't find the washing-machine prescription in many textbooks. But it helped her a lot. She was cured, she was brought back to health, she was made whole, if you will, by that prescription.

By taking the time to move beyond his patient's objective symptoms and signs of disease and enter into a discussion of her "reason for being"— her identity, purpose, and spiritual values—the doctor gave his patient permission to heal herself. Just the simple act of listening, paying attention, and acknowledging that life is stressful initiated the healing process. Another physician interviewed by Moyers tells a story of a miscommunication between a doctor and his patient that actually created a sickness of heart and soul.

> We once had a doctor on staff who told a Cambodian woman that she had a kidney infection. In her belief system the kidney is very important, so having a kidney infection is like having an infection of the soul. Now you can't have a little infection of your soul, that's a life-threatening thing. So she was very, very concerned. She went home and gave away her possessions, the family came in and wailed, but three days later she was still, miraculously, alive. So they called the doctor back and said, "Why is she still alive?" And he said, "Well, she's just got a little kidney infection, why shouldn't she be alive?"
>
> Meanwhile, of course, we had put enormous stress on this woman and her family because we didn't communicate or try to understand her value system.

In a very real sense, every illness infects the soul, for when our bodies are sick, our minds and spirits are also thrown out of balance. While modern technology is often extremely efficient at saving the critically ill (even participating in the occasional miracle of bringing the dead back to life), the more complicated, less easily quantified matters of mind and soul go untouched and unheeded. Modern medicine with its computerized diagnostic procedures, experimental drugs, and high-tech machines is so busy intervening in catastrophes that doctors don't have time to pursue strategies that could prevent people from getting sick in the first place.

Anthony Robbins, author of the best-seller *Awaken the Giant Within*, tells a wonderfully vivid story in his workshop presentations that serves as a metaphor to help people understand the demands and pressures on their doctors and the need to assume responsibility for preventing problems. Robbins is sensitive to the extraordinary pressures on modern doctors, whose superhuman efforts to save lives leaves them little time to spend on preventative strategies.

> Imagine you're outside and you're going by a river. All of a sudden you hear somebody screaming and you know they are drowning. . . . A few people are real leaders—they're called doctors—they put themselves on the line and jump in the river even though it's going really fast. This person is going down, and they use every ounce of their strength and ability to save him. They grab him out of the water, swimming against the river, fighting the whole time. They get the person out, pump the water out, give him mouth-to-mouth resuscitation, and just as that person is coming to life, guess what they hear? Two more screams out there. The doctor swims out and gets the first person, brings him in, swims out to the other one, pumps the water out of both of them, gives them both mouth-to-mouth resuscitation, and guess what? As soon as these two are just about to recover, four more screams. The doctor gets the next one, the next one, the next one, he's got all four, pumping like crazy, giving his all, he's about to collapse he's giving so much. And you know what? Eight more screams.
>
> That's a little stressful. Plus you know what happens? He's so busy saving these people, he never has time to go upstream to see who's throwing them in!

Traditional healers, trained to think in terms of prevention rather than cure, recognize the futility of pulling dead and dying bodies out of the water. Rather than expend their energies on heroic resuscitations, they wander upstream, searching for the cause of the problem, asking the essential question "Why are these people so sick?" Clearly we need both approaches, with doctors trained in "resurrection medicine" stationed downstream to rescue the helpless, and traditional healers upstream to prevent people from falling in in the first place. The obvious solution is for a partnership, with modern technological medicine providing heroic resuscitations for the critically ill while traditional healing methods offer preventative strategies designed to help the body/mind/spirit heal itself.

But many modern physicians and specialists would enter such a partnership with a handicap, which is the *hubris* of the linear, analytical mind. Practitioners of modern technological medicine are too often convinced that their way is the only way because it follows the rigors and discipline of the scientific method, with each technological intervention, diagnostic procedure, and pharmaceutical remedy carefully weighed, measured, and double-blind tested. Talk about the soul, values, family, community, and environment are considered outside the doctor's purview, and preventative measures focusing on meditation, relaxation, and spiritual "centering" are regarded with skepticism and disdain.

And yet this attention to body, mind, and spirit as an integrated whole and the concern with strengthening the connections between individuals, the community, and the cosmos have been among the most powerful tools available to traditional healers. Shamans and wise women have always understood that a distinction must be made between curing and healing. While modern science focuses on curing, which involves external methods used to intervene in the disease process and alter the body's basic functioning, traditional methods concentrate on the patient's inner resources and innate powers of self-healing. In the effort to cure disease, the focus is placed on the physical body, while healing considers the needs of heart and soul preeminent. When doctors seek a cure, they hope to prevent death; healing is concerned with the capacity to affirm and embrace life.

More than a thousand years ago, Al-Razi (865–925, also known as Rhazes or Ar-Razi), medical chief of the hospital of Baghdad, wrote a book on the limitations facing "men of science" in their attempts to cure diseases. The thirty-three–word title is priceless: *The Reason Why the Ignorant Physicians, the Common People, and the Women in Cities Are More Successful Than Men of Science in Treating Certain Diseases and the Excuses Which Physicians Make for This.*

A letter written by Dr. Al-Razi deals with the same basic subject and enjoys a slightly shorter but equally delightful title: *Why a Clever Physician Does Not Have the Power to Heal All Diseases, for That Is Not within the Realm of the Possible.* What is within the realm of the possible is the prevention of many diseases and disorders through various traditional healing techniques. Good nutrition, careful attention to hygiene, and "simple" medicines were recommended by Dr. Al-Razi, who advised his colleagues that when "a cure can be obtained by diet, use no drugs and avoid complex remedies where simple ones will suffice."

Doctoring with "simples"—crude plant extracts readily supplied by Mother Earth in cultivated gardens, tropical rain forests, and wild weed patches—has always been the mainstay of the "ignorant physician," but the art of herbal healing gradually lost its allure as the university-trained physicians were confronted with the challenge of wiping out the virulent plagues of civilized society. Any village wise woman could prescribe a handful of rosemary, sage, and hyssop for laryngitis, a mustard foot bath for a chest cold, or a distillation of cowslip for insomnia, but such homely remedies were powerless to halt the progression of the Black Death, typhoid, smallpox, cholera, and diphtheria.

When syphilis began its deadly spread through Europe in the late fifteenth century (picked up by French soldiers in Naples from prostitutes who had been unlucky enough to consort with Christopher Columbus's sailors returning from the West Indies), simple medicines were powerless to halt its horrific progression, and the lethal poison mercury was soon promoted as the only effective cure. Most sixteenth- and seventeenth-century physicians believed in the ancient Hippocratic humoral theory, in which disease is thought to result from an imbalance in one of the four "humours" of choler, bile, phlegm, and blood, and treatment is geared to righting the imbalance by promoting evacuation through sweat, vomit, urine, and bowel movements. Mercury impressively provokes evacuation through every one of these normal avenues, but because the poison is so toxic to the human body, another evacuation route is immediately employed: the saliva. Because of the syphilitics' constant, unrelieved salivating and spitting, the tongue and gums swelled; teeth loosened, turned black, or fell out; sores developed on the tongue and palate; ulcers infected the jaws and cheeks; and whole sections of the face, including the eyes, cheekbones, and jawbones, simply rotted away. That many syphilitics died from their treatment and many more suffered hideously from stomach cramps, bloody diarrhea, violent sweating, tremors, paralysis, and loss of sight and hearing did not dampen the enthusiasm of their physicians, who, in the absence of any other cure, reasoned that their patients would die anyway.

Antimony (lead) was another favorite chemical medicine, initially prescribed for virulent and often fatal diseases such as the plague, syphilis, typhoid fever, and smallpox, but eventually offered as a cure for such chronic disorders as asthma, colic, ulcers, stomach "weaknesses," and women's complaints. Immediately after ingestion of this powerful irritant poison, the patient experienced excruciating abdominal pain. Nausea, vomiting, convulsions, and violent cramping followed, and long-term effects included liver and kidney damage and, occasionally, heart failure. In France in 1650, M. d'Avaux, one of Louis XIV's finance advisers, became seriously ill with pulmonary problems and was unlucky enough to be treated by the king's private physician, who was enamored of the new "chemical" medicines. The patient's sufferings at the hands of his doctor are described by Barbara Griggs in *The Green Pharmacy*:

> He was getting perfectly acceptable medical treatment when a relative insisted that he should be seen by the King's physician, Vautier—who prescribed antimony, which he swallowed. An hour afterwards he began to cry that he was burning and that he saw he had been poisoned, that he was sorry that they had allowed him to take the remedy, and that he regretted that he had not made his will. Then the poison having ravished his entrails, he died vomiting, three hours after having taken it.

While the new chemical medicines were frequently lethal, the diseases for which these poisons were administered were also deadly. If a lucky patient happened to survive both his disease and its treatment, the doctor was credited with producing a miracle. When patients died, their deaths were attributed to the ravages of a fatal, untreatable disease and not to the heroic cure. Lesser diseases begat less-agonizing but nonetheless stomach-churning treatments. A prescription for pleurisy, still used in London hospitals in the early eighteenth century, contained six full ounces of fresh horse manure. Ingestion of white peacock's dung was promoted as a cure for epilepsy, while the gemstone topaz was considered just the tonic for diarrhea. A seventeenth-century remedy invented by M. Antoine d'Aquin, another of King Louis XIV's physicians, was composed of such exotic and bizarre (not to mention expensive) ingredients as "pearls, hyacinths, corals, male peony root gathered during the waning of the moon, scrapings from the skull of a man who had died a violent death, and the nails of the eland."

Nicholas Culpeper, a seventeenth-century Oxford-trained English herbalist and apothecary, could barely contain his contempt for such useless and frequently toxic treatments, advising his countrymen that these strong purges would "gnaw their bodies as fast as doctors gnaw their purses." Enraged by the supercilious attitude displayed by the wealthy doctors of England's College of Physicians (who catered almost exclusively to the upper classes), Culpeper took his colleagues to task for ignoring safe, inexpensive, and freely available herbal remedies. "I would they would consider," Culpeper wrote, "what infinite number of poor creatures perish daily who else might happily be preserved if they knew but what the Herbs in their own Gardens were good for."

But most apothecaries and regular (i.e., university-trained) physicians were so preoccupied with the challenge to cure fatal disease that they completely neglected the ancient healing arts. A feverish search was well under way for "magic bullet" medicines capable of wiping out the virulent scourges of an increasingly crowded, industrialized society, including pneumonia, puerperal fever, smallpox, typhoid, meningitis, polio, and tuberculosis. The science of alchemy, in which all manner of minerals and metals are combined, cooled, heated, distilled, brewed, and painstakingly prepared into complicated formulas, pointed the way to a brave new world where disease and disorder could be challenged, and perhaps even defeated, by mixing the alchemists' distilled powders into the morning's cup of tea. Little did people know that the chemical concoctions they took with such trust and faith were slowly sapping their strength, destroying their immune systems, and poisoning them to death.

By the end of the eighteenth century a powdered, crystallized preparation of mercury called calomel became one of the most popular alchemical preparations available in North America. Considered an all-purpose purge for expelling harmful impurities from the body, calomel was lauded by the most famous and successful physicians of the time, including Dr. Benjamin Rush of Philadelphia. A Princeton graduate and professor at Pennsylvania University (which at that time produced 75 percent of the university-trained physicians in North America), Dr. Rush praised calomel as a "safe and nearly an universal medicine."

Dr. Rush was not alone in his enthusiasm for calomel. In *Modern Domestic Medicine*, a home medicine book written for housewives by Dr. Thomas Graham early in the nineteenth century, readers are briefly warned about the "excessive" use of mercury and then informed about calomel's impressive ability to counteract the symptoms of forty-six different infirmities including asthma, jaundice, headaches, and indigestion. Newborn infants were regularly dosed with the poison, children with influenza were administered enormous quantities, and from puberty onward women were told to take calomel for menstrual problems ranging from cramps to "obstructed menses" to the many and diverse inconveniences of pregnancy.

Some keen observers questioned the wisdom of using such strong purges for minor ailments that would improve or disappear if left untreated, while others wondered aloud why the health of the once-vigorous American woman was steadily deteriorating. As Florence Nightingale wrote, it was not uncommon in those days to see "a great-grandmother, who was a tower of physical vigor, descending into a grandmother perhaps a little less vigorous, but still sound as a bell, and healthy to the core, into a mother languid and confined to her carriage and house, and lastly into a daughter sickly and confined to her bed."

Physician Oliver Wendell Holmes, appalled by the sickly state of the American population, suggested that physicians might ask themselves "why our young men and women so often break down." Could it be, he asked, that their medical treatment, specifically the drugs prescribed by their doctors, was weakening their resistance and slowly poisoning them to death? While addressing the Massachusetts Medical Society in 1860, Holmes uttered his famous line: "On the whole, more harm than good is done by medication. . . . I firmly believe that if the whole materia medica, as now used, could be sunk to the bottom of the sea, it would be all the better for mankind—and all the worse for the fishes."

A century later, social critic Ivan Illich echoed Holmes's sentiments. "The medical establishment has become a major threat to health," Illich boldly pronounced in his book *Medical Nemesis.* "The pain, dysfunction, disability, and anguish resulting from technical medical intervention now rival the morbidity due to traffic and industrial accidents and even war-related activities, and make the impact of medicine one of the most rapidly spreading epidemics of our time. Among murderous institutional torts, only modern malnutrition injures more people than iatrogenic disease in its various manifestations."

In the modern age, the epidemic of iatrogenesis (doctor-produced illnesses) continues. Medical interventions for even the most benign conditions have created life-threatening situations. In *Matters of Life and Death,*

Eugene Robin, M.D., tells the story of a young man who was lucky to escape alive from a simple operation to remove an ingrown toenail:

> Because the patient was apprehensive, it was decided to put him to sleep for the procedure. While the anesthesia was being administered, the patient's heart stopped. The surgeon opened the chest and succeeded in restarting the heart, but because haste was imperative, failed to take adequate sterile precautions. After resuscitation, while being wheeled to a hospital room, the patient suffered a fractured leg in an elevator accident. He was returned to surgery, where the fractured leg was placed in a cast.
>
> During the course of the next two days, he developed bacterial pericarditis, an infection of the membranes covering the heart, undoubtedly the result of inadequate sterilization at the time his chest was opened to restart his heart. An operation on the heart was now necessary to drain the infection. This was followed by treatment with antibiotics, during which the patient developed a pulmonary embolism or blood clot in the lung, a common complication both of major fractures of the leg and of prolonged bed rest. This in turn required treatment with an anticlotting drug, and massive bleeding from an ulcer in the stomach followed. The ulcer was probably the result of stress related to the numerous complications and treatments he had undergone, and the anticlotting drug increased the intensity of the bleeding.
>
> After some months, the patient was discharged from the hospital, his ingrown toenail still untreated. He left the hospital alive, a tribute to his youth and his indomitable spirit.

In hopes of dispelling the notion that such episodes are rare, Dr. Robin briefly describes twenty-four "iatroepidemics," epidemics or plagues caused by systematic, preventable errors in medical treatment. "The list," he writes, "is by no means complete." A few of his examples follow:

> *Diethylstilbestrol (DES) to prevent spontaneous abortions.* The drug DES was administered to millions of pregnant women to prevent abortion. It did not prevent abortion, but it did have another and unexpected effect: It exposed the children of the treated women to the development of genital cancer at relatively early ages.

High oxygen exposure and blindness in children. Although oxygen is known to be toxic to many tissues, numerous premature infants were treated with high oxygen concentrations without adequate precautions. The eyes of many were injured by a disease called retrolental fibroplasia. By the 1950s this disease was the leading cause of blindness in children.

Internal mammary artery ligation for coronary artery disease. An artery in the chest is tied to increase blood supply to the heart. Designed to protect patients from heart attacks, this operation proved to be of no value. Before this was demonstrated, huge numbers of patients underwent the procedure and suffered pain, disability, and, occasionally, death.

Ileal bypass and obesity. The last segment of the small intestine (the ileum) was bypassed by a surgical procedure to help patients lose weight. This procedure resulted in liver disease, arthritis, and even death in significant numbers of patients and has now been abandoned. Survivors still suffer from the complications of the surgery. Attempts to remove the bypass have created a second wave of complications.

Radiation for acne. A high incidence of cancer of the skin occurred among patients who had earlier been treated by x-ray to the skin.

The first example, the DES saga, is particularly disturbing, because the drug continued to be prescribed for nearly two decades after controlled studies proved it was ineffective. According to Robert Mendelsohn, M.D., author of *Confessions of a Medical Heretic*, control studies conducted at the University of Chicago and completed in 1952 convincingly demonstrated that DES didn't work, but the drug companies kept producing it, and doctors kept prescribing it. Between 1940 and 1980, six million women received prescriptions for DES, even though the drug was known to be highly toxic and capable of causing congenital malformation. "Now we have a generation of DES daughters with cancer of the vagina, DES sons with tumors of the testes," Mendelsohn writes. "The women who took DES have an increased incidence of cancer *eight times higher* than normal."

Even our "best friend" drugs have metamorphosed into our worst enemies. A 1994 *Newsweek* article titled "Antibiotics: The End of Miracle

Drugs?" describes in chilling detail the improper prescribing and resultant overuse of antibiotics. Studies cited by *Newsweek* show that antibiotic sales have doubled in this country in the last ten years, 50 to 60 percent of all outpatient prescriptions are "inappropriate," and seven out of ten Americans who seek treatment for colds receive antibiotics—even though these drugs are powerless against viral infections such as colds and flus.

In our quest for the quick fix, which includes a willingness to take powerful but ineffective drugs for relatively mild illnesses, we are in the process of creating superbugs capable of protecting their genetic material from invasion by antibiotics. Every time we take an antibiotic, we send a signal to the body's bacteria (described by Stanford University microbiologist Stanley Falkow as "clever little devils") to look for ways of staying alive and protecting their offspring by mutating into a drug-resistant strain. How can we clean up the mess we've made? "Maybe what we need is not more technological fixes," the *Newsweek* article concludes, "but some plain common sense. Like not tossing the hand grenade of powerful antibiotics at the mosquito of a minor infection."

But even when the howitzer-power of an antibiotic is used appropriately, it can create mayhem. John Shen, a practitioner and teacher of Traditional Chinese Medicine, uses a vivid metaphor to help us imagine the havoc we have created by overuse of antibiotics. When germs invade the "home" of our being, doctors send in the antibiotic storm troops, which blaze away with their machine guns, shooting everything in sight—even the benevolent "house detective" bacteria. After the massacre, the storm troops board up all the windows and doors, leaving the carcasses to rot inside. While this may seem like a good idea, remember that this "house" is your body, and somehow you will have to find a way to coexist with the rotting bacteria and with the fact that there are no healthy bugs left to clean up the mess.

The potentially grim consequences of modern interventions are well-known to medical professionals, who sometimes tell jokes as a way of coping with disturbing topics:

> *The doctor took a week off and went hunting in Maine. When he got back to the hospital, a nurse asked, "How was your trip?"*
> *"I didn't kill a thing," he complained.*
> *"Hmph!" she said. "You'd have been better off staying here."*

How far we have strayed from the ancient practice and philosophy of medicine, which considered healers the servants of nature, revered the human body as self-healing and innately balancing, and treasured simple herbal remedies for their gentle, supportive actions. If we listen, we can hear the ancient voices calling out to us. Hippocrates (468–377 B.C.), the Greek healer who is considered the father of modern medicine, taught that "natural forces are the healers of disease" and "whenever a doctor cannot do good, he must be kept from doing harm." Five centuries later, Galen (131–200 A.D.), a native of Pergamom in Asia Minor, argued that "the physician is Nature's assistant." More than a millennium after Galen, the Swiss-German doctor known as Paracelsus (1493–1541) declared that "the physician is only the servant of nature, not her master. Therefore it behooves medicine to follow the will of nature." And the eighteenth-century French philosopher Voltaire insisted that "the art of medicine consists in amusing the patient while nature cures the disease."

These are the same basic messages repeated by modern healers and shamans such as Rolling Thunder who believe that "the most basic principle of all is that of not harming others" and who understand the gentle healing power of herbs, freely provided by Mother Earth for those who understand both the "need and the purpose." Herbs work their magic slowly and gently, helping to restore balance and harmony to the body, mind, and spirit. The plant's healing powers come from the "whole" package, a philosophy at extreme odds with the ancient alchemical and modern pharmaceutical view that "al the vertue is separated from the substance of the medicine, so that the more pure and subtil part of every remedy or medicine, maye be drawn out from the grosse and erthy part."

We are enamored in the modern age with the "pure and subtil" parts, while we are suspicious of the "grosse and erthy." Doctoring with simples is scoffed at by many physicians, who proclaim that someone has to protect amateurs from themselves and who tend to be highly skeptical about the value of herbal remedies, which they regard as quaint, homely, harmless, or at worst, a dangerous form of quackery. "A mountain of prejudice stands between today's doctors and the use of simple plant medicine," writes Griggs in *The Green Pharmacy*, "while the hostility, the amused contempt, or even the outrage that the very idea of doctoring people with plants evokes in medical circles has to be experienced to be believed."

Witness the curious response of the entrenched scientific community to the astonishing protective effects of a simple herbal yeast tonic called Bio-Strath. In double-blind trials conducted in the Netherlands with 123 mentally retarded children, significant improvements were noted in the subjects' ability to concentrate and express themslves. In a study conducted at Zurich University, white mice were subjected to x-ray treatments; those fed Bio-Strath produced larger litters, more litters, and bigger babies. In a double-blind research study conducted at a leading Swiss cancer hospital, patients recovering from surgery and receiving radiation treatment were given Bio-Strath; they experienced dramatic improvements in appetite, physical activity, and general well-being and, on average, gained seven pounds more than the control patients. For several years, Bio-Strath was available for sale in the United States with FDA approval. Then, inexplicably, the FDA banned the herbal preparation, refusing to reveal its reasons. When Bio-Strath's Swiss manufacturer challenged the ban, the FDA admitted that it had no evidence to support its decision, and Bio-Strath was once again freely available in the United States.

The FDA expends a prodigious amount of time and energy guarding the public against the imagined perils of simple herbal remedies. In 1960, the federal agency banned sales of sassafras tea and the use of sassafras in soft drinks after a number of rats given massive doses of safrole, a constituent of the essential oil of sassafras, developed liver cancer. The FDA's decision didn't take into consideration the fact that because safrole is largely insoluble in water, a cup of sassafras tea contains only trace amounts; in fact, not one recorded case of sassafras poisoning or sassafras-related cancer has ever been recorded. Another perplexing aspect of the ban on sassafras is the fact that the FDA didn't forbid the sale of nutmeg, pepper, star anise, or ordinary tea, all of which contain equally infinitesimal amounts of safrole.

The healing plant comfrey has been used for centuries as a food and medicine for treating stomach complaints, mending broken bones, and healing lung disorders. But when pyrrolizidine alkaloids were identified and isolated in the leaves and roots of the plant and then fed to laboratory rats in absurdly high doses (comprising 30 to 50 percent of their basic diet), tumors developed on the animals' livers. Attempts were made to locate cases linking the use of comfrey with the later development of liver disease, but only three highly questionable cases were identified. Nevertheless, comfrey was banned in Canada, and the FDA is presently considering a ban on the herb.

In a "Special Communication" of the *Journal of the American Medical Association* (August 2, 1976), herbal teas were listed as "potential health hazards." The tannins in the teas, it was revealed, could interfere with the biochemical actions of prescription drugs the tea drinker might be taking. Physicians were advised to evaluate their patients' herbal-tea drinking and "discourage these practices whenever feasible" in order to ensure safe and effective drug therapy." Barbara Griggs points out the ludicrous implications of such admonitions:

> The logical inference is that doctors should tell their patients that on no account should they drink ordinary tea—rich in these ominous tannins—when they are taking drugs. Or, if the action of complex modern drugs can be distorted by one simple biological factor, maybe patients taking drugs should stop eating and drinking altogether?

The openly hostile attitude of the medical profession toward herbal remedies makes little sense when we consider the fact that fully one-fourth of the prescription drugs sold in U.S. pharmacies contain active herbal (plant) constituents. Many of these drugs have been packaged and marketed in such a way to disguise their lowly plant origins, but the main ingredients are indeed "grosse and erthy":

- Syrup of Ipepac, which can be found in most family medicine cabinets and is used to induce vomiting in poison cases, is produced from *ipecacuanha*, a South American herb.
- Aspirin, which reduces fever and swelling and has been used to reduce the risk of heart attacks and strokes, is synthesized from willow bark.
- Ephedrine and drugs such as theophilin, which are commonly used for asthma, are derived from the Chinese herb *ma huang* (also known as herb ephedra).
- Antimalarials are manufactured from quinine, an alkaloid from the bark of the cinchona tree found in Peru and Ecuador.
- The dried latex extracted from the unripened fruit of the opium plant is the major constituent of morphine and codeine.
- Curare, a powerful poison extracted from an Amazonian plant, is used as a muscle relaxant during abdominal, rectal, and throat surgeries.
- The rosy periwinkle, native to southeastern Madagascar, contains at least six alkaloids with cancer-fighting properties that have been used to fight lymphoma, Hodgkins disease, and leukemia.
- Digitalis, one of the most effective and commonly used modern remedies for cardiac disease, is obtained from the foxglove plant native to Europe.

In *Tales of a Shaman's Apprentice*, Harvard ethnobotanist Mark Plotkin discusses the untapped potential of the rain forests and bemoans the ignorance of the modern scientific world regarding lowly plant remedies:

> There exists no shortage of "wonder drugs" waiting to be found in the rain forests, yet we in the industrialized world are woefully ignorant about the chemical—and, therefore, medicinal—potential of most tropical plants. . . . In fact, only about 5,000 of the world's 250,000 species have been extensively screened in the laboratory to determine their therapeutic potential, and the approximately 120 plant-based precription drugs on the market today are derived from only 95 species. A quarter of all prescription drugs sold in the United States have plant chemicals as active ingredients. About half of those drugs contain compounds from temperate plants, while the other half have chemicals from tropical species. According to one recent study, the value of medicines derived from tropical plants—that is the amount consumers in the United States spend on them—is more than $6 billion a year.

Despite the countless lives saved (not to mention the enormous profits reaped by the pharmaceutical companies), herbal therapy continues to be regarded with suspicion and outright hostility. Plants are apparently too messy, too muddy, too impossibly complex, and so prejudice against herbal medicines persists, as does skepticism about the value of doctoring with simples. Even when physicians have the opportunity to observe firsthand the healing effects of herbal remedies, they often refuse to seek out additional knowledge or expertise. The following story is told from my own experience.

> Several years ago I was diagnosed with an inguinal hernia. Surgery, I knew, was my only option, but I wanted to complement my treatment by using certain Chinese and Native American herbs to promote healing and recovery. After my surgeon assured himself that the herbs were completely nontoxic (and insisted that I sign a release form), he agreed to allow me to pursue this "experimental" approach to healing. Three weeks after the surgery, the doctor inspected the incision and regarded me with amazement. "I've done thousands of these operations,"

he told me, "but this is the first time I've detected no swelling or bruising."

I was delighted by the impression the herbal therapy made on my doctor, and I offered to write up a brief description of the various herbs so that he could recommend them to other patients.

"Oh, no, no," he said, shifting uncomfortably in his chair. "I really don't care to know anything more about these herbs. They just don't fit into my practice."

Few and far between are the doctors willing to admit that simple herbs may be more effective (and significantly less toxic) than synthetic chemicals. Fewer still would risk the ridicule of their colleagues by offering their patients herbal remedies available without prescription in any health food store. But the problem does not reside only with doctors, for we are all part of a culture that reveres the scientific method and values the quick fix, believing that for every problem there is an instant solution.

When we visit a doctor with symptoms of a cold or the flu, we want to have our illnesses treated seriously, and we expect to leave the doctor's office with some official evidence that we have been treated seriously—most notably, a prescription, which serves to validate the decision to visit a doctor in the first place. If the doctor informs us that antibiotics are useless for flus and colds and suggests instead that we take time to rest and recuperate, most of us respond with impatient bewilderment. Where, we would like to ask, can we find the time "to rest and recuperate"? Who will get the work done, who will take care of the kids, who will pay the bills, answer the mail, run the errands? The ancient healing prescriptions seem not to fit the demands of the modern world.

At the same time, however, we are beginning to understand the risks and perils of the modern technological approach. Our doctors seem cold and aloof, literally out of touch with what is happening inside us. As our relationship with our health care providers becomes increasingly mechanical and impersonal, feelings of hopelessness and helplessness pervade. We feel dissatisfied, unhappy, ill at ease. Something is wrong, and we are beginning to understand that the problem is not with individual doctors but with a system that has lost its connection to the feminine spirit of healing.

As we search for ways to make our health care system less systematic and more caring, many of us are turning to alternative treatments, believing that if nothing else, such treatments will do no harm. An unparalleled opportunity exists to admit our shared ignorance and create a synthesis of the old and the new, in which modern technological medicine would continue to devote its technological brilliance and impressive diagnostic skills to crisis situations and life-threatening diseases, while the ancient art of mind/body healing would be applied to prevention of disease and treatment of chronic, debilitating illnesses.

As in any partnership, the excesses and limitations of each side must be appreciated by both parties. Herbal remedies can't set a broken leg, and antibiotics can't treat the common cold. Surgery may be the only option for an inflamed appendix or bulging hernia, but recovery from surgical procedures can be expedited by herbal treatments. Modern and traditional medicines each have something to offer the other, but we can't realize the potential benefits of cooperation unless both participants admit that they don't have all the answers. It is time to be humble, to recognize, as Dag Hammerskjöld put it in *Markings*, that "humility is just as much the opposite of self-abasement as it is of self-exultation. To be humble is *not to make comparisons*. Secure in its reality, the self is neither better nor worse, bigger nor smaller, than anything else in the universe. It *is*—is nothing, yet at the same time one with everything."

To be humble is not to make comparisons. Modern medicine is "neither better nor worse, bigger nor smaller" than traditional medicine. The ancient insight that we are each the source of the other and that male and female energies must combine for balance and harmony to be achieved underscores the need to search for wisdom elsewhere while remaining open to any and all opportunities to share our wisdom with others. But sharing cannot take place within the competitive mind-set that one method is necessarily superior to another or that modern medicine by itself is enough. As Native American medicine man and wisdom-seeker Rolling Thunder reminds us, there is too much knowledge in the world to be captured in any one theoretical framework; the pathway to wisdom requires that we unite our efforts and work together for the common good. "Not all of the knowledge can be put into books," says Rolling Thunder. "It includes all nature, all of life, and there's too much of it. But I will say that we Indians do know some things the same as other people know some things, and that's why we should share. We would be better off if we could share. We do not look for contests, and we do not believe in competition. We flow with nature and we are guided by the Spirit—the spirit of brotherhood and sharing in all things."

We would be better off if we could share, but we can't share unless we first admit that we don't have all the answers. No one individual or system of thought has a corner on all the wisdom available in the world. Wisdom comes from experience; it is revealed only when we have prepared ourselves to receive it. Once again the feminine spirit of healing guides us, confirming that our strength comes not from self-absorption but from acknowledging our need for each other.

> *As a youth the great master Mat-su was a zealot who would sit in meditation for many hours at a time. One day the disciple Huai-jang approached him.*
>
> *"What on earth do you hope to attain by this fanatic addiction to cross-legged sitting?" Huai-jang asked his friend.*
>
> *"Buddhahood," Mat-su responded serenely.*
>
> *Huai-jang sat down next to Mat-su, picked up a brick, and began to polish it with great effort and care. Annoyed by the interruption in his routine, Mat-su asked his friend what on earth he was doing.*
>
> *"Why, I'm making a mirror out of my brick."*
>
> *"You can polish it until the end of time," chided Mat-su, "but you'll never make a mirror out of a brick."*
>
> *"Aha!" Huai-jang smiled, setting down his brick. "Perhaps you are beginning to understand that you can sit with your legs crossed until the end of time but it won't make you into a Buddha."*

Polishing the brick of our own ignorance won't make us into great healers or sages, but it may be the first step toward developing the humility that underlies true wisdom. For only when we are humble and willing to acknowledge our own ignorance will we be able to see the deep connections that bind us each to the other, an interdependence that extends in ever-expanding circles beyond ourselves to our families, our communities, and the all-forgiving, ever-embracing earth—the mother of all.

> *Teach your children*
> *what we have taught our children—*
> *that the earth is our mother.*
> *Whatever befalls the earth*
> *befalls the sons and daughters of the earth.*
> *If men spit upon the ground,*
> *they spit upon themselves.*

This we know.
The earth does not belong to us;
we belong to the earth.
This we know.
All things are connected
like the blood which unites one family.
All things are connected.

Whatever befalls the earth
befalls the sons and daughters of the earth.
We did not weave the web of life;
We are merely a strand in it.
Whatever we do to the web,
we do to ourselves.

                                   —Chief Seattle

PART II

THE MEANING OF HEAVEN AND EARTH

CHAPTER 5

THE STREAM OF LIFE

After a time of decay comes the turning point. The powerful light that has been banished returns. There is movement, but it is not brought about by force. . . . Everything comes of itself at the appointed time. This is the meaning of heaven and earth.

—The I Ching

When we experience consciousness of the unity in which we are embedded, the sacred whole that is in and around us, we exist in a state of grace.

—Charlene Spretnak

The waters on the surface of the earth flow together wherever they can, as for example in the ocean, where all the rivers come together. . . . What is required is that we unite with others, in order that all may complement and aid one another through holding together.

—The I Ching

For every ending there is a new beginning; after a period of death and decay comes a time for renewal and regeneration. Controlled for thousands of years by a predominantly male energy that has emphasized linear thought rather than intuitive wisdom, competition rather than cooperation, and war rather than peace, our civilization has sustained deep and abiding wounds. Destruction and domination determine the course of our lives. Nuclear weapons, capable of destroying all life on earth, await a moment of anger or a desire for revenge to release their awesome destructive power. Toxic chemicals poison the air we breathe, the food we eat, and the water we drink. Tens of millions of people are starving. Hundreds of millions, most of them children, are undernourished. More than a third of the earth's population lacks safe drinking water.

Those of us who are blessed by luck and circumstance with material luxuries have discovered an emptiness at our core. Our lives are filled with activity and material possessions but devoid of meaning and purpose. We crave a return to a remote but remembered past when a sense of the sacred permeated the relationship between human beings, the earth, and the universe. Cut off from the rest of the natural world, we long to be embedded again in its larger, enfolding reality.

The intensity of our need and our longing signal that the turning point has arrived. The appointed time is upon us when heaven and earth can once again share their powers, when the moon's dark power is honored as an equal to the stronger, light-giving energy of the sun, and when peace and harmony govern relationships between human beings. The powerful light of age-old wisdom offers a way to heal our wounds and become whole again. This wisdom is all around us, in the sun, moon, and stars of the heavens and in the mountains, rivers, and green, growing life on earth. To grasp the meaning of heaven and earth, we need only look into our own hearts, as the Chinese philosopher Lao-tzu wrote thousands of years ago:

> There is no need to run outside
> For better seeing. . . .
> Rather abide
> At the core of your being;
> For the more you leave it, the less you learn.
> Search your heart and see. . . .
> The way to do is to be.

The laws of the natural world are written within our own souls; if we look within, we can perceive the intricate splendor of all that lies without, for every human being is a microcosm of the universe, and inside each individual consciousness can be discovered a sense of the unity and indivisibility of life.

> *God created the world and was happy. On the seventh day he decided it was time to rest, but Adam called out: "God, I've got a problem, Eve is trying to feed me this apple, what should I do?"*
>
> *And then Eve called with troubles of her own: "God, Adam keeps telling me I have to take care of him and attend to his every need— how do I make him respect my rights as a human being?"*
>
> *And then that quarrelsome twosome had dozens of children, who had hundreds of children, who had thousands of children, and it did not take long before God was thoroughly exhausted with all their problems and demands for his time. Calling a meeting of his angels and advisers, God expressed a desire for some peace and quiet.*
>
> *"I'm afraid I've created a monster," God said, "and I must find a place to hide."*
>
> *"Perhaps you could hide out at the top of the Himalayas," one of the angels suggested.*
>
> *"No," God replied, "I'm afraid you don't understand what I've created. In just a few moments measured by my time, they will be there, too."*
>
> *"What about the moon?" suggested one of his advisers.*
>
> *"No," God replied wearily, "in just a few minutes more they will be there, too."*
>
> *They sat together, heads in hands, wings folded, wondering how to proceed. Suddenly a smile spread over God's face. "I know where they will never look!" he pronounced, looking very pleased with himself. "I'll hide inside human beings themselves."*
>
> *And to this day, that is where God is hiding.*

Inside each of us resides the wisdom of the world. When peace and harmony prevail, we are guided by an intuitive sense of the spiritual meaning of life, but when we are thrown off balance by stress or illness, we may lose touch with our internal wisdom. At those times wisdom-seekers from many different cultures suggest that we look for guidance and inspiration in the ongoing cycles of change taking place in the natural world. Our internal wisdom is mirrored in the world around us, and when we look beyond ourselves, we can often see ourselves more clearly.

My travels and studies have immersed me in many diverse healing traditions, but I've found no system of thought that is as lyrically beautiful and profoundly pragmatic as Traditional Chinese Medicine. More than three thousand years ago, Chinese sages and scholars devoted their energies to understanding and describing the vital, life-giving connections between the universe, the earth, and the human being. Over many hundreds of years, they created an elaborate philosophy aimed at a higher awareness of the grand unity of the cosmos, with the eminently practical goal of helping people to lead a healthy, happy, highly moral life.

Traditional Chinese Medicine is one of the most widely used systems of thought and practice that honor the feminine spirit of healing. At the root of this uniquely practical approach to life and health is the philosophy of Taoism, which is most eloquently described in *The I Ching, or Book of Changes*. The Chinese believe that in order to truly understand the philosophical heart of Traditional Chinese Medicine, you must immerse yourself in this ancient text, which sets forth in rich metaphorical prose the central concepts of balance, harmony, and wholeness. In the introduction to his modern-day translation of *The I Ching*, Richard Wilhelm comments:

> The Book of Changes opens to the reader the richest treasure of Chinese wisdom; at the same time it affords her[1] a comprehensive view of the varieties of human experience, enabling her thereby to shape her life of her own sovereign will into an organic whole and so to direct it that it comes into accord with the ultimate Tao lying at the root of all that exists.

Tao is synonymous with the Native American image of the sacred hoop, for it is imagined as an invisible web of interconnections that supports life, infusing all of nature with balance and harmony. In *The I Ching*, tao is described as the ultimate source of all life and creativity:

> There is nothing that tao may not possess, for it is omnipresent; everything that exists, exists in and through it. But it is not lifeless possessing; by reason of its eternal power, it continually renews everything, so that each day the world becomes as glorious again as it was on the first day of creation.

---

[1]In this and other quoted material, we have taken the liberty of changing the gender from male to female.

The concept of tao was first elaborated by Lao-tzu, a Chinese sage living around the time of Confucius (551– 479 B.C.). Stephen Mitchell's modern translation of Lao-tzu's book of wisdom, *Tao te Ching*, emphasizes the inherently female nature of tao, "the mother of the universe":

> *There was something formless and perfect*
> *before the universe was born.*
> *It is serene. Empty.*
> *Solitary. Unchanging.*
> *Infinite. Eternally present.*
> *It is the mother of the universe.*
> *For lack of a better name,*
> *I call it the Tao.*
>
> *It flows through all things,*
> *inside and outside, and returns*
> *to the origin of all things.*

The question many modern people ask about God can also be directed to tao. If tao can't be seen, touched, felt, heard, or directly experienced, how can we say that it exists at all? If tao existed before the world itself came into being, thus transcending the mortal world of space and time, how can we ever hope to penetrate its deepest mysteries? From *The I Ching* and the *Tao te Ching*, we learn that tao unfolds around us in every moment of every day. Because tao "flows through all things, inside and outside," we can begin to understand its meaning in our own lives by observing its effects on the natural world. Nature is the clay that is continually shaped by the artistry of tao, and the most fundamental law underlying all natural processes is the law of change. As *The I Ching* puts it: "Everything on earth is subject to change. Prosperity is followed by decline: this is the eternal law on earth."

In the natural, ongoing process of change, we can witness the reality of tao, for if the living world did not adapt, grow, and become, life itself could not exist. Thus we can see tao in the changes unfolding in the natural world; its gentle, yielding spirit is revealed in the bend and flow of living things, which by their example teach us how to adapt to the vicissitudes and unpredictable circumstances of life. As Lao-tzu wrote:

> *Men are born soft and supple;*
> *dead, they are stiff and hard.*

Plants are born tender and pliant;
dead, they are brittle and dry.

Thus whoever is stiff and inflexible
is a disciple of death.
Whoever is soft and yielding
is a disciple of life.

The hard and stiff will be broken.
The soft and supple will prevail.

The feminine spirit of receptivity and adaptability underlies the most basic activities of the natural world. From careful observation of nature, we learn that we have the power to shape our fate by softly bending and adapting to circumstances, thus altering the influence of benevolent or destructive forces. When we understand the meaning of tao, we begin to grasp the essence of our own nature. For we are the sun, moon, and stars. We are the earth, trees, soil, and minerals; the seas, rivers, and lakes; the wind, rain, thunder, and fire. Our lives are governed by the same eternal forces that rule all of nature. If we carefully observe the natural world and strive to live in harmony with her laws, Taoist philosophy teaches, we will find peace, serenity, and happiness; if we deviate from these fundamental principles, we will experience tension, frustration, and misfortune.

We become one with nature not by attempting to master her, but by letting go of any desire to be in control. We learn to accept what is, because what is *is* tao. In the story that follows, the essential nature of change and the necessity of surrender, or letting go, are explored. Though true in its nature to Taoist philosophy, this version of the story comes from Awad Afifi, a Tunisian Sufi master who died in 1870.

A stream, from its source in far-off mountains, passing through every kind and description of countryside, at last reached the sands of the desert. Just as it had crossed every other barrier, the stream tried to cross this one, but it found that as fast as it ran into the sand, its waters disappeared.

It was convinced, however, that its destiny was to cross this desert, and yet there was no way. Now a hidden voice, coming from the desert itself, whispered: "The wind crosses the desert, and so can the stream."

The stream objected that it was dashing itself against the sand,

and only getting absorbed: that the wind could fly, and this was why it could cross a desert.

"By hurtling in your own accustomed way you cannot get across. You will either disappear or become a marsh. You must allow the wind to carry you over, to your destination."

But how could this happen? "By allowing yourself to be absorbed in the wind."

This idea was not acceptable to the stream. After all, she had never been absorbed before. She did not want to lose her individuality. And, once having lost it, how was she to know that it could ever be regained?

"The wind," said the sand, "performs this function. It takes up water, carries it over the desert, and then lets it fall again. Falling as rain, the water again becomes a river."

"How can I know that this is true?"

"It is so, and if you do not believe it, you cannot become more than a quagmire, and even that could take many, many years; and it certainly is not the same as a stream."

"But can I not remain the same stream that I am today?"

"You cannot in either case remain so," the whisper said. "Your essential part is carried away and forms a stream again. You are called what you are even today because you do not know which part of you is the essential one."

When she heard this, certain echoes began to arise in the thoughts of the stream. Dimly, she remembered a state in which she—or some part of her, was it?—had been held in the arms of the wind. She also remembered—or did she?—that this was the real thing, not necessarily the obvious thing, to do.

And the stream raised her vapour into the welcoming arms of the wind, which gently and easily bore her upwards and along, letting her fall softly as soon as they reached the roof of a mountain, many, many miles away. And because she had had her doubts, the stream was able to remember and record more strongly in her mind the details of the experience. She reflected, "Yes, now I have learned my true identity."

The stream was learning. But the sands whispered: "We know, because we see it happen day after day: and because we, the sands, extend from the riverside all the way to the mountain."

And that is why it is said that the way in which the Stream of Life is to continue on its journey is written in the Sands.

Like the stream, which entrusted her fate to the wisdom of the sands and lifted up her arms to the wind, we learn how to continue our journey through life by listening to the whispered messages of nature and surrendering to her greater wisdom. Guided and inspired by our connections to the natural world, we begin to understand that we are participants in an ongoing, ever-changing process, which is nothing less than the unfolding power of the universe. If we look beyond ourselves, we can see the universe expanding; we are not only of it but inside it, part of the rhythmic dance of life, death, and rebirth.

All around us the wisdom of tao can be discerned; on earth and in the heavens, in every natural law and in every living thing, tao expresses its wisdom. Thus from the moon we learn the meaning of humility, for as *The I Ching* notes, when "the moon becomes full and stands directly opposite the sun, it begins to wane." Like the moon, "we must be humble and reverent when face to face with the source of enlightenment."

As majestic mountains erode away, filling up the lowly valleys, we discover that "it is the law of fate to undermine what is full and to prosper the modest."

From thunderstorms we learn about forgiveness, for just as thunder clears the air and "water washes everything clean," so should we act quickly and decisively to purge ourselves of resentment and pardon transgressions.

When clouds rise in the sky and a storm threatens, we learn about patience and destiny. "We should not worry and seek to shape the future by interfering in things before the time is right," *The I Ching* counsels, but fortify our bodies with food and drink and our minds with joy, for "fate comes when it will, and thus we are ready."

In every word and image, we discover the importance of self-knowledge and self-examination. *The I Ching* advises a "holy seriousness" when we contemplate "the divine meaning underlying the workings of the universe," for only through deep and persistent concentration can we hope to bring our thoughts and actions into harmony with tao. Self-knowledge and self-examination are synonymous with concern for the web of being itself, for every action we take, every thought we have, every emotion that courses through us impacts the whole. Concern for the web of the universe, the earth, and our fellow human beings constitutes the basis of all moral thought and action. As *The I Ching* notes, "Self-knowledge does not mean preoccupation with one's own thoughts; rather, it means concern about the effects one creates."

From constant reflection and careful observation of the natural world, we learn how to keep our vision fixed on the whole. As we begin to see ourselves as participants in the unfolding mystery of the universe, our spirit expands and our wisdom grows. Looking outward from within and inward from without, we see the same principles repeated and the same patterns evolving. The world is never static, never wholly at rest or wholly at peace, for the whole is governed by the law of change, which dictates that fullness must be followed by emptiness, prosperity by decay, and gathering by dispersion. In its continual transformation from one state to another, the world is exactly as it should be.

> *Many years ago a woman called Sono lived in a little town in Japan. Her devout heart and compassionate spirit had won her the respect and admiration of many followers, and fellow Buddhists often travelled long distances to seek her advice. One day a weary traveller approached Sono to ask what he could do to put his mind at peace and his heart at rest.*
>
> *Sono's advice was simple and straightforward. "In the morning and in the evening, whenever anything occurs to you, keep on saying, 'Thanks for everything. I have no complaint whatsoever!' "*
>
> *For an entire year the man faithfully followed her advice, repeating from morning until evening, "Thanks for everything. I have no complaint whatsoever." But still his mind was not at peace nor was his heart at rest. Thoroughly discouraged he again made the long journey to see Sono. "I've done everything you suggested," he said, "but my mind is not at peace and my heart is not at rest. Tell me—what should I do now?"*
>
> *At once Sono replied, "Thanks for everything. I have no complaint whatsoever!" Hearing these words, the traveller was enlightened and returned home, his mind at peace and his heart at rest.*

We are human beings, part of the world of change, and thus eternal peace and perfect tranquillity are not within our grasp. Life necessarily consists of both good and evil, heaven and earth, light and dark, tension and release. Accepting this truth and learning how to be grateful for life just as it is—*Thanks for everything. I have no complaints whatsoever*—is the only way to put our minds at peace and our hearts at rest, for in this insight, the enduring truth of the universe is recognized and celebrated. Tao is unity—the one, the source, the center—but out of the oneness that is tao emerge the two primal powers, yin and yang, which alternate in the continual process of change between increase and decrease, expansion and contraction, fullness and emptiness. Yin and yang are not opposites or contradictions, for Taoist philosophy teaches that everything in life literally and figuratively contains its opposite. Over time, each half is transformed into the other in a continual cycle of change. "The secret of tao in this world of the mutable," according to *The I Ching*, "is to keep the changes in motion in such a manner that no stasis occurs and an unbroken coherence is maintained."

According to Taoist philosophy, which forms the philosophical heart and soul of Traditional Chinese Medicine, we cannot say that something is good or evil, dark or light, night or day, heaven or earth, male or female. Such either-or categories do not exist, because all of reality is both this *and* that, good *and* evil, black *and* white, night *and* day, heaven *and* earth, male *and* female. When the complementary powers of yin and yang flow and interact in harmony, balance is achieved, tao is honored, and life's energy force flows unimpeded. When the balance between yin and yang is unequal, the two primal powers conflict with, rather than complement, each other, and the world is thrown into chaos.

Numerous images from nature are offered to help us imagine the relationship between yin and yang. While most moderns consider night and day to be distinct and separate realities, the Chinese imagine them as ever-changing aspects of a unified whole—the daily cycle. Night is conceived as yin (the dark, reflective, contractive power), while day is yang (the light, active, expansive power). At the moment when night emerges from day (twilight) or day arises from night (dawn), near-perfect balance is achieved, and for a few moments the world is exquisitely poised between the two primal powers as one becomes the other, fusing their natures so that night and day, dark and light, ending and beginning are indistinguishable.

The images of heaven and earth offer another way to imagine the ever-changing interdependence of yin and yang. Heaven, it is said, "moves" with the light-giving, divine (yang) energy, which gives birth to the spiritual longings that we call soul. Earth in her tolerance and humility permits the creative powers of heaven to be felt and experienced through her receptive, yielding (yin) nature. As the earth opens her arms to heaven, *The I Ching* explains, she "allows the divine light to enter, and by means of this light illuminates everything."

> The earth is still. It does not act of itself but is constantly receptive to the influences of heaven. Thus its life becomes

inexhaustible and eternal. Woman likewise attains eternity if she does not strive vaingloriously to achieve everything of her own strength but quietly keeps herself receptive to the impulses flowing to her from the creative forces.

In the modern age, we feel compelled to attach a value judgment to the two primal powers, conceiving of yang energy as superior, for it is active rather than passive, full of movement rather than infused with potential. But while the creative energy of the yang is revered as divine, the Chinese would insist that the yielding, receptive way of the yin offers the greatest source of wisdom for human beings. Because we are human and therefore mortal, our powers pale in comparison to the forces of nature around us. We cannot alter the seasonal cycles of the earth, stop a hurricane from forming, or prevent a river from overflowing. We are both powerful and powerless, magnificent and humble, divine and earthly, imbued by the yin and constrained by the yang.

Our limited powers become manifest only when we are receptive to the unchanging laws of the universe. From the yin energy we learn the way of suppleness and yielding, patience and calm, receptivity and humility. As the moon is sister to the sun, as earth is daughter to heaven, as night is mother of day, the dark-giving powers of the female (yin) energy keep the world in harmonious balance. As the natural world reveals, the gentle feminine energy of the yin consistently outlasts the harsh masculine energy of the yang. "The gentlest thing in the world overcomes the hardest thing in the world," wrote Lao-tzu; and in another passage, quoted earlier in this chapter, he noted, "The hard and stiff will be broken. The soft and supple will prevail."

In life, as in philosophy, our good fortune depends on gentleness, patience, steadfastness, and a yielding to tao, "the way." Taoist thought is eminently practical, for the goal is to become healthy, happy, and wise, with the understanding that wisdom is the essential first step leading to both health and happiness. Wisdom depends on balance, for if we can learn to balance within ourselves the yin and yang energies, so that one flows into the other in a constant, never-ending cycle, with neither over-powering the other, we will ensure a continuous flow of energy known as *chi*—the vital, animating force essential to life. *Chi* energy, like the concepts of tao and yin/yang, is a spiritual reality in the sense that we cannot see it, touch it, or possess it; we know it only when we experience its effects.

When the master entered the room the disciples were engrossed in a conversation about Lao-tzu's words:

> *"One who knows does not speak*
> *One who speaks does not know."*

"What do the words mean?" asked the disciples.
"Who among you knows the fragrance of a rose?" the master responded.
They all knew.
"Who among you can put this knowledge into words?"
They were all silent.

Like the attempt to describe the fragrance of a rose, when we attempt to define *chi*, we discover not its limitations but our own. Another story permits us to look at the phenomenon of *chi* energy from a slightly different perspective.

> *Two monks were arguing about a flag. One said: "The flag is moving."*
> *The other said: "The wind is moving."*
> *Master Eno overheard them and said, "It is not the wind nor the flag, but your mind that moves."*
> *The monks were speechless.*
>
> *Wind, flag, mind moves,*
> *The same understanding.*
> *When the mouth opens*
> *All are wrong.*

What is *chi*? *Chi* is the energy in the atmosphere that moved the flag. *Chi* is the force that enabled the observers to perceive that the flag moved. *Chi* is the power that prompted the observers to ask whether it was the flag or the wind that moved. *Chi* is the wisdom that understood that the flag and the wind moved only when the mind moved.

Chi is simply a name for the dynamic pattern of interactions that occur within the individual and between the individual and her environment. But by giving this principle of underlying energy a name and a distinct relationship to both internal and external forces, we begin to understand that life is not static or wholly predictable, but a vigorous, ever-changing adaptive process in which a state of balance determines health, vitality, and vigor, while loss of balance results in lethargy, depression, and illness. *Chi* is not just a reservoir of energy that we draw on and gradually deplete as we live our lives, but also a stream fed by numerous underground springs that ebb and flow in response to both internal and external forces.

The vital life force of *chi*, which allows us to stand up straight, walk, talk, think, move, feel, and react, can be nurtured or squandered depending on how we live our lives. We can keep the flow of *chi* strong and pure by carefully following the rules of nature, which insist on moderation, balance, and harmonious relationships. Our health, we learn, is influenced by the way we treat others as surely as it is affected by the way we care for our bodies, minds, and spirits. Anger, frustration, greed, fear, selfishness, pride, and intolerance are considered as dangerous to our well-being as eating unhealthy foods, drinking too much or too little, or not getting enough exercise, rest, or sleep. In fact, practitioners of Traditional Chinese Medicine teach that it is possible to be "angry to death"—filled up with so much wrath and rancor that these hostile emotions devour the stores of *chi* and damage the Liver (in Chinese medicine, the organ system where anger is stored). The emotion of sympathy, it is believed, can counteract the ill effects of excessive anger. And while happiness is undoubtedly good for the body, mind, and spirit, unrestrained joy can damage the Heart.

Any physical, mental, or spiritual imbalance threatens health and happiness by obstructing the flow of *chi*. But we do not have to wait until illness occurs before imbalances in *chi* energy can be detected. In fact, in the old days a Chinese doctor would receive a fee only if the patient remained in good health—payments stopped when the patient became sick. According to an ancient Chinese proverb, treating a patient who is already sick is like digging a well after you're dying of thirst; the maxim originated in a section of *The Yellow Emperor's Classic of Internal Medicine*, written more than two thousand years ago:

> The sages did not treat those who were already ill; they instructed those who were not yet ill. . . . To administer medicines to diseases which have already developed and to suppress revolts which have already developed is comparable to the behavior of those persons who begin to dig a well after they have become thirsty and of those who begin to cast weapons after they have already engaged in battle. Would these actions not be too late? . . . The superior physician helps before the earliest budding of

disease. . . . The inferior physician begins to help when the disease has already set in. And since his help comes when the disease has already developed, it is said of him that he is ignorant.

A superior physician is able to recognize the signs and symptoms of an imbalance in *chi* before it results in illness or disease. Chinese medical treatments stimulate the body's innate self-healing capabilities by manipulating *chi* energy in three basic ways:

1. Acupuncture or acupressure, ancient techniques that involve stimulating specific trigger points, also known as acupoints, along the meridians—energy pathways that connect to deeper channels feeding *chi* and blood into the vital organs.
2. Herbal remedies, which work gently to remove an excess or correct a deficiency in *chi* energy.
3. Advice about modifying behavior through good nutrition, regular exercise, and stress reduction techniques. (Doctors schooled in Traditional Chinese Medicine often tell their patients that the most essential requirement for maintaining good health is to lead a happy life.)

When a patient visits a doctor of Traditional Chinese Medicine, she will be asked many of the same questions posed by Western medical practitioners. "What are your major problems and complaints?" the doctor might begin. "Do you have any history of chronic and degenerative diseases in your family? Have you had any recent accidents or hospitalizations?"

But before long the questions begin to veer off into unfamiliar territory. "How is your general energy level?" the doctor continues. "What about your sexual energy? What emotions do you have difficulty expressing? Tell me about your skin—do you tend to bruise easily, do you have dry skin, do you feel that you are thin- or thick-skinned? What is your favorite color? What season do you most enjoy? At what time of day do you feel at your best or worst? Are there any tastes that you particularly like or dislike? What foods attract or repel you? Do you have a favorite number? What symbols and themes recur in your dreams?"

All these questions, and many more, are intended to reveal underlying physical, emotional, and spiritual patterns that will provide the doctor, acupuncturist, or herbalist with information about your basic nature and constitution. The Chinese believe that five elements or phases interact to create your unique personality, emotional character, spiritual nature, and physical attributes. Taken together these patterns form the system known as *Wu Hsing*, frequently referred to as "Five-Phase Theory" or the "Five Elements"; we have created the expression the "Five Transforming Powers" to emphasize the Taoist philosophy of dynamic potential and eternal change.

In the complex system of correspondences and affinities embraced by the Five Transforming Powers, the pragmatic nature of Traditional Chinese Medicine becomes abundantly clear. For while the esoteric concepts of tao, yin/yang, and *chi* may seem only remotely connected to real life, the Five Transforming Powers—Wood, Fire, Earth, Metal, and Water—are tangible and immediately recognizable, providing a comprehensive guide for understanding the cycles of growth, maturity, and decay that occur in our daily, monthly, seasonal, yearly, and lifetime cycles.

Beyond the lyrical beauty and penetrating wisdom of Taoist philosophy lies a uniquely practical approach to life. As Fritjof Capra states in *The Turning Point*, "When the Five Phase theory was fused with the yin/yang cycles, the result was an elaborate system in which every aspect of the universe was described as a well-defined part of a dynamically patterned whole." According to Chinese philosophy, the Five Transforming Powers are not only outside us, generating change in the external world, but they are also inside us, governing the strength and vitality of our bodies, minds, and spirits. As we come to understand the unique characteristics and common boundaries of these powers, we learn how to live in harmony with the universe and its inherently moral laws. Wood, Fire, Earth, Metal, and Water act as a mirror that reflects back a vision of the self and its temporary resting place in the universe. When we look in that mirror and reflect on the images contained within its ever-expanding borders, we gain a deeper understanding of the interconnections between body, mind, and spirit, the kinship between human beings and the earth, and the unity of earth and heaven.

As our vision expands, we perceive that the whole of nature is reflected in every one of its parts, just as every one of the parts reflects the whole. We sense that the cycles of change taking place in the external world are repeated in the inner world of our bodies, minds, and spirits, and we begin to comprehend the pragmatic meaning of tao: if Wood, Fire, Earth, Metal, and Water are the basic elements that give structure and meaning to the world of both inner and outer experience, then we are not only inseparable from nature, but permanently and irrevocably bonded to her.

CHAPTER 6

AFFINITIES

Things that accord in tone, vibrate together. Things that have affinity in their inmost natures seek one another. Water flows to what is wet, fire turns to what is dry. . . . What is born of heaven feels related to what is above. What is born of earth feels related to what is below. Each follows its kind.

—*Confucius*

The interaction of the Five Elements brings harmony and everything is in order. At the end of one year the sun has completed its course and everything starts anew with the first season, which is the beginning of Spring. This system is comparable to a ring which has neither beginning or end.

—**The Yellow Emperor's Classic**

Wood, Fire, Earth, Metal, or Water . . . which of the five transforming powers most clearly defines your basic nature? In the process of asking the question "Who am I?" and determining your basic affinity with one of these essential powers, you will gain valuable insights into your physical ailments, emotional imbalances, psychological problems, and spiritual yearnings.

As you learn to recognize how the powers work within you, expanding and contracting your nature in the same way in which they exert their influence in the natural world, you will experience a kinship and connectedness to all of nature that extends beyond metaphor into a deep and abiding appreciation for the delicate balance and indivisible harmony of life.

According to *The Yellow Emperor's Classic,* "The sages combined Water, Fire, Wood, Metal, and Earth . . . and they held them as inseparable and constant." These five powers ebb and flow within every one of us, each power contributing to the fundamental integrity of the body, mind, and spirit. No one single element is sufficient unto itself, for in order to manifest itself, each power relies on the energy generated by the other four powers.

Thus in the natural world, soil, for example, is composed primarily of Earth, but its essential nature is not complete without Water (moisture), Metal (minerals), Fire (ash), and Wood (decaying leaves and twigs). So it is with the human being. While you may be predominantly influenced by the power of Metal, the strength of your Metal is dependent on the corresponding strengths or weaknesses of your Earth, Fire, Water, and Wood energies.

Each of the powers is central to the whole, for life as we know it could not exist without all Five Transforming Powers. Each power generates and sustains the others, and a surge or decrease in any one power will send ripples of meaning throughout the whole body. Truly you are a river fed by many streams and tributaries, each of which nourishes your spirit, expanding and contracting your flow of energy to correspond to your present needs, and assisting you to move through life with agility and grace.

THE GENERATION CYCLE
Supporting Sequence: *Sheng*

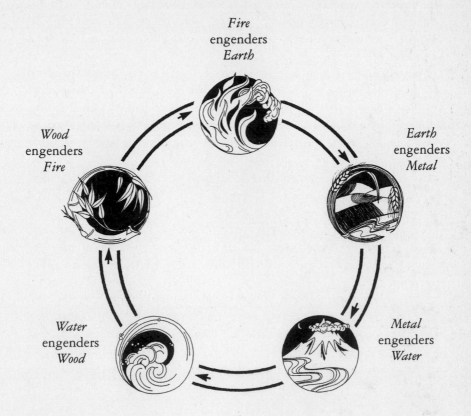

Fire
engenders
Earth

Earth
engenders
Metal

Wood
engenders
Fire

Metal
engenders
Water

Water
engenders
Wood

The Generation Cycle, depicted by the clockwise arrows in the illustration above, is also called the Mother/Child Cycle, for the Five Transforming Powers generate and support each other in the same way that a mother gives birth to her children and then nourishes and sustains them in the process of growth and maturity. Fire is considered the mother or generator of Earth; Earth is the mother to Metal; Metal nourishes Water; Water creates Wood; Wood gives birth to Fire; and so on.

According to classical Chinese theory, the universe was formed by a massive ball of Fire, which eventually cooled down to create Earth. As the cooling Process continued, Earth's core solidified into minerals and precious ores (Metal), which permeated Water and strengthened its life-giving qualities. Water then contributed to the proliferation of plant material (Wood), which burned to create Fire, which created more ash (Earth), which solidified into Metal, which enhanced Water, and so on as the cycle continues through eternity.

THE CONTROL CYCLE
Restraining Sequence: *Ke*

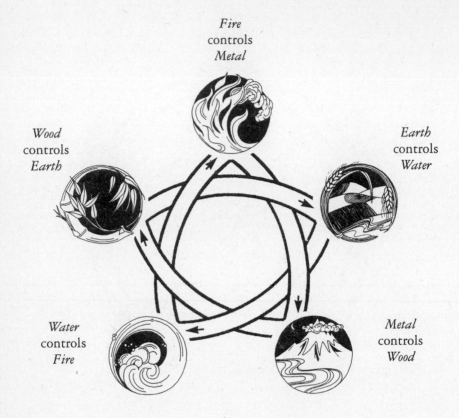

Fire
controls
Metal

Wood
controls
Earth

Earth
controls
Water

Water
controls
Fire

Metal
controls
Wood

Just as a mother sets the boundaries and limits for her children, so do each of the Five Transforming Powers restrain and inhibit the others, ensuring that no one power rages out of control or becomes predominant. Water controls Fire by quenching it; Fire restrains Metal by melting it, allowing it to be shaped and molded; Metal inhibits Wood by cutting it (symbolized by the axe chopping the tree); Wood restrains Earth by covering it, literally rooting the Earth in place and preventing erosion; and Earth controls Water by absorbing it and forming natural dams and riverbanks to keep it within bounds.

THE CONTROL CYCLE AND
GENERATION CYCLE COMBINED

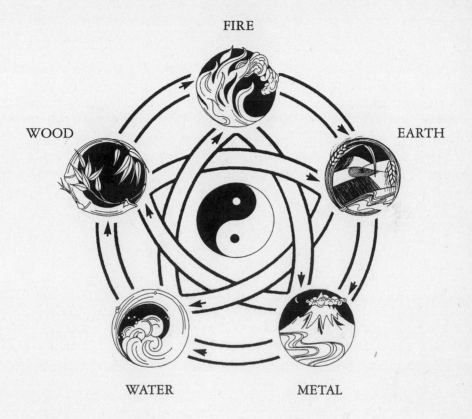

The Generation and Control Cycles demonstrate the interdependence and inter-connectedness of the Five Transforming Powers. These cycles work in concert to ensure that balance and harmony are maintained.

Because all of life is characterized by change, in one day you will feel the advance and retreat of each of these powers. At various times during the day, your natural affinity to a particular power will rise and fall, building up energy, gradually weakening, then gathering in strength once again. In every month, in every season, in every year, countless changes take place as the powers of Wood, Fire, Earth, Metal, and Water expand and contract.

Women have a natural, intuitive understanding of these rhythmic, ever-changing cycles of life because from puberty onward, they feel the force and sway of the powers within them. From her monthly cycle a woman learns that tension is followed by release, ebbing by flowing, waxing by waning. She feels the pull of the moon as it works its magic on her inner tides, creating cycles of fullness and emptiness. She senses the shifts and alterations in energy from one month to the next, and she experiences the corresponding adjustments in her body, mind, and spirit. She is privileged to understand these truths through her body's innate physiology; she does not have to sit at the window looking out at the moon, for the moon is radiating from within. She is the window reflecting its light, its meaning, and its message.

In each stage of a woman's life, the powers of nature touch her spirit, as the wind caresses the surface of the lake, making the invisible visible. As she moves from one stage of her life to the next, she feels the ebb and flow of Wood, Fire, Earth, Metal, and Water within her body, mind, and spirit. In puberty, the supple, radiating power of Wood predominates, teaching her how to move forward with gentle pressure and strength of purpose. In her childbearing years, passionate Fire infuses her being with warmth and sexuality, while Earth's yearning for harmony and balance creates a stable foundation for nurturing her creative energies. In the years that mark the change of life, she is most strongly influenced by Metal's focus on depth, substance, and quality of experience. In the waning years of her life, Water fills her with trembling anticipation as she comes to understand the potential depths of her spirit and her power to contribute to the ongoing cycle of life, death, and rebirth.

While all five powers exist within every human being, each individual has an affinity to one particular power that predominates and energizes her identity, even her destiny. How can you discover which power surges most strongly within you? According to the ancient texts, specifically *The I Ching* and *The Yellow Emperor's Classic of Internal Medicine*, each of the

Five Transforming Powers expresses itself in a pattern of characteristics called correspondences, or affinities. A specific emotion with both positive and negative aspects is associated with each power, as is a distinct season, climate, direction, time of day, color, odor, taste, sound, body type, personality style, and spiritual attribute. Five distinct organ networks, each of which involves an elaborate system of tissues, channels, meridians, and acupoints, govern the physiological, psychological, and spiritual functions corresponding with a particular power.

In the next five chapters, we will explore the basic nature and unique expression of each of the Five Transforming Powers. As you search for the power that most clearly defines your temperament and personality, be aware of the minor attractions and aversions that you experience with the other powers. With a firm understanding of your basic nature and an appreciation for the combined influence of the five elements on your body, mind, and spirit, you will gain essential philosophical and practical information. Once you have identified the power primarily responsible for creating and sustaining your basic nature, you will have a better understanding of the risks you take or avoid, the goals you set, the innate talents that drive you, the fears and doubts that threaten you, the situations that cause you stress or conflict, the talents you have (or have neglected), the values that motivate you, and the dreams that inspire you.

Through the elaborate, functional system of the Five Transforming Powers, we are given an opportunity to journey deep into the very heart and soul of the universe, where we learn to see ourselves as microcosms of nature and to read our symptoms as messages indicating a state of harmony or disharmony with nature's unchanging laws. Our wisdom becomes three-dimensional, our connections strengthen, our sense of being at home in the world gains depth and breadth as we learn to seek answers to our physical, mental, and spiritual problems in the way we fit or fail to fit into the natural world. From the sun, moon, and stars above and the earth below, from the buds bursting forth in spring and the rigid ice floes forming in the dead of winter, from wind, thunder, and rain, from raging rivers and stagnant pools, from the majestic mountains and the lowly valleys, we discover a new perspective on the obstacles and adversities that face us in our daily lives.

Imagine the Five Transforming Powers, then, as five rivers flowing from a central, inexhaustible source high atop a majestic peak. The rivers follow their nature downward, moving easily and gracefully through the pebbled streambeds, meeting the unmovable boulders by gently parting and flowing around, mixing their waters with other tributaries but always remaining true to their essential nature. A sense of direction and purpose guides the waters toward the sea, where they reach the end of their journey and merge to become one.

We are like these rivers, arising from a central source and flowing with direction and purpose toward our ultimate destination. Our entire journey leads to that joining together that is experienced as home, wholeness, unity, the one—that place where the individual is enfolded into the soul of the universe, and the universe is enclosed within each individual soul.

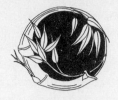

CHAPTER 7

WOOD: THE VISIONARY

The supernatural [powers] create wind in Heaven and they create wood upon earth. Within the body they create muscles and of the five viscera they create the liver. Of the colors they create the green color and of the musical notes they create the tone chio; and they give to the human voice the ability to form a shouting sound. In times of excitement and change they grant the capacity for control. Of the orifices they create the eyes, of the flavors they create the sour flavor, and of the emotions they create anger.

—**The Yellow Emperor's Classic**

The power of Wood is gentle, persistent, and filled with creative potential. This is the power of both being and becoming—being true to your own nature and becoming more yourself by clearly expressing your inner needs and desires to the world. Wood gently penetrates the earth to bring forth water, the source of all life. Like the simple plant, our basic needs are satisfied by sinking our roots deep into the inexhaustible springs of the earth. There, in the still, silent center, the water of life nourishes our bodies, minds, and spirits. Drawing from the roots, we find the energy to push forward with strength and firmness of purpose, always remaining supple, yielding, and true to our own nature.

If you are energized by Wood, you are driven by the need to stay in motion. You know when to move forward with resolution, when to wait patiently, and when to retreat gracefully. Challenges are approached with confidence, and decisions are made with care and deliberation. When it is time to act, you intuitively know how to achieve your goals. You understand who you are and where your inner potential can take you, and you have no difficulty deciding how to reach your destination.

Firm and strong of purpose, you rely on gentle but persistent pressure to achieve your goals. Like the warm breezes of spring, you encounter rigidity with tender persuasion, dissolving the rigid and the hard with your supple but sturdy nature. When you are free to move with purpose and resolve into the world, health and happiness abound. But when your energy is blocked or diverted, you will experience tension and mounting frustration as your need to express yourself is thwarted.

In the ancient Chinese texts, this inner state of tension and increasing pressure is symbolized by the image of thunder. "A thunderstorm brings relief from tension, and all things breathe easily again," advises *The I Ching*. Nature is refreshed after a spring thunderstorm, tension is resolved, and relief is experienced. Because it is in your nature to be direct and forceful like thunder, you are capable of expressing your feelings to the world in an honest, persuasive manner while maintaining a clear vision of where your emotions are destined to take you. You are always in control, using your passionate energy to make a point or remove the obstacles blocking your progress.

Anger is the emotion that energizes Wood types. In its balanced state, anger is a healthy emotion, for it can be understood as a natural reaction to stress, frustration, or injustice. When expressed with gentle control, anger acts like thunder to clear the air, dispel tension, and restore balance.

A young female disciple spent many hours sitting in her room, meditating on the meaning of loving-kindness and striving to fill her heart with love and compassion for all living creatures. Her discipline was sorely tested, however, when she went to the marketplace to buy food, for one particular shopkeeper constantly followed her around and tried to caress her. One day she reached the end of her patience. Brandishing her umbrella she angrily chased the shopkeeper around the marketplace, until she noticed her teacher standing on the side of the road observing the scene. Thoroughly ashamed of herself and expecting a severe reprimand, she went to stand before him.

He regarded her kindly and then offered this advice. "What you should do is to fill your heart with loving-kindness and then, with as much energy and enthusiasm as you can command, hit that ill-mannered fellow over the head with your umbrella."

The gentle, vibrant energy of Wood serves to "make things flow into their forms, to make them develop and grow into the shapes prefigured in the seed," says *The I Ching*. This vital, life-giving energy is experienced most strongly in spring, the season of renewal and regeneration.

In springtime when thunder, life energy, begins to move again under the heavens, everything sprouts and grows, and all beings receive from the creative activity of nature the childlike innocence of their original state.

Wood's climate is windy, its direction is east ("Beginning and creation come from the East"), and its power is experienced most intensely between 11:00 P.M. and 3:00 A.M.

The color associated with Wood is green; a subtle, greenish hue often can be detected around the Wood type's mouth and eyes. If you feel a natural attraction to the color green, you may be expressing your affinity with Wood. A strong dislike or aversion to the color green may indicate an imbalance in this power.

A rancid odor, similar to the sour-sweet smell of urine or sweat, or the rank aroma of meat and cheese in a butcher shop, is connected with Wood. The taste is sour, and a strong attraction or repulsion to acidic, caustic, or tangy foods (vinegar, sour pickles, lemons) often indicates a correspondence to Wood.

The sound correlating with Wood is shouting. Wood types tend to shout out their words in an aggressive, forceful way; a lack of dynamic energy in the voice, resulting in a monotonous vocal tone with little or no inflection, may reveal an imbalance in Wood energy.

A well-proportioned, muscular (but naturally supple) body type with broad shoulders and a distinctly square physique is typical of Wood types.

Hands tend to be strong, slim, and well proportioned, with palms and fingers of equal length; a slight bulging around the knuckles is common. Feet and toes are generally long, thin, and powerful. Wood types tend to tan easily and maintain the bronzed, healthy look of being vigorously active even in the winter months. The skin is often thick and somewhat rough to the touch; over time, a naturally tawny or dark-skinned complexion may take on a leathery appearance.

Constant movement and regular exercise are critical for the Wood type, who needs to move upward and outward, forcefully expressing her thoughts and emotions to the world at large. This natural need to be in motion is balanced by an innate ability to judge when it is time to proceed with purpose and resolution and when it is best to stay still and gather strength. The balanced interaction between movement and decision making is ruled by the sister/brother organs the Liver and the Gallbladder. (In Western medicine the body's organs are viewed as fixed anatomical structures with specific functional duties. The Chinese emphasize function rather than structure [one of the Chinese organs, the Triple Heater, does not even exist as an anatomical structure] and extend the organs' influence to include emotional and spiritual manifestations.) Working harmoniously together, the Liver and the Gallbladder enable the power of Wood to circulate internally and manifest itself externally in a creative interaction between the individual and her environment.

The Liver is viewed in Chinese medicine as the seer or visionary, which "has the functions of a military leader who excels in his strategic planning." Plans are carefully developed and carried out by the Liver, which is responsible for maintaining homeostasis and balance within the entire organism, thus ensuring that all the various organ systems interact and cooperate to create a harmonious whole. The Liver is said to rule flowing and spreading, creating a smooth, even movement of *chi* and blood throughout the entire body. When the energy in this organ is blocked or impeded, symptoms associated with obstruction (migraine headaches, high blood pressure, constipation, and heartburn) may occur. Because the Liver also balances the emotions, stagnant Liver *chi* can create a chronic state of anger and emotional frustration.

The Gallbladder, also known as the Wise Decision Maker, "occupies the position of an important and upright official who excels through his decisions and judgement." Knowing when to store and when to release bile (the bitter fluid necessary for digestion) is one of the most important decisions governed by the Gallbladder. In emotional and spiritual terms, this organ is thought to moderate impulsive or reckless behavior. If a person consistently makes rash decisions, an excess of Gallbladder *chi* is suspected; indecisive behavior points to a deficiency of energy in this organ.

IMBALANCES IN WOOD ENERGY

EXCESS

While Wood types tend to push themselves to the limit and function well under pressure, an excess of Wood energy results in "overly yang" behavior—pushing ahead without adequate planning. The classic image associated with such headstrong behavior is a wooden pole stressed to the breaking point:

> The load is too heavy for the strength of the supports. The ridgepole, on which the whole roof rests, sags to the breaking point, because its supporting ends are too weak for the load they bear.

The problem is intensified by a natural tendency to stay in motion and push through any obstacles in your way. Ignoring the strain (and refusing to heed the advice of others), you recklessly continue onward.

> She accepts no advice from others, and therefore they in turn are not willing to lend her support. Because of this the burden grows, until the structure of things bends or breaks. Plunging willfully ahead in times of danger only hastens the catastrophe.

Excess Wood energy also contributes to insensitivity to the needs of others. Stubborn and strong-willed, you tend to exert your authority in an obstinate, defiant, know-it-all way. Believing that you know the precise boundaries separating right from wrong, you are determined to let the rest of the world hear your thoughts. Quick to anger, you shout out your demands in impulsive, volatile outbursts. Tension results when others

ignore you or stubbornly cling to their own opinions, refusing to bow
down before your greater wisdom.

You are, in short, driven by an internal compulsion to succeed, to win,
to become the best, the brightest, the number one shining star. If you
are not always on the move, pushing ahead (while often shoving others
aside), you experience frustration and anxiety. While you may accomplish
a great deal and win grudging respect from others for your lack of fear
and restraint, you will undoubtedly make many mistakes and encounter
numerous enemies along the way.

> *The master Bankei always spoke straight from the heart, and his
> simple speeches would attract many followers. A priest from a rival
> Buddhist sect was envious of the master's reputation, and he arrived
> at the temple determined to debate with his perceived rival.*
>
> *As Bankei began to speak, the priest called out, "Hey, Zen teacher!
> Those who respect you will obey you, but I have no respect for you. Can
> you force me to obey you?"*
>
> *"Come up here and stand next to me," said Bankei, "and I will
> show you."*
>
> *The priest pushed through the crowd to stand next to the teacher.
> "Come over here to my left side," Bankei said, and the priest obeyed
> him.*
>
> *Bankei stroked his chin. "No, that is not right," he said, "we can
> talk better if you stand on my right side."*
>
> *The priest did as he was told.*
>
> *"I can see that you are a very gentle person," Bankei smiled, "for
> you have obeyed me well. Now, please, sit down and listen to what I
> have to say."*

The excess Wood type refuses to sit down and listen to what others
have to say. Eventually the strain becomes too much to bear, as the burden
grows and "the structure of things bends or breaks." Headaches, muscle
spasms, tendon injuries, and high blood pressure signal the underlying
tension in your body, mind, and spirit. Because it is part of your nature
as Wood to be self-reliant, you will resist seeking help for your increasingly
distressing problems. Only when your symptoms become too painful or
too obvious to ignore will you turn to an expert for help, but even then
you tend to be curt and domineering. "Fix me up quick," you might say,

"because I have too much to do, and I can't afford to slack off for one minute."

If your doctor offers medications, you will gratefully accept them, for you can't bear the idea of taking time out of your busy schedule for rest and recuperation. But treating the symptoms of a Wood imbalance with drugs only drives the disharmony even deeper, and as time goes by, your physical, emotional, and spiritual problems will intensify. With excess Wood types, treatment must focus on teaching the wisdom of "the middle path"—balancing advance with retreat, and spontaneity with deliberation.

> She who pushes upward blindly deludes herself. She knows only advance, not retreat. But this means exhaustion. In such a case it is important to be constantly mindful that one must be conscientious and consistent and must remain so. Only thus does one become free of blind impulse, which is always harmful.

Symptoms Associated with Excess Wood Energy

- Muscular tension with cramps and spasm, usually in the head, neck, and shoulders, but also in the hips, legs, hands, and feet
- Tendon injuries
- Sciatica (radiating pain following the course of the sciatic nerve from the lower back through the buttock and down the leg)
- Headaches, especially migraines
- Irritability and violent outbursts of anger
- Visual disturbances
- Ringing in the ears
- Menstrual irregularities, particularly PMS, with emotional instability and spasm
- Digestive disturbances, including heartburn, constipation with cramps and spasm, hiatal hernias, and ulcers
- Cysts and growths of all kinds that, if left untreated, can become cancerous
- High blood pressure, with tendencies toward atherosclerosis
- Chinese wind syndrome (The Chinese believe that the wind is "the cause of a hundred diseases," capable of depleting the body/mind/spirit's energy reserves and resulting in serious, even fatal illnesses ranging from minor tics to grand mal seizures and strokes.)

DEFICIENCY

While excess Wood energy often leads to a rigid mind-set and reckless plunging ahead, a deficiency inevitably contributes to internal collapse. With Wood, as with the other transforming powers, a deficiency generally follows a prolonged period of excess, during which the *chi* energy is gradually depleted and sources of renewal and regeneration are drained. Anger is turned inward, and feelings of shame, embarrassment, and humiliation begin to invade the body/mind/spirit. Lack of self-worth is an issue for both types of Wood imbalance, but while the excess type ignores her feelings and asserts herself in a boisterous manner, the deficient type inhibits her emotions due to fear of ridicule.

A danger of stagnation exists, for you no longer have the energy to move forward out of the standstill you find yourself in. Your creative energy is blocked, and you feel stuck in the mud, unable to send your roots deep into the fertile soil to nourish yourself with the restoring waters of life. The longer these patterns continue and remain untreated, the greater your exhaustion and the more despondent your mood. As your ability to focus clearly and make quick decisions is impeded, fatigue and lethargy set in. As time goes by, your power dwindles and eventually collapses.

You may become dependent on external sources of stimulation such as drugs, coffee, soda, and sugar, or sources of sedation such as alcohol, tranquilizers, and cigarettes. These unnatural stimulants and sedatives further deplete your natural resources, and as the cycle continues, you become more withdrawn, anxious, indecisive, and irritable.

> When adversity befalls a woman, it is important above all things for her to be strong and to overcome the trouble inwardly. If she is weak, the trouble overwhelms her. Instead of proceeding on her way, she remains sitting under a bare tree and falls ever more deeply into gloom and melancholy. This makes the situation only more and more hopeless. Such an attitude comes from an inner delusion that she must by all means overcome.

The "inner delusion" that must be overcome is the belief that she can meet all obstacles by simply pushing them aside. When she encounters obstructions, she "butts her head against a wall" and "leans on things that have in themselves no stability and that are merely a hazard for her who leans on them." This is clearly a precarious state, for Wood types are accustomed to unlimited reserves of energy and an active, productive life. If you do not seek help for your underlying problems and continue to use external, unnatural supports, your Liver orb will be seriously stressed, creating even more fear, guilt, and frustration. As time goes on, feelings of depression and hopelessness take over the body/mind/spirit. Without outside assistance and appropriate guidance, the symptoms of pain and distress will intensify.

Symptoms Associated with Deficient Wood Energy

- Anxiety and restlessness
- Free-floating tension and nervous energy
- Premenstrual syndrome (PMS)
- Irregularities in the menstrual cycle
- Chronic tension in neck and shoulders
- Insomnia, including difficulty falling asleep as well as fitful sleep
- Hypersensitivities, including allergies of all kinds, from hay fever to food sensitivities to dermatological allergies
- Itchy eyes, urethra, anus
- Visual disturbances, including blurry vision and extreme sensitivity to light (photophobia)
- Muscle spasms and tics, such as eye twitches and restless leg syndrome
- Digestive problems, including gas, bloating, irritable colon, and hiatal hernias
- Fatigue, lethargy, lack of energy
- Unstable blood pressure (fluctuating between high and low blood pressure)

THE WISDOM OF WOOD

Wood in the earth grows upward. . . . The pushing upward is made possible not by violence but by modesty and adaptability. . . . Adapting itself to obstacles and bending around them, wood in the earth grows upward without haste and without rest. Thus too the superior woman is devoted in character and never pauses in her progress.

—*The I Ching*

WOOD: THE VISIONARY

An individual with an affinity to Wood is driven by the need for action, movement, and fulfillment. She has deep and abundant resources that enable her to view challenges as adventures, always pushing herself to the limit and performing well under pressure. Her love of adventure and her desire to be the first and the best help her to translate her dreams into realities.

NATURAL QUALITY: Solid yet supple; growing, spreading

SPIRITUAL QUALITY: Creativity

EMOTION: Anger
   BALANCED: Assertive, confident, decisive
   IMBALANCED
      Excess: Aggressive, arrogant, pretentious, tyrannical, compulsive
      Deficiency: Ambivalent, passive, ineffectual, intolerant, erratic

SEASON: Spring

CLIMATE: Windy

DIRECTION: East (rising sun)

TIME OF DAY: 11:00 P.M.–3:00 A.M.

COLOR: Green

SMELL: Sour-sweet (urine, sweat, meat, cheese)

TASTE: Sour

SOUND: Shout

ORGANS
   YIN: Liver
   YANG: Gallbladder

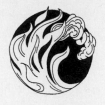

CHAPTER 8

FIRE:
THE COMMUNICATOR

The supernatural [powers] of Summer create heat in Heaven and fire upon Earth. They create the pulse within the body and the heat within the viscera. Of the colors they create the red color and of the musical notes they create chih and they give to the human voice the ability to express joy.

—The Yellow Emperor's Classic

Fire is the power of radiant passion. If you are infused with the warm, luminous energy of Fire, you attract others to your light and warmth as the flame draws the moth. You are ablaze with a contagious enthusiasm and passionate love for the earth beneath your feet, the sun, moon, and stars in the heavens, and the community of human beings whom you long to enfold in your embrace.

You feel a need to be in touch, both literally and figuratively. You will touch your partner when you talk, rest your hand on an acquaintance's shoulder, and freely offer hugs to both friends and strangers and be delighted to receive them in return. When deprived of touch, you suffer physically, emotionally, and spiritually.

A forty-year-old woman who was separated from her young children for a week complained that her hands ached. "I miss touching my children," she explained. Her need to touch and her penetrating insight into the nature of her distress are characteristic of the healthy Fire type, who is known for her intuition, empathy, and intense craving for intimate relationships.

The ability to create relationships and the energy to sustain them is part of Fire's natural power. Fire fills us up with its passion for life, but this passion is too intense to be contained internally, and so you continually reach outward, hoping to extend your boundaries in order to share your fervent emotions with others. This all-consuming need to be "one with everything" characterizes the essential spiritual nature of the Fire type. Separation creates pain, for you believe that two belong as one and that it is within your power to fuse your nature with others, creating new life. With all your heart you believe that fusion—the union of two souls into one—is the quintessential experience of life.

Because your desire to melt and merge with others is so strong and compelling, at times in your life you may have difficulty separating yourself from those you love. What others feel, you feel; what they experience, you experience. Highly intuitive and empathic, you often know what your loved ones are thinking or feeling before they do. Your perception is acute, your heart is wide open, your joy is boundless. A story, as always, helps to make the point.

> *Rumi knocked on his lover's door.*
> *"Who is there?" asked his beloved.*
> *"It is I, Rumi," he responded.*
> *"Go away," her voice came back to him, "for there is not enough room for the two of us here."*
> *Rumi went away to meditate and pray. Returning later he knocked on his lover's door.*
> *"Who is there?" she asked.*
> *"It is you," Rumi answered.*
> *The door was thrown open, and the lovers passionately embraced.*

The abundant, spirited enthusiasm for life that we call joy is the emotional manifestation of a healthy Fire. As with all emotions, however, balance is crucial, for excessive joy (mania or hyperexcitability) is as harmful to the body/mind/spirit as lack of joy (selfishness, apathy, and indifference). In *The I Ching*, the desired state of balanced joy is artfully described:

> A quiet, wordless, self-contained joy, desiring nothing from without and resting content with everything, remains free of all egotistic likes and dislikes. In this freedom lies good fortune, because it harbors the quiet security of a heart fortified within itself.

The Fire type must always be aware of the steady and consistent flame—more like a pilot light than a fire fed by wood or straw—that feeds and nourishes her basic nature. The need and capacity to merge with others is both your greatest strength and your greatest weakness, for the potential exists to consume yourself with your own passion.

> Fire clings to wood, but also consumes it. . . . Here the image used is that of a meteor or a straw fire. A woman who is excitable and restless may rise quickly to prominence but produces no lasting effects. Thus matters end badly when a woman spends herself too rapidly and consumes herself like a meteor.

When the Buddha was enlightened, it is said that he laughed out loud with passionate and abundant joy. But immediately afterward he was overcome with grief, for at the moment of his enlightenment, he understood that he was intimately joined with all other sentient beings, each of whom would have to achieve enlightenment to gain entrance into paradise. The Buddha's balanced expression of passionate joy and compassionate sorrow define the secure boundaries of the Fire personality. The Buddha would have enjoyed a deep belly laugh at the story of the Zen master who approached a New York City hot dog vendor. "Please," he said, "make me one with everything."

The color associated with Fire is red. A woman infused with this power has a rosy, even ruddy complexion; a slight red hue can be seen emanating from the area around the eyes and temples. If the energy of Fire becomes excessively powerful or is severely diminished, the facial texture and quality of the skin will serve as a strong guide to the condition of the Heart, one of the organ systems connected with Fire. As *The Yellow Emperor's Classic* explains, "the complexion of a person shows when the heart is in a splendid condition." An excessive attraction or repulsion to the color red may also signify an imbalance in Fire.

The power of Fire is felt most intensely in the season of summer, that "period of luxurious growth" when the "breaths of Heaven and Earth intermingle and are beneficial." The climate is hot; the direction is South; and the time of day when Fire is most powerful is between 11:00 A.M. and 3:00 P.M.

A scorched odor, similar to the smell of burned toast or of clothing just removed from the dryer, corresponds to Fire. When this scent can be detected on a person's body, it indicates an imbalance of Fire energy. The taste or flavor corresponding to Fire is bitterness. According to *The Yellow Emperor's Classic*, "the heart craves the bitter flavor," which "has a strengthening effect." The bitterness of coffee, tea, unsweetened chocolate, barbecued foods, and green, leafy vegetables (spinach, kale, dandelion greens) appeals to the Fire type; an extreme distaste or preference for such foods indicates an imbalance in Fire.

The sound associated with Fire is laughing. A warm voice with a good sense of humor indicates a healthy Fire. Inappropriate laughter or excessive giggling may suggest an excess of Fire, while a lack of humor often points to a deficiency in Fire.

The Fire body type is reflected more in vivacity and intensity than in a distinct constitutional tendency. If you are infused with this power, you may be thin and delicate, with fine features and fragile bones, or you may be stocky and compact, with a strong frame and well-developed muscles. A long neck, arms, and legs, and graceful hands and feet are characteristic of the Fire type.

When the energy of Fire is healthy and strong, your skin will be soft, moist, and warm, ranging in color from rosy to bronzed to bright red. Fire types tend to blush easily. A strong, bright red skin color indicates an excess of Fire, while an ashen, pale complexion points to a deficiency.

Fire is unusual in that it is associated with two yin and two yang organ systems or orbs; because this power is so intimately bound up with relationships, each of these orbs is thought to govern a particular type of relationship. The yin orbs are the Heart and Circulation Sex. Located at our core or center, the Heart represents firmness and strength within, expressed outwardly in a gentle, yielding nature.

> The joyous mood is infectious and therefore brings success. But
> joy must be based on steadfastness if it is not to degenerate

into uncontrolled mirth. Truth and strength must dwell in the heart, while gentleness reveals itself in social intercourse.

In the ancient texts, the Heart is compared to a supreme monarch responsible for maintaining internal peace and harmony. By controlling and circulating the blood, the Heart makes sure that all organs receive their fair share of blood, *chi*, and nutrients. Spirit *(shen)* resides in the Heart, and the names of the acupuncture points along the Heart meridian—Spirit Path, Spirit Gate—attest to the central relationship between the Heart and the spirit.

Circulation Sex, which is associated with the pericardium (the muscle surrounding the heart), is primarily responsible for blood flow and sexual secretions. Also called the Heart Protector, Circulation Sex functions as a trusted adviser that guards the inner sanctum of the Heart by carefully screening out "undesirable" ideas, thoughts, and images. Intimate relationships with lovers, friends, children, and parents are guided by this energetic function, and numerous psychological disorders, especially those reflecting a problem with boundaries, can be viewed as imbalances within this orb. Acupoints along the Circulation Sex meridian (Heavenly Pond, Heavenly Spring, Palace of Weariness, and Inner Gate) attest to this orb's power and influence.

The yang organ systems associated with Fire include the Triple Heater (also known as San Jiao, the Three Warming Spaces, or the Official of the Bursting Water Dam) and the Small Intestine. The Triple Heater is the only organ within the Chinese classification system that is solely functional and has no structural counterpart; however, it is considered an extremely powerful component of the body/mind/spirit, responsible for heating and cooling the entire system. The Three Heaters include the misting, the factory (or churning), and the swamp. The misting rules the upper part of the body from the rib cage to the neck, housing the Heart and Lungs and ruling over the refinement and distribution of *chi* and blood. The factory governs the middle part of the body, from the umbilicus to the rib cage; its duties of digestion and assimilation are carried out by the Stomach, Spleen, Pancreas, Liver, and Gallbladder. The lower heater, the dredging or swamp, supervises the area from the pubic bone to the belly button and is responsible for gynecological functions and the storage of wastes in the bowels and bladder.

Metaphorically, the Triple Heater rules over three different levels of consciousness. The swamp is said to rule sensuality and sexual response;

the factory governs practical matters; and the misting controls the spiritual domain. Working together to keep the body/mind/spirit in harmonious balance, the three heaters are responsible for maintaining peaceful, stable relationships with self, family, society, church, country, and various ideological groups.

Although Westerners may find the names of these organ systems nonsensical and their lack of anatomical correspondence unscientific, many modern and traditional medical practitioners consider this elaborate system, which includes functional patterns as well as anatomical structures, a more highly developed and practical framework for understanding the complex interactions between body, mind, and spirit. Acupuncturist Dianne Connelly, for example, considers the recognition of Circulation Sex and the Triple Heater as "perhaps the greatest gift traditional Chinese medicine has to offer the Western world of therapies and the ailments of sick people."

The final yang orb associated with Fire is the Small Intestine, also known as the Sorter or the Separator of the Pure from the Impure. In the Small Intestine, a fine filtration system sorts out the pure nutrients from food and drink, transporting them to the Spleen, where they are transformed into *chi* and blood, and then directing the impure parts downward to the Large Intestine for elimination. On a mental and spiritual level, a similar process takes place, for we are constantly being fed psychic energy through our relationships, and this energy needs to be sorted and filtered so that we absorb only the digestible material and eliminate from consciousness the extra garbage. When our emotional Small Intestine malfunctions, we are unable to discriminate between the healthy and hurtful parts of our relationships. As a result, our psychic waters become clogged with debris, and confusion reigns in the body/mind/spirit.

IMBALANCES IN THE POWER OF FIRE

EXCESS

The hyperexcitability of an excess in Fire power can be compared to a 110-volt electric line being forced to channel 220 volts: it's only a matter of time before the wires burn out. A state of overstimulation is taking place inside the excess Fire type's body/mind/spirit, causing generalized anxiety that can lead to panic attacks with palpitations and speeded-up heart rate (the Heart energy is constricted); cold and/or sweaty extremities (the Heart is unable to circulate the blood freely); indigestion (the Heart's mother/daughter relationship with the Spleen has been disrupted); and/or a state of inactivity and apathy (Fire is consuming itself).

If you suffer from an excess of Fire, you feel a desperate need to be noticed, and you will go to extremes to get praise and attention. The hyperexcitability associated with excess Fire energy inevitably leads to restlessness and manic behavior. You tend to jump from one project to the next without the ability to concentrate on the details and finish what you've begun. As your energy channels gradually burn out, your creative juices dry up, and depression ensues. Your despondency is intensified by difficulties in relationships, for the mania and extreme excitability of excess Fire is exhausting to others, who feel overwhelmed by your intensity and obsessive need for intimacy. While friends and acquaintances often enjoy a short period of intense conversation or activity with an excess Fire type, they will avoid prolonged exposure.

A passionate sex life is characteristic of a healthy Fire, but passion in excess is rapidly transformed into preoccupation and obsession. The Fire has broken through its boundaries and threatens to consume everything within reach. If it is allowed to rage out of control, confusion reigns, depression deepens, and internal collapse is imminent.

Symptoms Associated with Excess Fire Energy

- Inappropriate, loud, and annoying laughter
- Irrational thinking, confused thought patterns, forgetfulness, inability to focus
- Extreme anxiety or restlessness, often bordering on mania
- Hysteria, delirium, and various forms of depressive illness
- Excessive perspiration and/or a tendency to overheat
- Flushed complexion, ranging from bright red to purple
- Insomnia
- Disturbing dreams
- Skin irritations or eruptions, including sores on mouth, tongue, and lips
- Eczema and psoriasis
- Lack of appetite when agitated or depressed

- Obsession with intimate relationships
- Irregular or rapid heartbeat with palpitations and angina (pain in the chest or radiating down the left arm). (These symptoms are serious and must be attended to immediately.)

Deficiency

In contrast to the manic, overexcitable nature of excess Fire, a deficiency creates feelings of indifference and apathy. Unable to generate warmth and affection, you have difficulty experiencing or expressing joy, your voice tends to drone on in monotony, and a conspicuous lack of humor pervades your relationships. It isn't that you don't have feelings—you just can't summon up the energy or the confidence to express them. In metaphorical terms, your internal pilot light is wavering and unsteady; as time goes by, the flame is in danger of flickering out.

"What's the point of living?" you might ask. And truly, there seems to be no point, for you have lost your spark—your spirit—and you feel empty and chilled inside. As your Heart fire cools down, feelings of melancholy and depression invade your body/mind/spirit. Depression is not to be confused with sadness, which is characterized by a deep and profound longing for reconnection with a relationship that has been lost or broken. If you are depressed, your energy and enthusiasm are seriously depleted, the darkness of melancholy gradually overshadows the light of joy, and feelings of emptiness and hopelessness pervade.

While you may seem cold and unemotional on the outside, your interior life consists of inventing fantasies and creating unrealistic hopes for the future. Over time, as you come to realize that your idle imaginings will not materialize, your depression deepens, and you wander as if lost, seeking in external pleasures and vain indulgences the passionate intensity that was once such a secure part of your inner nature.

> If a woman is unstable within, the pleasures of the world that she does not shun have so powerful an influence that she is swept along by them. Here it is no longer a question of danger, of good fortune or misfortune. She has given up direction of her own life, and what becomes of her depends upon chance and external influences.

Symptoms Associated with Deficient Fire Energy

- Insomnia and free-floating anxiety, reflecting restless (in contrast to excited) agitation
- Forgetfulness and confused thinking
- Heart irregularities and palpitations, including tachycardia (heart rhythm is too fast) and arrhythmia (irregular heartbeat or missed beats)
- Hypertension
- Cardiac insufficiency or congestive heart failure
- Malaise and other signs of classical depression, including fatigue and lack of appetite
- Chronic fatigue syndrome, typically experienced as a general sense of lethargy and lack of vitality
- Digestive problems, including constipation, gas, and heartburn

THE WISDOM OF FIRE

What is dark clings to what is light and so enhances the brightness of the latter. A luminous thing giving out light must have within itself something that perseveres; otherwise it will in time burn out. Everything that gives light is dependent on something to which it clings, in order that it may continue to shine.

—*The I Ching*

FIRE: THE COMMUNICATOR

An individual with an affinity to Fire has the capacity for great joy, which can be used to forge strong and enduring relationships. Intuitive and empathic, she longs to fuse her nature with others and suffers intensely when she is separated from those she loves.

NATURAL QUALITY: Heating, warming, attracting

EMOTION: Joy
  BALANCED: Happy, lively, passionate, compassionate
  IMBALANCED
    Excess: Excitable, hypersensitive, manic
    Deficiency: Selfish, cold, forgetful

SPIRITUAL QUALITY: An open heart, desire for union, capacity for intimacy

SEASON: Summer

CLIMATE: Hot

DIRECTION: South

TIME OF DAY: 11:00 A.M.–3:00 P.M.; 7:00 P.M.–11:00 P.M.

COLOR: Red

SMELL: Scorched

TASTE: Bitterness

SOUND: Laughing

ORGANS
  YIN: Heart/Circulation Sex (pericardium)
  YANG: Small Intestine/Triple Heater

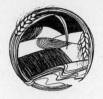

CHAPTER 9

EARTH: THE PEACEMAKER

The [mysterious] powers of the earth create humidity in Heaven and fertile soil upon earth. They create the flesh within the body, and of the viscera they create the stomach. Of the colors they create the yellow color . . . and they give the human voice the ability to sing . . . of the flavors they create the sweet flavor, and of the emotions they create consideration and sympathy.

—**The Yellow Emperor's Classic**

When we think of the earth, we imagine a globe or sphere, but in the ancient Chinese texts, heaven is represented by the circle while the earth is symbolized by the square. Squareness is considered a primary quality of Earth; in its verb form, this seems absolutely right, for "to square" something means to reconcile, conciliate, harmonize, adapt, and adjust— activities and states of being that are governed by the power of Earth.

The symbol of heaven is the circle, and that of earth is the
square. Thus squareness is a primary quality of the earth. . . .
Nature creates all beings without erring: this is its straightness.
It is calm and still: this is its foursquareness. It tolerates all
creatures equally: this is its greatness. Therefore it attains what
is right for all without artifice or special intentions. Woman
achieves the height of wisdom when all that she does is as self-
evident as what nature does.

Earth is mother, peacemaker, and lover of harmony; her devoted,
receptive nature is the perfect complement to the creative powers of heaven.
One complete revolution of the heavens makes a day, one day is followed
by another, and in this cycle is created the idea of time, which is the
"untiring power" inherent in the image of heaven. Earth does not attempt
to compete with heaven's power—her great and enduring wisdom resides
in the realization that she cannot compete—but through her yielding,
receptive nature, she ensures that a sense of wonder will find its way into
earthly affairs. By conforming her nature to the impulses and creative
potential of heaven, Earth allows herself to be guided by divine energies.
Through her tangible, spatial energy, Earth permits the spiritual potential
of heaven to be experienced. For only through the visible (Earth) can the
invisible (heaven) be perceived: "The wind blows over the lake and stirs
the surface of the water. Thus visible effects of the invisible manifest
themselves."

Humility is a central quality of Earth, but not in the modern-day sense
of the word, which focuses on self-abnegation and servility. To the ancients,
humility connoted mildness, modesty, patience of spirit, and a willingness
to remove oneself from the center of the universe. This is the nature of
Earth's humility, for she has an unerring sense of her limitations and she
is keenly aware of the place where she fits and feels at home.

The image of a soaring bird is offered in *The I Ching* to help us understand
the nature of home, that place where we do not strain or stray from the
way of our own nature. Just as a bird invites misfortune by attempting
to transcend its limitations and fly directly into the sun, so should we
follow the dictates of our own nature and keep our feet firmly grounded
on Earth.

A bird should not try to surpass itself and fly into the sun; it
should descend to the earth, where its nest is. . . . If a bird will

not come to its nest but flies higher and higher, it eventually
falls into the hunter's net. She who in times of extraordinary
salience of small things does not know how to call a halt, but
restlessly seeks to press on and on, draws upon herself misfortune
. . . because she deviates from the order of nature.

Earth calls us back home, offering a safe haven where we can rest and
refresh our spirits. Earth's power reminds us that we are just flesh and
blood, but she also understands that we are sparked with spirit and yearn
to fly into the heavens, hoping to penetrate the mysteries of the unknown.
As we struggle with our limitations and imperfections, the power of Earth
reminds us who we are and where we belong: "When a woman seeks to
climb so high that she loses touch with the rest of humankind, she becomes
isolated, and this necessarily leads to failure."

If Earth is the primary power that molds and shapes your nature, you
are naturally tolerant and forgiving. People feel safe with you, for you accept
all of life in all its glorious diversity, making no attempt to discriminate,
categorize, or judge others. All fit within your embrace, all belong, all
are accepted, for you do not ask others to be anything but themselves.
By following Earth's example, we learn how to be tolerant: "Just as the
earth is boundlessly wide, sustaining and caring for all creatures on it, so
the sage sustains and cares for all people and excludes no part of humanity."

If you are energized by the power of Earth, you are a natural mediator,
for Earth types thrive on peace and harmony and are thrown off balance
by discord and dissension. You dislike quarreling, and you naturally avoid
conflicts—not because you fear the airing of differences but because you
would rather be stripped of your possessions (including pride and the
desire to have the last word) than see someone else deprived.

*Two old men had lived together a very long time and always treated
each other with great respect. In fact, never once had they quarreled.
But after a lifetime of watching other people argue and fight over their
possessions, one of the old men suggested to his friend that perhaps they
should learn how to quarrel as others did.*

"But I don't know how to quarrel," the other replied.

*"This is the way to create a quarrel," the first explained, for he
had observed well. "I will put a brick between us and say, 'This is
mine.' Then it is your turn to say, 'No it is mine.' And then the
quarrel will begin."*

So they put a brick between them and one said, "This is mine," after which the other dutifully said, "No, it is mine." But then the first said, "Yes, of course, it is all yours, you must have it." And as soon as the quarrel had begun, it was over.

Earth helps us to find a center between opposing forces, teaching us how to resolve our differences and find sensible solutions to even the most difficult problems. Earth's wisdom is contained in a maxim from *Tao te Ching*, which advises that we "just stay at the center of the circle and let all things take their course."

Like the moon, who turns her face to the sun and is contentedly illuminated by its powerful, light-giving energy, Earth gratefully accepts divine inspiration from higher sources. Earth intuitively understands the moon's cyclic nature, for just at the moment when the moon becomes full and stands directly opposite the sun, her powers begin to wane. Following the moon's example, Earth prepares for a waning after every waxing, instinctively knowing when it is time to retreat and store up her energy in preparation for the responsibilities that await her. It is in Earth's nature to be prepared.

If your Earth energies are strong and your affinities are here, you experience great joy in giving and receiving. Because you know that the most precious possessions in life cannot be given or taken away, you are content to live simply, experiencing deep gratitude for the abundant gifts of life— gifts that can never wholly be possessed.

In a little hut at the foot of a majestic mountain the Zen master Ryokan lived very simply. One autumn night when Ryokan was taking a walk in the moonlight, a thief entered his hut only to find that there was nothing of value to steal. When Ryokan returned, he found the disappointed thief preparing to leave empty-handed.

"My dear fellow," he said, "you have come a long way to visit me, and you must have something to show for your troubles." Ryokan stripped naked and removed the blanket from his bed, offering these gifts to the bewildered thief, who quickly ran off with them.

Sitting down naked in the moonlight, Ryokan found himself wishing that he could have given the thief the lovely harvest moon. In the silver silence beneath the moon he composed this Haiku poem:

The moon out the window!
Left by the thief unstolen.

A sense of kinship and connectedness to other human beings is essential to your health and happiness, and you have a gift for creating loving communities. In contrast to the Fire type, who fascinates others with her charismatic charm, people are attracted to you because you accept them for who they are and do not attempt to change them to suit your needs or preferences.

Stable, quiet, compassionate, and well-grounded, you can move out of yourself to experience another person's pain or joy and, with equal ease, come back home to yourself. Your sense of self is so secure and your boundaries so well defined that you can step into another person's shoes without becoming confused about whose shoes you are wearing. You are able to practice in your daily life the wisdom contained in this Native American prayer: "Great Spirit, grant that I may not criticize my neighbor until I have walked a mile in his moccasins."

Earth corresponds to the season known as Indian summer, that intense, glorious period when all four seasons combine to create a feeling of heaven on earth. In the ancient Chinese texts, the season of Earth was described as the twilight period at the end of each season in which the forces of nature are in near-perfect balance. But as Earth knows (perhaps better than any of the other powers), the eternal, immutable laws of nature decree that all of life is subject to change—prosperity is followed by decline, gathering by dispersion, growth by decay. Thus, one of the secrets hidden in the magic of Earth's season is the knowledge that periods of harmony and prosperity inevitably will be followed by times of discord and degeneration.

The climate corresponding to Earth's power is dampness and humidity; excess dampness or humidity are considered harmful to Earth types. Earth's power is at its peak between 7:00 A.M. and 11 A.M.

The direction of Earth is the center. According to *The Yellow Emperor's Classic*, "Everything that is created by the Universe meets in the center and is absorbed by the Earth." Earth's color is yellow, for yellow is the color of the middle, indicating, as *The I Ching* explains, "that which is correct and in line with duty." In its healthy state, yellow is an impartial color, unbiased and coolly neutral. A pale, sickly yellow or an intense orange hue around the eyes or temples may suggest an imbalance within Earth.

Earth's odor is fragrant; if your Earth powers are out of balance, a sickening-sweet smell similar to rotting, overripe fruit indicates the malfunction. Earth's flavor is sweet, similar to the subtle sweetness of ripening fruit; an addiction to (or intense dislike of) sweets may indicate an Earth imbalance. Singing is the sound of Earth, and a monotonous, singsong voice or an overly melodious voice may indicate a disharmony in this power.

The organ orbs corresponding to the power of Earth are the Spleen/ Pancreas and Stomach. The Spleen has been called the Official in Charge of Distribution and the Transporter of Energy. Its primary function is to extract the pure nutrients from food and fluids and alchemize these elements into *chi*, blood, and waste products, which are then transported to the organs that govern elimination and circulation. Thus, the Spleen is the center of a massive distribution center, supplying the body/mind/spirit with sufficient energy, blood, and nutrients. The Spleen is also thought to keep the blood flowing within its proper channels. If the Spleen *chi* is deficient or weak, the blood is in danger of moving recklessly and overflowing its pathways, leading to symptoms such as nosebleeds, spotting between menstrual periods, flooding, hemorrhaging, vomiting blood, or blood in the stools.

The Stomach (the Official of Rotting and Ripening or the Sea of Food and Fluid) is responsible for the active (yang) functions of receiving food, sifting and sorting for nutrients, and then transporting the pure nutritive energy to the Spleen, where it is transformed into *chi* and blood. The Stomach is thought to rule descending (forcing nutrients downward), while the Spleen governs ascending (distributing nutrients to vital organs). When the Stomach orb is not functioning properly, we are unable to assimilate the nutrients needed to strengthen our body/mind/spirit, and our energy level gradually weakens. Nausea, gastrointestinal pain, distention, belching, and vomiting are considered to be signs of disharmony and weakness in the Stomach orb.

IMBALANCES IN THE POWER OF EARTH

EXCESS

"Where do I end and you begin?" This is a question an excess Earth type might ask, for an all-consuming need to please others and win their approval leaves little time or energy for the fulfillment of your own needs.

Your innate need to nurture others has been transformed into a smothering overprotectiveness. You are literally off center; the squareness of "I know who I am" has become blurred, and the boundary separating self from others is no longer clearly defined.

If the center remains unoccupied, feelings of emptiness begin to influence your thoughts and emotions. Supportive behavior turns meddlesome, and a natural concern for the welfare of others degenerates into constant fretting. The Chinese believe that Earth's tendency to become "sick with worry" stagnates the yang energies in the Stomach, creating conditions of heat and decay that can contribute to the development of ulcers.

The worst fear of the excess Earth type is deprivation, which is typically experienced as a severing of connections with other human beings. Feeling empty, lonely, undernourished, hungry for love and attention, you attempt to fill yourself with those foods associated with the power of Earth— sweets. Eating sweets temporarily soothes your fears and helps you to feel nourished and rewarded for being a good person, but you feel full only when you are literally gorged with food, and even then you are unable to fill up your center. An excess of Earth energy contributes to such intense feelings of emptiness and off-centeredness that the constant craving for more continues unabated.

With so much stress placed on the Stomach orb, metabolism falters, food and nutrients can't be assimilated properly, and intestinal and digestive problems result. As your metabolism slows down, you are prone to rapid weight gain, and the internal feeling of off-centeredness manifests externally as a seesaw battle between strict dieting and compulsive overeating.

Symptoms Associated with Excess Earth Energy

- Excess appetite
- Water retention
- Irregular bowel movements and urination
- Tender gums
- Premenstrual syndrome (PMS) with lethargy, bloating, soreness, hunger, and swelling
- Aching, heavy-feeling head and eyes
- Thick mucus in nose, throat, and mouth
- Mental bogginess, cloudiness, heaviness
- Heavy limbs that make moving around an effort

- Heaviness of consciousness
- Metabolic problems, including sluggish metabolism and difficulty losing weight
- Tendency to thyroid problems, especially hypothyroidism (deficient thyroid)
- Bowel and digestive disturbances, including loose stools, diarrhea
- Lethargy, lack of energy, heavy spirit

Deficiency

Deficiencies in Earth energy typically begin in childhood, for Earth types need constant support and nourishment in order to develop feelings of self-worth. If your emotional supports were somehow strained or ruptured in childhood, you may have learned to cover up your real needs with an outward display of detachment and indifference. Whereas an excess in Earth power translates into difficulty asking for what is rightfully yours, a deficiency typically leads to deep feelings of inadequacy and an inability to care for yourself. The squareness of Earth, which connotes solidity, firm boundaries, and the ability to maneuver around sharp corners, disintegrates into a wobbly roundness, like a tire that is slowly losing air and deflating and cannot sustain its burden.

The first symptom of a deficiency in Earth is an ever-increasing dependence on others for your emotional and physical needs. A constant craving for attention, appreciation, and love defines every one of your relationships. Fear of abandonment organizes your energies, and you cling possessively to relatives and friends, smothering them with constant demands for attention and love. The need to be nourished is felt so acutely that you can no longer move out of yourself to appreciate other people's needs or problems.

> She who seeks nourishment that does not nourish reels from desire to gratification and in gratification craves desire. Mad pursuit of pleasure for the satisfaction of the senses never brings one to the goal. One should never . . . follow this path, for nothing good can come of it.

When the power of Earth is deficient, the functions of the Spleen and Stomach orbs are inhibited. Because the Spleen is responsible for transforming food and fluids into energy, blood, and waste products and then transporting these materials to the appropriate organs, a deficiency in Earth energy inevitably creates problems with digestion, which leads to symptoms of fatigue and lethargy. The Chinese believe that when the power of Earth is out of balance, food and fluids are not broken down or eliminated properly, and a watery sludge begins to pond up in the system, eventually coagulating into a mucoid substance called *tan*. A buildup of *tan* creates an overall quality of excessive dampness, which manifests physically with loose stools, arthritis (which is aggravated by dampness in the atmosphere and/or barometric pressure changes), and edema (a buildup of fluid, especially in the abdomen). In the mind and spirit, a buildup of *tan* is experienced as lethargy, heaviness of spirit, a sense of being sodden or weighed down ("The weight of the world is on my shoulders"), and increasing pressure in the head, which results in foggy thinking, difficulty concentrating, absentmindedness, and forgetfulness.

The Spleen is also responsible for creating upright *chi*, the energy that sustains and supports the body/mind/spirit and keeps the organs in their proper places. When Earth's energy is deficient, the Spleen can no longer produce a sufficient amount of upright *chi*. Hemorrhoids and bladder or uterine prolapses are thought to signify a weakness or deficiency in Spleen energy; bloody noses, bleeding gums, a tendency to bruise easily, and breakthrough bleeding between menstrual periods indicate a breakdown in the Spleen's ability to hold blood within the vessels. The spiritual counterpart of this physical process of caving in involves feelings of being weighed down by problems or unable to hold yourself up, a sensation of your energy leaking out at a steady rate, an inability to maintain proper boundaries, and a general feeling of loss of control.

Symptoms Associated with Deficient Earth Energy

- Constant hunger, with indecision about what to eat
- Difficulty losing weight
- Bloating, fluid retention
- Poor muscle tone
- Prolapse of stomach, intestine, uterus
- Varicose veins
- Slow healing of cuts
- Tendency to bruise easily

- Bleeding gums
- Tooth decay
- Swollen glands

THE WISDOM OF EARTH

The earth in its devotion carries all things, good and evil, without exception. In the same way the superior woman gives to her character breadth, purity, and sustaining power, so that she is able to support and to bear with people and things.

—*The I Ching*

EARTH: THE PEACEMAKER

———

An individual with an affinity to Earth has the capacity to nurture herself and others, mediate disputes, and create loving communities. Earth types thrive on peace and harmony and are thrown off balance by disagreement and discord.

NATURAL QUALITY: Fertile, nourishing, solid, restful

EMOTION: Caring and concern
   BALANCED: Supportive, relaxed, considerate, centered
   IMBALANCED
     Excess: Overprotective, worried, meddlesome
     Deficiency: Vacillating, hungry for nourishment (attention, love)

SPIRITUAL QUALITY: Centeredness

SEASON: Indian summer, or the transition period between seasons

CLIMATE: Dampness, thunder

DIRECTION: Center

TIME OF DAY: 7:00 A.M.–11:00 A.M.

COLOR: Yellow

SMELL: Fragrant (ripe, sweet fruits)

TASTE: Subtle sweetness (simple foods)

SOUND: Singing

ORGANS
   YIN: Spleen/Pancreas
   YANG: Stomach

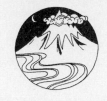

CHAPTER 10

METAL:
THE ARTIST

The [mysterious] powers of Fall create dryness in Heaven and they create metal upon Earth. Upon the body they create skin and hair, and of the viscera they create the lungs. Of the colors they create the white color . . . and they give to the human voice the ability to weep and to wail. . . . And among the emotions they create grief.

—**The Yellow Emperor's Classic**

The power of Metal finds its natural metaphor in a majestic mountain rising toward heaven. Both deep and broad, the mountain owes its stability and endurance to its firm foundation on the earth:

> The mountain rests on the earth. When it is steep and narrow, lacking a broad base, it must topple over. Its position is strong only when it rises out of the earth broad and great, not proud and steep.

At the center of the earth, we discover the metallic ores that give our planet its structural integrity. If you are guided by the power of Metal, you feel drawn to the core issues, the essential structures and guiding principles of life. Small talk bores you, for you crave discussions with depth and substance. Blessed with a fine aesthetic sense, you are attracted by beauty and surround yourself with valuable objects and sophisticated, erudite friends. Proportions concern you, symmetry pleases you, purity inspires you. Your environment is extremely important to your sense of harmony and balance, and when you encounter an aesthetically jarring or unpleasant situation, you experience intense distress and discomfort.

Grounded by earth and inspired by heaven, you feel impelled to extend yourself upward, reaching toward the higher truths and the moral imperatives of art and philosophy. Strict formalities and unnecessary embellishments irritate you, for in your eyes, they cover up the essential substance. You believe that beauty of form is both exalting and life-changing and that simplicity of design is more ennobling than external brilliance.

> Here at the highest stage of development all ornament is discarded. Form no longer conceals content but brings out its value to the full. Perfect grace consists not in exterior ornamentation of the substance, but in the simple fitness of its form.

Your spiritual powers depend on inner concentration and mental clarity. Through contemplation and careful reflection, you achieve inner composure. Just as it is in the nature of the mountain to keep still, if you are ruled by Metal, you discover inspiration when you achieve "tranquil beauty—clarity within, quiet without."

> When desire is silenced and the will comes to rest, the world-as-idea becomes manifest. In this aspect the world is beautiful and removed from the struggle for existence. This is the world of art.

You are most powerfully drawn to the emotion of grief, experiencing with penetrating sharpness the anguish of the passing of time. Your grief is not a passing mood indicating self-pity or remorse, but an adaptive, flexible response to the immutable laws of change. With keen insight, you understand the temporary, transitory nature of life, in which night succeeds day, the waxing of the moon follows its waning, the mountains erode while the valleys fill up, and decay follows luxuriant growth. Your grief, pure and undistorted, is an expression of appreciation for the temporary nature of all that is beautiful and exquisitely formed.

You understand with special poignancy the transitory nature of life, but by focusing on the enduring meaning of life, you know that within every ending is contained the promise of a new beginning. While the seasons and cycles of life change around you, you stand firm like a mountain in its tranquillity, silently grieving for what is gone while gratefully embracing what arrives in replacement. Detachment comes easily to you, for you know that what endures is the inner substance and not the outer form.

"Which is the right way, rabbi—that of joy or that of sorrow?" asked one of the disciples.

"There are two kinds of joy and two kinds of sorrow," the rabbi responded. "If a man grieves over his pains and woes, secluding himself and refusing all offers of help, that is a bad kind of sorrow, for it is said that the Divine Presence will not reside in a place of rejection. But when a man understands what he has lost and grieves with a pure heart, that is a good kind of sorrow.

"In the same way," the rabbi continued, "a man who is so caught up in the pursuit of empty pleasures that he does not recognize his lack of inner substance deceives himself. True joy is experienced deep within the soul and is not dependent upon external circumstances or material possessions. A man whose house has burned down does not spend his time grieving over his losses, but begins to build anew. With every stone that he puts into place, his heart expands with joy."

The season of Metal is autumn, the time to begin the process of shutting down and eliminating all that is unnecessary and extraneous. In autumn, we compress and contract our energies, letting go and settling in, pruning back in order to nourish and invigorate the root system. Flexibility and adaptability are crucial, for the energy of Metal, expressed in the sharp chill of an autumn day, foreshadows the season of death and decay that lies ahead.

A dry climate is associated with Metal; if you feel an affinity (or an aversion) to dryness and desertlike conditions, you may be expressing an imbalance in your Metal energies. Extremely dry skin may also be a sign of an imbalance in Metal.

The direction corresponding to Metal is west, for as *The Yellow Emperor's Classic* notes, "Precious metals and jade come from the regions of the

West." The power of Metal is most keenly felt between 3:00 A.M. and 7:00 A.M.

The color associated with Metal is white, which in traditional Chinese texts is associated with simplicity. A healthy white glow to the skin indicates well-balanced Metal energies, while a dull, pale hue suggests depletion and illness. A sharp, pungent smell similar to the odor of old garbage cans or the metallic scent associated with antique coins is connected with Metal energy. The sound of Metal is weeping; if you sound as if you are constantly on the verge of tears, even when discussing happy events or experiences, you may be expressing a disharmony in Metal.

Metal types tend to be thin, tall, and angular, with narrow shoulders and hips, and fine, sharp features. The excess Metal type often has a full and stiff but constricted chest, while the deficient type is generally underdeveloped, with a sunken-in or deflated chest and rounded shoulders, giving an overall impression of tight, stiff muscles. Hands are typically long and narrow, with fingers approximately the same length as the palms and rectangular fingernails. The skin tends to be on the dry side, and the complexion is pale or milky.

The organ functions associated with Metal—the Lung and Large Intestine—reflect this power's essential spiritual nature of refinement and purity. The Lung—called the Tender Organ because it is most directly affected by "external pernicious influences"—oversees the relationship between the interior and exterior world. Joining the *chi* of heaven (air) with the *chi* of earth (nutrients), the Lungs create additional sources of energy responsible for vitalizing and sustaining life processes. The Lungs are directly responsible for the formation and distribution of *ching chi*, the energy needed to supply the organ systems, and *wei chi*, the defensive or immune energy of the body/mind/spirit.

Wei chi protects us from invasions by exogenous pathogens such as colds and viruses. Wei chi also ensures that the internal treasures of blood, *chi*, and spirit are not lost to the outside world through "the third Lung"— the skin. The skin's semipermeable membrane defines the boundary between the body/mind/spirit and the outside world, selectively permitting nutrients and oxygen to enter while simultaneously allowing toxins to be eliminated through perspiration.

Expanding and contracting, the Lungs are both yielding and demanding, at once self-contained and self-renewing. Through the restrained and delicate movements of inhalation and exhalation, they instill the body/mind/spirit with a sense of rhythm and order based on the understanding that for every ending there is a new beginning.

The end is reached by inward movement, by inhalation, systole, contraction, and this movement turns into a new beginning, in which the movement is directed outward, in exhalation, diastole, expansion.

As the Officials of Rhythmic Order, the Lungs balance the inhalation and exhalation of air by ruling the expansion and contraction phases of breath and heartbeat, and of receiving and letting go in emotional and spiritual terms. The yin (contractive) and yang (expansive) qualities within Metal are forever giving and taking, and a healthy Metal type is able to balance the gathering up of air with the letting out of breath. Thus, it can be said that the organs associated with Metal "know" when to let substances in and when to let them go, a wisdom that is considered essential for health and happiness.

The Large Intestine, known as the Dust Bin Collector or the Drainer of the Dregs, is responsible for absorbing water from food and fluids, storing waste materials, and eliminating solid wastes. In the Chinese point of view, these functions are not automatic or in any sense routine, for the Large Intestine, like all other organ systems, is exquisitely sensitive to balance and harmony within the entire organism. Relaxation and flexibility are central to the healthy functioning of the Large Intestine, which must do its work in order to create the necessary space for the Lungs to disseminate the *chi* energy.

When we are under stress, the Large Intestine's decision-making skills become extremely important. Before it can eliminate waste products, the Large Intestine must be able to make distinctions between the harmless and the harmful, the useless and the useful. This ability to discriminate ensures a clear and uncluttered work space, while a breakdown in this power leads to overcrowding and congestion, creating symptoms of abdominal pain, cramping, diarrhea, and/or constipation, all of which deplete the vital energy circulating through the body/mind/spirit.

IMBALANCES IN THE POWER OF METAL

EXCESS

If the power of Metal becomes dominant or exaggerated, your natural flexibility and adaptability gradually erode into rigidity and dogmatism.

The more unbalanced your energies, the more extreme your need for order and discipline. An immaculate home and office reflect your need to have everything organized. If a pen is left on the table, you will immediately pick it up and put it where it belongs; if the kitchen counter is covered with dishes or food scraps, you will not be able to relax until you have cleaned up the mess. Any deviation from your normal routine creates intense physical anxiety, which inevitably affects your emotional and spiritual balance.

As you become more uncompromising and unyielding, you tend to attach yourself to various dogmas and philosophies. The excess Metal type is the religious convert who follows the only "true" path to grace and salvation, the political dogmatist who insists that all other doctrines are misguided, or the teacher who is convinced that her method of discipline is the only way. It is almost as if the pores of the skin (which Metal governs) close off, refusing to let anything in from the outside. Deprived of fresh ideas and energy, the body/mind/spirit begins to congeal and stagnate, like a pool of water that has been isolated from its source.

Locked inside the psyche of your self-righteous stoicism is a basic lack of self-esteem and self-respect. An excess of Metal has created a hardening effect, in which your naturally molten nature cools down, becoming solid and unyielding. As you lose sight of the need to balance your inward contraction with outward expansion, you begin to concentrate more and more on hoarding and retaining your possessions. You become possessive of all that you own, for in your eyes, these possessions reflect the measure of your worth. Over time, you become possessed with possessions. The material world is so central to your sense of self that you feel naked without these external symbols of beauty and brilliance.

Relationships also become possessive, for you have forgotten the basic wisdom intrinsic to Metal: quality emanates from within, and simplicity of form is superior to external ornamentation. Having lost your focus, you become obsessed with the superficial manifestations of quality (beauty, breeding, wealth, culture, and refinement). Threatened by the idea of disorder, you demand agreement and conformity from your relatives and friends, and anyone who deviates from your expectations is harshly judged and bitterly resented.

As you become more attached to your relationships and material possessions, your natural tendency to grieve becomes exaggerated, metamorphosing into misery over perceived losses. Grief generally occurs in response to loss, and when Metal types carry through with this emotion, they are able to let go of losses and thus create the space for the new to enter and replace the old. But when an excess of Metal contributes to a tendency to hold on to grief, or to a refusal to let yourself express this emotion, natural feelings of loss and mourning are transformed into envy, jealousy, and greed. When you perceive that you no longer possess beauty, wealth, or influence, you begin to crave these qualities in others, and your craving gradually develops into obsession.

As the power of Metal hardens, your character becomes rigid and immobile. You have forgotten the wisdom of the way of the yin, which is expressed in Lao-tzu's words: "If you want to be given everything, you must first give everything up." Unable to let go and grieve for what you no longer have, you cling possessively to all tnat you own, whether it be material possessions or rigid adherence to a fixed set of beliefs.

> *On their way to the monastery two Buddhist monks came to the shore of a river and prepared to wade across. A beautiful woman was standing on the embankment, unable to cross because the water was too high. Without a word, one of the monks lifted the woman onto his back and carried her to the other side.*
>
> *As they continued on their way to the monastery the monk received a severe reprimand from his brother. "What were you thinking about?" asked the horrified monk. "Were you so blinded by her beauty that you forgot your vows? How dare you touch a woman? Not only did you touch her, but you carried her on your back! What if someone had seen you? Did you ever consider what the consequences might be for the brotherhood?"*
>
> *On and on the monk continued, filled with his own self-righteousness. After listening patiently to the interminable harangue, the offending monk finally spoke up. "Brother, I left that woman at the riverbank. Why are you still carrying her?"*

Symptoms Associated with Excess Metal Energy

- Rigidity of musculature, with a tendency to move in a stiff, clumsy manner
- Stiff spine, neck, and posture
- Spine and joint problems
- Chronic sinus infections, with sinus headaches

- Shortness of breath, chronic dry cough, tight chest, and tendency to develop asthma
- Intestinal difficulties including constipation, diarrhea, colitis, and irritable bowel syndrome
- Dry skin, hair, nails, lips, nasal passages, and other mucous membranes
- Nasal polyps
- Lack of perspiration

DEFICIENCY

If you are deficient in Metal, your boundaries gradually blur and become obscured. In a figurative sense, your power is liquefying and spilling out of your pores. The need for approval dominates your thoughts and actions, for your self-confidence is so depleted that you feel good about yourself only when others are openly and consistently approving of your behavior. Friends and relatives are often uncomfortable offering constructive advice or criticism, for you are so soft that they fear wounding you. Casual comments are often taken personally, resulting in persistent hurt feelings and damage to self-esteem. As the authors of the book *Between Heaven and Earth* explain it, you are "like old Jell-O, stiff on the surface and gooey at the core."

Because the power of Metal rules rhythm, order, and synchrony, a deficiency results in difficulties with letting go. Whereas an excess in Metal results in a tendency to hold on to objects or possessions, a deficiency creates an obsession with relationships. You cling tenaciously to your loved ones, even if they are abusive; rather than confront them, you modify your behavior to fall in line with their expectations, thus increasing your sense of inferiority and intensifying your fear of letting go. You tend to give of yourself too easily, putting people on pedestals and then experiencing great disillusionment when they disappoint you or fail to meet your expectations.

Filled with confusion and self-doubt, you no longer know what is right and what is wrong. Lacking inner resolve, you rely on the outer constraints imposed by social convention or political correctness. Good manners, proper etiquette, and superficial beauty have come to mean more to you than inner quality and substance.

When forced into a situation with people you perceive as gross or coarse, you experience a strong visceral sensation of disgust or repulsion. You are hypersensitive to your environment and may suffer from allergic reactions and environmental sensitivities. Allergies almost always involve a disharmony in the power of Metal and correspond to those body areas and organ systems ruled by Metal—the sinuses, skin, and Lungs. Your breathing tends to be shallow and constricted, leading to shortness of breath and chronic congestion of the nose, throat, and sinuses. Food allergies create disturbances in the bowel and intestinal tract and can lead to irritable bowel syndrome, colitis, and Crohn's disease.

Symptoms Associated with Deficient Metal Energy

- Shortness of breath and tendency to bronchial spasm, especially when under stress
- Congested nose, throat, sinuses
- Food and environmental allergies, including hay fever, allergic reactions to cats, dust, chemicals, dairy products, etc.
- Asthma, especially allergic asthma
- Dry skin, hair, lips, nails, and nasal passages
- Moles and warts
- Loss of body hair
- Cracked, dry, or soft nails
- Headaches, typically experienced in reaction to loss or disappointment
- Varicose veins
- Bowel disturbances: constipation, loose stools, or irritable bowel syndrome (alternating diarrhea and constipation)
- Depleted immune function, characterized by persistent colds and flus, a tendency to sinus congestion and postnasal drip, and immunodeficient disorders such as chronic fatigue syndrome and Lupus

THE WISDOM OF METAL

We cannot lose what really belongs to us, even if we throw it away. Therefore we need have no anxiety. All that need concern us is that we should remain true to our own natures and not listen to others.

—The I Ching

METAL: THE ARTIST

An individual with an affinity to Metal has a strong sense of aesthetics and a deep and abiding interest in spiritual matters. Grounded by earth and inspired by heaven, she feels impelled to reach upward toward the higher truths of art and philosophy. Metal types tend to have difficulty with letting go.

NATURAL QUALITY: Malleable, strong, aesthetically inclined

EMOTION: Grief, sadness
  BALANCED: Accepting, disciplined, calm
  IMBALANCED
    Excess: Hypercritical, dogmatic, perfectionistic, self-righteous
    Deficiency: Needy for approval, clinging, self-doubting, hypersensitive

SPIRITUAL QUALITY: Inspiration

SEASON: Autumn

CLIMATE: Dry

DIRECTION: West (setting sun)

TIME OF DAY: 3:00 A.M.—7:00 A.M.

COLOR: White

SMELL: Raw flesh, fish

TASTE: Pungent, spicy

SOUND: Weeping

ORGANS
  YIN: Lungs
  YANG: Large Intestine

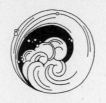

CHAPTER 11

WATER:
THE SAGE

The [mysterious] powers of Winter create the extreme cold in Heaven and they create water upon earth. Within the body they create the bones, and of the orifices they create the kidneys (testicles). Of the colors they create the black color. . . . They give to the human voice the ability to groan and hum. In times of excitement and change they create trembling, and among the emotions they create fear.

—**The Yellow Emperor's Classic**

From the power of Water, we learn how to adapt to unusual or demanding situations, remaining steady and constant while never losing sight of our goal. Dependable and infinitely adaptable, Water holds firm to its course and flows on. When it encounters a rock or boulder, Water does not attempt to remove the obstacle in order to continue on in a straight line, but chooses instead to flow around. Water is content to separate, knowing that through such division its power is multiplied: "In order to find one's place in the infinity of being, one must be able both to separate and to unite."

The power of Water does not fret over setbacks, nor does it seek to shape the future by imposing its will on the world. Every action Water takes, even the nonaction of pooling up and reserving strength, is filled with potential and readiness to continue onward toward the goal.

> If a person encounters a hindrance at the beginning of an enter-
> prise, she must not try to force an advance but must pause and
> take thought. However, nothing should put her off her course;
> she must persevere and constantly keep the goal in sight.

Water knows its limitations; it can only flow downward, toward earth. If its natural movement is interrupted or impeded, it yields by retreating, refusing to expend its energy in vain pursuits, biding its time, and awaiting the right moment. When danger threatens, Water does not shrink in fear or give up the struggle in hopeless resignation; it remains true to its basic nature, knowing when to hold back and collect its energies in preparation for the journey ahead, and when to continue on with force and determination. When the time is right, Water does not hesitate but follows its course with strength and purpose.

> Water on top of a mountain cannot flow down in accordance
> with its nature, because rocks hinder it. It must stand still.
> This causes it to increase, and the inner accumulation finally
> becomes so great that it overflows the barriers. The way of
> overcoming obstacles lies in turning inward and raising one's
> own being to a higher level.

Water understands that there are many pathways leading to her destination. Along the way hazards will present themselves, and risks must be taken, but as long as she respects her limitations and remains true to her basic nature, she will meet with good fortune.

> "What is the true path to God?" one disciple asked another, who
> began to explain that the true path to God relies on inner strength and
> constant struggle. "Praying, paying attention, living rightly, giving
> yourself wholly and completely to the task of following the Law—this
> is the true path," he insisted.

"But that is the way of ego, not true effort," asserted the other disciple. "To truly follow the way, one must surrender completely, letting go of all need and desire and committing oneself to proclaiming at all times, 'Not my will but thine.' "

The argument continued for many hours until a third disciple suggested that they seek the master's advice. After eloquently describing the way of wholehearted effort, the first disciple to speak asked the master if this was not the true path of God. "Yes," said the master, nodding thoughtfully. "You are right."

The other disciple, who had initiated the whole discussion, was quite upset that judgment had been pronounced before he had been able to offer his argument. "But master," he said, "doesn't the true path of God involve surrender and letting go of one's egotistical needs and desires?"

"Why, yes," said the master, after listening carefully. "You're right."

The third disciple who had been listening with great interest to the debate suddenly spoke up. "But master, they can't both be right!"

The master stroked his chin and smiled. "Why, you're right, too!"

Water has the strength of mind to know that the right way is her way, wherever that way happens to lead. Following her nature and instincts, she continues onward, disregarding the advice of those who would suggest that her path is not the right path. She understands both the wisdom and the warning contained in Antonio Porchia's words: "They will say that you are on the wrong road, if it is your own."

If Water defines your nature, your energy is naturally abundant, powerful, and directed. Casual meandering and aimless wandering are not your style, for you know where you are going, and you have the inner resources, mental determination, and courage to move forward without hesitation or doubt. You are insatiably curious, and the world of ideas appeals to your basically introspective, reflective nature. But you intuitively understand that prolonged isolation will diminish your strength and vitality, and so you periodically unite with others to pool your wisdom and refresh your spirit.

A lake evaporates upward and thus gradually dries up; but when two lakes are joined they do not dry up so readily, for one replenishes the other. It is the same in the field of knowledge. Knowledge should be a refreshing and vitalizing force. It becomes so only through stimulating intercourse with congenial friends with whom one holds discussion and practices application of the truths of life. In this way learning becomes many-sided and takes on a cheerful lightness, whereas there is always something ponderous and one-sided about the learning of the self-taught.

Your relationships are based on honesty and trust. Your sense of self— I know who I am—is well balanced, and you do not pretend to be either less or more than you are. You feel no need to look back and brood on what once was or could have been. The past is over and done with; it is the present that absorbs you, and the future that draws you forward. Imagination rather than history fascinates you; science fiction, poetry, mysteries, and riddles engage your curious mind.

Your primary spiritual quality is the ability to *be*, for while activity (doing) is the expression of your abundant energy, a reflective stillness (being) informs your spirit. You live in the moment, content to be exactly who you are but always mindful of the fact that circumstances might force you to change your direction. You continue on, refusing to look backward to gloat over difficult obstacles overcome. Your spirit is captivated by the urgency of the here and now. "I am in the present," said the composer Igor Stravinsky, surely a Water type. "I cannot know what tomorrow will bring forth. I can know only what the truth is for me today. That is what I am called upon to serve, and I serve it in all lucidity."

Fear is the emotion that moves and directs you. In its healthy, balanced state, fear allows you to remain alert and attentive. When you are confronted with danger, fear guides you along with its message of caution and restraint. Obstacles and detours predictably interrupt the course of every life, and even seemingly benign situations are often fraught with danger. With fear as your guide, you do not tremble with terror, nor are you waylaid by panic. Instead, you are filled with readiness and the courage to face whatever situation might present itself. You use your fear like a ladder to surmount your difficulties, setting it aside when you no longer require its services.

A community leader came to see Jacob, hoping to find peace of mind, an ease for his burden.

The man was troubled by a repetitive dream that he did not understand.

"Jacob, in my dream, I have traveled a long distance and am finally arriving at a great city. But, at the entrance to the city, I am met by a tall soldier who says that I must answer two questions before I am admitted. Will you help me?"

Jacob nodded.

"The first question the soldier asks is 'What supports the walls of a city?' "

"That is easy," said Jacob. "Fear supports the walls of a city."

"But what supports the fear?" asked the man. "For that is the second question."

"The walls," answered Jacob. "The fears we cannot climb become our walls."

The season of Water is winter, when the natural world withdraws and pulls inward, conserving its energy for the time of renewal and regeneration that lies ahead. In winter, Water is content to fill up with passive energy, changing its fluid nature and becoming solid. If you dread the coming of winter and suffer from agitated, restless, pent-up energy during this season, you may be experiencing an imbalance in Water. *The I Ching* advises that in winter, we should devote our energies to restoring and renewing our body/mind/spirit.

In winter the life energy, symbolized by thunder, the Arousing, is still underground. Movement is just at its beginning; therefore it must be strengthened by rest, so that it will not be dissipated by being used prematurely. This principle, i.e., of allowing energy that is renewing itself to be reinforced by rest, applies to all similar situations. The return of health after illness, the return of understanding after an estrangement; everything must be treated tenderly and with care at the beginning, so that the return may lead to a flowering.

A cold climate is associated with Water, and the direction is north. The peak time of day for this power is between 3:00 P.M. and 7:00 P.M.

Blue and black are the colors associated with Water, and a bluish-black hue around the eyes and temples or a strong attraction or repulsion to these colors may indicate an imbalance.

A putrid, acrid smell, which could be compared to the odor of an infrequently cleaned public restroom, is associated with an imbalance in Water. The stagnant, decomposing quality of an imbalance can also be detected in the scent of flowers left to rot in a vase of stale water.

The sound governed by Water is groaning or moaning; in its exaggerated form, this is characterized by an unconscious, persistent tone of whining. While a child whines to accomplish an end, the moaning sound of Water is unintended and unconnected to problems or frustrations taking place in daily life. When the power of Water is out of balance, this vocal quality becomes pervasive and exaggerated.

The Water body type tends to be sturdy, with a strong but lean physique, large bones, and narrow shoulders with wider hips. Features are clearly defined, with chiseled cheekbones, a prominent nose, deep-set eyes, strong jaw bones, and a long forehead. Hands are generally small, with short fingers and delicate fingernails. The skin tends to be soft and a bit puffy, which may signify a tendency to water retention. Excess Water types tend to be tall, sinewy, and powerfully built, while the deficient type is fleshier and tends to slump over.

The power of Water nourishes the body/mind/spirit with *chi* energy, both real and potential, which is stored in the Kidneys. *Ching chi* is an acquired energy produced from the nutritive elements distilled from the foods and fluids we ingest, the air we breathe, and the various relationships we engage in. *Yuan chi*, or *jing*, is inherited from our parents, especially our mother, and rules the entire life cycle of birth, growth, maturation, and death; thus it is believed that the quality of your inherited *jing* determines your individual destiny. The primordial source responsible for infusing the egg and sperm with the life force of reproductive power, *jing* contributes to sexual energy and desire. Problems with sexual function such as impotence, frigidity, premature ejaculation, and infertility are considered symptoms of Water imbalance in general and *jing* deficiency in particular; premature aging is associated with a Kidney *jing* deficiency.

The Chinese believe that the Kidneys (called the Storehouse of the Vital Essence) are the pilot light of the body/mind/spirit. Kidney fire, or ming men-huo, sparks the system, separating the pure aspects of Water from the impure. The contaminated parts are transported to the Bladder for storage and elimination, while the pure parts are transformed into a mist, which is circulated freely throughout the body. In metaphorical terms, Kidney fire provides the driving energy and resolute will-power needed to press forward, overcome obstacles, and reach our goals in life.

Life Gate Fire is an acupuncture point that epitomizes the Kidneys' function of sparking activity in all other parts of the body/mind/spirit. Other acupoints along the Kidney pathway attest to its role in sexual function (Bubbling Spring, Great Cup, Greater Mountain Stream), and still others underscore the spiritual nature of Kidney energy (Spirit Seal, Spirit Wilderness, and Spirit Storehouse). "When the Kidneys are deficient," pronounces *The Yellow Emperor's Classic*, "the spirit becomes easily provoked."

The power of Water is also responsible for maintaining healthy teeth, bones, and bone marrow. Because the ancient Chinese medical scholars considered the brain and spinal cord as extensions of the bone marrow, Water is thought to rule over skeletal structure and function as well as intelligence, reason, perception, and memory. Lethargy, disturbed sensory and motor functioning, indecisive behavior, sluggish responses, and memory problems are all associated with deficient Kidney energy.

Four thousand years ago when the Chinese elaborated on the functional duties of the Kidneys, they had no knowledge of the adrenal gland, a small endocrine gland that rests on top of each kidney. Yet the functions attributed to the Kidneys by the ancient sages and scholars correspond directly to modern-day descriptions of adrenal function. The adrenal cortex (the outer shell of the gland) manufactures the corticosteroid hormones, which control the metabolism of protein, fat, and carbohydrates and balance fluid and electrolyte levels in the body. The medulla (the inner core of the gland) secretes the stress hormones adrenaline and noradrenaline, which directly affect automatic responses such as cardiac activity, gastrointestinal actions, and various metabolic functions.

The yang organ associated with Water is the Urinary Bladder (the Official in Charge of Eliminating Fluid Waste). This flexible, adaptable organ is compared to a reservoir that holds the vital *chi* energy until it is needed. When the Bladder is not functioning properly, the entire body/mind/spirit is in danger of slowing down and filling up with toxic wastes.

The Bladder meridian is the largest meridian of the body, containing sixty-seven acupuncture points with names like Spirit Hall, Thought Dwelling, and Penetrating the Valley, which attest to this organ's extensive influence throughout the body/mind/spirit. Depression, coping difficulties, inability to adapt to new or unusual circumstances, and a general sense of foreboding may indicate an energy imbalance in the Bladder orb. Chronic fatigue is often considered a symptom of a "leaky" bladder.

IMBALANCES IN THE POWER OF WATER

EXCESS

If you are an excess Water type, inflexibility rules your body/mind/spirit. Your posture is stiff and erect, your movements lack grace and flexibility, and you tend to be opinionated and intolerant of viewpoints that diverge from your own. The world revolves around you (or so you believe), and you are convinced that you know what is best for everyone else. If your opinions are challenged, your resentment is deep and long-lasting. Competitive by nature, you focus on winning for the sake of winning; when you lose, you create elaborate excuses to justify what you perceive as a failure.

When dealing with authority figures, you tend to be defiant. "Nobody tells *me* what to do!" you might say, or "What do those stupid, incompetent, inefficient idiots know, anyway?" Your belligerent behavior is a thin cover-up for a mounting sensation of fear; strong feelings of inadequacy are generating anxiety and a presentiment of impending disaster. Forceful and defiant on the outside, you are filled with trepidation on the inside. Over time, you become suspicious of others, imagining that they are talking about you and conspiring behind your back. (In your self-centeredness, you can't imagine who else they would be talking about.) Paranoid tendencies and a fear of persecution become pronounced if the imbalance continues undetected and untreated.

Water types are naturally intelligent, but as excess Water energy accumulates, you will begin to lose a sense of the joy of learning and become obsessed with accumulating scattered bits of knowledge in order to present yourself as an expert on numerous and diverse subjects. You have trouble discriminating between important and trivial facts, and your innate sense of timing is off—you pause when you should continue, and you push ahead when it is time to rest and reflect. You are in such a hurry to advance yourself and achieve something measurable and worthwhile that you often exceed your boundaries, depleting your natural energies and wasting your time on vain pursuits.

Symptoms Associated with Excess Water Energy

- Requires little sleep
- Lack of sweat and urine
- Arthritis (both osteo- and rheumatoid) and stiffness in the joints
- Severe low back pain
- Knee problems
- Urinary infections, kidney and bladder stones
- High blood pressure, with a tendency toward heart attacks and strokes
- Hypersexuality, but with a tendency to be detached and uninvolved
- Headaches, typically severe behind the eyes or in the occiput, where the skull and neck meet
- Tendency to neurological disturbances or diseases

DEFICIENCY

Whereas an excess in the power of Water leads to an engorged sense of self (like a river at flood stage overflowing its boundaries), a deficiency creates a gradual condensation or contraction of self. The deficient Water phase begins with feelings of fatigue and lethargy. The introverted part of your nature, which craves isolation and introspection, takes over, crowding out the complementary need for fellowship and companionship.

As you continue to pull into yourself and away from others, feelings of disconnectedness and isolation intensify. You feel arid and empty, and you fear that you are drying up inside, slowly evaporating into nothingness. As your fear grows, your creative ability deteriorates, leading to a persistent state of depression and despair. You begin to feel as if everything you do is a chore, with no meaning or inherent value. "Since nothing I do makes a difference, why do anything?" you ask yourself, over and over again. As time passes and your Water energy continues to dissipate, you lose the ability to interact naturally and spontaneously with others. Relationships are difficult to maintain, for you lack the deep reserves of concern and compassion that are necessary for true friendship and love.

If you are a deficient Water type, you tend to slouch over, indicating by your posture that you're not quite sure how to stand up for yourself. In your fear, you have lost the essential wisdom of Water: to hold together, refuse to shrink from danger, and stand firm against all temptations to stray from your true nature.

Abbot Pastor was approached by a brother who asked for his advice. "I am plagued by many negative and unpleasant thoughts, and I feel that I am in danger," said the brother. "Tell me, what can I do to protect myself?"

The old man asked his brother to step outside. "Open up your robe and seize the wind," he commanded.

"This I cannot do," replied the brother.

"It is so," the old man said. "You cannot take hold of the wind and neither can you prevent these thoughts from entering your mind. But just as you can stand steadfast against even the most powerful wind, so can you stand firm against the thoughts that tempt and torment you."

Symptoms Associated with Deficient Water Energy

- Fatigue, lethargy, lack of energy or stamina
- Loss of appetite
- Prematurely thin, gray hair
- Wrinkled skin
- Weak, stiff spine with degeneration of disks and cartilage
- Osteoporosis
- Weak abdominal muscles
- Sore lower back and achy, weak knees
- Tendency to ear infections or tinnitus (ringing in the ears)
- An aversion to winter, particularly to the cold
- A dark hue around the eyes indicating a weakness in kidney and adrenal functions (If the shade is very dark, almost black, and can be seen underneath the eyes, it indicates adrenal exhaustion.)
- Urinary problems, including frequent urination and chronic urinary infections
- Vaginal and yeast infections
- Amenorrhea (unusual menstrual bleeding, e.g., menstruation has never occurred, or a woman stops menstruating after years of regular bleeding)
- Frigidity, impotence, infertility

THE WISDOM OF WATER

Water . . . flows on and on, and merely fills up all the places through which it flows; it does not shrink from any dangerous spot nor from any plunge, and nothing can make it lose its own essential nature. It remains true to itself under all conditions.

—The I Ching

WATER: THE SAGE

An individual with an affinity to Water contains within herself a deep sense of the power of silence, patience, and introspection. She knows how to live in the moment, filling herself with potential and readiness for whatever challenges and adventures life might present.

NATURAL QUALITY: Yielding, fluid, tending to stillness, full of potential

EMOTION: Fear
  BALANCED: Candid, curious, watchful, ingenious, willful
  IMBALANCED
    Excess: Inflexible, suspicious, opinionated
    Deficiency: Lethargic, isolated, cynical

SPIRITUAL QUALITY: The ability to be

SEASON: Winter

CLIMATE: Cold

DIRECTION: North

TIME OF DAY: 3:00 P.M.–7:00 P.M.

COLOR: Blue and black

SMELL: Rotting, putrefaction

TASTE: Salty

SOUND: Moaning

ORGANS
  YIN: Kidneys
  YANG: Bladder

PART III

THE SEASONS OF LIFE

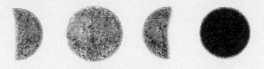

CHAPTER 12

A CIRCLE WITH NO BEGINNING OR END

Like the day or the year in nature, so every life, indeed every cycle of experience, is a continuity by which old and new are linked together.
—**The I Ching**

The transformative stages of a woman's life can be imagined as the seasons of spring, summer, autumn, and winter. With each passing month, a woman's wisdom deepens; with each new season her spirit expands. In the season of spring, the child/woman shares with the budding world a sense of her explosive power and potential. Touched by the magic of metamorphosis, she is forever altered by the mysterious energies coming to life within her. In summer, her passion is kindled; over time, the intensity of her devotion is directed toward the life-giving powers of her womb and the deeply creative energies of the female spirit. In the autumn of her life, she focuses inward, condensing, pruning back, concentrating on the roots—the core issues and essential substance of life. And in winter, she directs her attention to matters of heart and soul, seeking ways to unite that which has been separated and preparing for the ultimate transformation from body to soul.

While we present the pivotal stages of a woman's life in a sequence beginning with youth and ending in old age, we do not intend to convey a linear ascension (or as our culture has come to imagine the aging process, an accelerating descension). Just as the four seasons ebb and flow into each other, each representing a distinct period of time but all essential to the yearly cycle, so do the major transformations of a woman's life ebb and flow into each other to exchange vital energy. The innocence of the child is firmly rooted in the soul of the white-haired woman, just as the grandmother's powers of perception are seeded in the passions of her youth.

As a woman matures, she learns how to draw on each and every part of her female nature—the inquisitive child, the passionate lover, the nurturing mother, and the wise grandmother—for balance and harmony. She feels free to roam between these stages as a pilgrim wanders, looping, backtracking, crisscrossing, and sidestepping, knowing that life is in balance only when it is in transition.

As these seasonal metamorphoses are a natural and, indeed, a crucial part of life, the ability to move through them gracefully and with relative ease indicates a state of health and balance. When the flow of energy is obstructed, resulting in disharmonies throughout the body, mind, and spirit, many healing methods are available to help the individual move through the impediments and continue on her journey. In my practice, I emphasize the basic principles of Traditional Chinese Medicine, using acupuncture and Chinese herbal medicine, but I also rely on my training in Western herbal medicine, nutrition, body work, and psychology. I use all my senses in the diagnostic process, respecting each individual's history and experience and reminding myself at all times that there is never one right way leading to wholeness, but rather many divergent pathways.

At every stage of treatment, I seek to tap into a deeper level of healing, one that extends beyond an understanding of the individual and her specific energy imbalances to recreate a sense of the basic unity and commonality of the female life experience. To penetrate this realm of heart and soul, I rely on stories, myths, legends, and parables. While I draw from many different cultures and traditions, the stories that never fail to elicit a spontaneous, heartfelt response are borrowed from the Native American tradition.

In their wisdom stories and healing rituals, the Native Americans emphasize spiritual values, respect for the earth, and harmony with others—the basic underlying tenets of the feminine spirit of healing. From puberty onward, Native American women were taught to look upon their bleeding as their "moon time," an extraordinary interlude when the world of intuition and spirit unveiled its deepest mysteries. When the moon—the radiant symbol of the female life cycle—began to surrender its light, women followed its example and prepared to shed their blood, retreating into the Moon Lodge to rest, reflect, and gather wisdom. In the House of the Moon, women of all ages gathered together to celebrate the life-giving, life-sustaining powers of their blood and to strengthen their connections with the natural rhythms and cycles of life.

Perhaps the greatest wisdom healers in any tradition can bring to their art is a sense of humility and an appreciation of their limitations. We cannot heal all wounds or cure all diseases; we can only hope to work with the individual to unearth her innate powers of self-healing. The journey to wholeness is both self-directed and self-fulfilling; while we can learn from others along the way, the changes must emanate from within. The inevitability of change and the wisdom gained by experience are celebrated in a wonderful story found in numerous spiritual traditions. This version features our old friend Nasrudin, the "wise fool" of the Sufis.

When Nasrudin was an old man, he sat in a tea shop telling the story of his life to his friends.

"When I was young," he recalled, "I was filled with passion and the desire to enlighten everyone around me. I would pray to Allah to give me the energy and devotion needed to change the world.

"Then, when I reached middle age and realized I had changed no one, I prayed to Allah to give me the energy and devotion needed to change those close to me who, I believed, desperately needed my help.

"But now that I am older and wiser"—Nasrudin smiled and winked at his friends—"my prayer is much simpler. 'Allah,' I implore, 'please give me the energy and devotion needed to at least change myself.'"

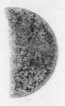

CHAPTER 13

SPRING: FROM CHILD TO WOMAN

Know the male
Yet keep to the female:
receive the world in your arms.
If you receive the world,
the Tao will never leave you,
and you will be like a little child.
                    —Tao te Ching

It is said in Native ways that this first blood is the richest and the most powerful a woman will ever have. On this day, she is very special and is so honored, for she is becoming like her Mother the Earth: able to renew and nurture life.

                    —*Brooke Medicine Eagle*

The passage from child to woman marked by the onset of menstruation is the first and most important metamorphosis in the female life cycle. This is the season of spring, when the earth enfolds the swelling seed within its ample breast, and the seedling sleeps, nourished by the mother. Swirling above, unheard and unfelt, gentle winds caress earth's frozen surface, and the melting begins. Leafless trees shudder as the warming sap flows upward and outward, filling the veined limbs with the fluid of life. As the warmth penetrates deep into earth, the seedling stirs, sending forth slender, snakelike shoots to grab hold of the soil and drink from its inexhaustible springs. Strengthened and renewed, the greening stem pushes upward, bending around obstacles, yielding, adapting, doing everything within its power to follow the compelling impulses of mysterious inner forces. At last it bursts forth, opening up to embrace the luminous light of the newly awakened world.

Sweet spring, when the air goes soft, the wind gentles down, and fragrant flowers carpet the earth, is the season when a child becomes a woman, experiencing, in the poet Dylan Thomas's words, "the force that through the green fuse drives the flower." With her first blood, the child/woman enters a mysterious new world. As the rich, red blood pools up within her, building in power until it overflows, she experiences with throbbing intensity the ebb and flow of earth's cyclical rhythms. Her joy is edged with pain and her celebration with grief, for with the shedding of her blood, she leaves behind a stage of life when she was cradled and nurtured by the mother. Her first blood signals that it is time to stand alone and begin the challenging process of discovering who she is and what she is yet to become.

For many months, the child/woman will live in a world precariously balanced between the carefree, joy-filled days of childhood and the challenges and deeper wisdom of womanhood. Her roots are buried deep within the mother; drawing from the core, she feels earth's fire rising up within her, charging her blood with passionate energy and intuitive wisdom. The phases of the moon guide her spirit; as she comes to know the moon's cycles, she gathers wisdom about herself. Each month she follows the moon's lead, learning from its waxing and waning how to concentrate her energies and refine her spirit. The waning moon tells her to turn inward and take time to reflect, remember, and dream. As the moon fills with light, she begins to feel restless, for this is the time to move outward into the world, transforming the energy gained during rest and reflection into creative work. When the moon begins to empty itself of light, she knows the time has come to discharge her energy in preparation for the new moon, when she will feel once again the pulling inward toward the dark, mysterious powers that open her soul to wisdom and healing.

A woman's monthly bleeding symbolizes the power of renewal and the mysterious, ongoing cycle of life, death, and rebirth. Blood *is* power. In many Native American cultures, a menstruating woman is considered even more powerful than the medicine men and warriors. The Lakota tribe would not permit a menstruating woman near a *yuwipi* man, or psychic healer, because they believed that her blood endowed her with such intense, concentrated energy that her mere presence interfered with the healer's skills. The Crows forbid women who were menstruating to venture into the same vicinity as wounded men or warriors preparing for battle, because they feared that her powers would weaken the men's physical and spiritual strength.

In other cultures, the life- and death-giving potential of menstrual blood sometimes became a source of contention between men and women, as a popular Chinese myth illustrates:

> *The goddess Chang-O guards the menstrual blood. When Chang-O lived on earth, men attacked her. They envied her bleeding, for it meant that she possessed the power of life, death, and rebirth, and these were mysteries to them. She became so angry at the men's jealous attacks that she withdrew to the moon and forbade men to take part in her festivals from that time on. So it came to be in China that the women celebrate full-moon festivals only among themselves, with songs and praise to honor women, Chang-O, and menstrual blood—the blood of life and death.*

As time passed the feminine spirit of healing lost power and influence, and "the blood of life and death" came to be cursed rather than praised. Today, we no longer honor the female monthly cycle as a time of special powers and privileges, when a woman is most sensitive to the rhythms and cycles of the natural world. We have lost a sense of the healing power of women's blood and accepted a different interpretation of the monthly cycle, which emphasizes pollution rather than cleansing, death and decay rather than renewal and regeneration. Through the centuries, in diverse religious codes, philosophical dicta, and cultural traditions, menstrual blood has been reinterpreted as "unclean" and invested with fearsome, repulsive energy.

The polluting nature of female blood is clearly stated in the Bible. In Leviticus 15:19–30, it is proposed that anyone who touches a menstruating women is contaminated and that animal sacrifices should be offered as penance in atonement for the female's bloody "sin":

> And if a woman have an issue, and her issue in her flesh be blood, she shall be put apart seven days: and whosoever toucheth her shall be unclean until the evening. . . .
>
> And if any man lie with her at all, and her flowers be upon him, he shall be unclean seven days, and all the bed whereon he lieth shall be unclean. . . .
>
> But if she be cleansed of her issue, then she shall number to herself seven days, and after she shall be clean.
>
> And on the eighth day she shall take unto her two turtles, or two pigeons, and bring them unto the priest, to the door of the tabernacle of the congregation.
>
> And the priest shall offer the one for a sin offering, and the other for a burnt offering; and the priest shall make an atonement for her before the Lord for the issue of her uncleanness.

In 65 A.D., the Roman naturalist Pliny the Elder described the fearful powers of "the monthly flux," which he claimed could destroy crops, kill insects, and poison animals:

> Contact with it turns new wine sour, crops touched by it become barren, seeds in gardens dry up, the fruit of trees fall off. The bright surface of mirrors in which it is merely reflected is dimmed, the edge of steel and the gleam of ivory are dulled. Hives of bees will die. Even bronze and iron are at once seized by rust and a horrible smell fills the air. To taste it drives dogs mad and affects their bite with an incurable poison.

Jewish scholars warn in the Talmud that a menstruating woman can kill a man by her mere presence. In the Eastern European Jewish tradition, when a young woman menstruates for the first time, her mother slaps her hard on the face, hoping to impress her daughter with the grim importance of the occasion.

"I first got my period on my birthday," one young woman remembers. "I went and told my mother and she SLAPPED me! What a surprise!"

Another woman recalls the reactions of her family members when she started menstruating: "I was 10 when I got my period. My brother smirked and said, 'Here comes the Kotex kid,' my father said (leeringly), 'Now you're a woman' (I wanted to die), and my mother said, 'Well, you'll only have it another 40 years.'"

Even when a young woman experiences stirrings of excitement and pride at this unmistakable sign of maturity, her initiation into womanhood is often so cold and unfeeling that any joy she might feel is immediately undermined by embarrassment. In *Her Blood Is Gold*, Lara Owen describes the conflicting emotions she experienced at menarche:

> My first period came in August—a month after my fourteenth birthday. I had a bath one evening and I looked down and there was a thin trickle of red on the inside of my thigh. I went downstairs. My mother was in the hall. Still on the stairs, holding the stair-rail, clutching the towel around me, feeling a hole where my stomach used to be, I said, "There's some blood on my leg." My mother said, "It must be your period. Oh dear, I used those pads myself last month when I ran out." She held out her hands in apology. "I'd kept them for so long." It was a Sunday. The shops were closed. I don't remember what happened; we must have found a pad somewhere. She was very kind but somehow I felt like a nuisance. I felt empty. Then I felt very excited. I felt special. No one said very much. I carried on bleeding. I felt empty again.
>
> When school started again I told my friend Nina. "I had my period," I said, trying to sound casual. She looked at me angrily. "I suppose you think that makes you something special," she hissed. I stepped back, shocked. Well, yes, it did, but I didn't want to upset her. The fragile little balloon that was my pride in my womanhood deflated even more. I was just having a period. It was nothing special. Who did I think I was anyway? . . . As the months went by, I felt more and more the shame and embarrassment and less and less the excitement and the pride that had glimmered for a moment with the first blood.

In our modern, sanitized society, menstruation is viewed as a bothersome and embarrassing nuisance that is best camouflaged with deodorized pads and strong douches. Tampons stem the tidal flow, pushing the blood back inside where it can be ignored, even forgotten. Young women are not taught how to celebrate the dark mysteries evoked by their menstrual blood; without the proper initiations, they come to believe that they are "cursed" rather than "blessed" with the blood. The old ways, in which women intuitively understood that the physical changes in their bodies signaled a time to retreat inward and reflect on their emotional and spiritual needs, seem archaic and antiquated. Taking time to sit still and pay attention, listening to the rhythms of the earth and exploring the varying energies of the moon, strikes the modern mind as silly and self-indulgent.

Many middle-aged women (the mothers of adolescents today) grew up with messages like this one from a 1963 insert in a Tampax box:

WHEN YOU'RE A WIFE

Don't take advantage of your husband. That's an old rule of good marriage behavior that's just as sensible now as it ever was. Of course, you'll not try to take advantage, but sometimes ways of taking advantage aren't obvious.

You wouldn't connect it with menstruation, for instance. Yet, if you neglect the simple rules that make menstruation a normal time of month, and retire for a few days each month, as though you were ill, you're taking advantage of your husband's good nature. He married a full-time wife, not a part-time one. So you should be active, peppy, and cheerful every day.

Don't take advantage. Menstruation is normal. Be active, peppy, and cheerful. Gently but firmly, women are reminded of their duty at this time of month: *Stuff it.* Stuff the blood back inside, stuff the wild, fluctuating emotions away where they won't have a negative impact on others, stuff the power and the dark mysteries and pretend that everything is normal and nothing has changed. Change itself is given a negative cast, for *every day* should be the same, day after day after day. Forcing yourself to be active, peppy, and cheerful is a *full-time* activity.

Contrast this modern interpretation of menstruation with the traditions practiced by the Yurok tribe of Northern California:

A menstruating woman should isolate herself because this is the time when she is at the height of her powers. Thus the time should not be wasted in mundane tasks and social distractions, nor should one's concentration be broken by concerns with the opposite sex. Rather, all of one's energies should be applied in concentrated meditation "to find out the purpose of your life" and toward the "accumulation" of spiritual energy. The menstrual shelter, or room, is "like the men's sweathouse," a place where you "go into yourself and make yourself stronger." . . . The blood that flows serves to "purify" the woman, preparing her for spiritual accomplishment.

During the time of their bleeding, Yurok women bathed and cleansed themselves in a sacred moon-time pond. Every month, they participated in rituals celebrating the power of their blood and the intimate connections that they shared with the earth, whose waters also ebb and flow with the phases of the moon. As their connections to the natural world strengthened with each monthly cycle, so did their pride in their womanhood.

In the Lakota tribe, a woman retreated into the Moon Lodge during the days of her bleeding. In the House of the Moon, she gathered with other menstruating women to celebrate the wild and untamed emotions that joined them to the mysteries and creative energies of the universe. Observing the moon's cycles, she came to know how the moon affected her body, mind, and spirit. Feeling the moon's cool, pulsing energy coursing through her deepest veins, pulling on her inner tides, she understood that she and the earth were sisters, for every month they shared this sacred "moon time."

In her book *Buffalo Woman Comes Singing*, Brooke Medicine Eagle offers a lyrical description of the cycles of "Grandmother Moon." By following the moon's example, women can learn how to open their souls to the great mysteries of the universe:

Let me take you around and around the cycle of Grandmother Moon, so that you may begin to know her as she lives within you. Ideally, we begin with Grandmother at her brightest and most open: the full Moon. This is a time of outward activity and high energy. If you sleep where the moonlight touches you you will often find yourself quite wide-eyed until very late on these magnificent, luminous nights. . . . Magic seems to touch everything as the silver light shimmers upon it.

Then Grandmother begins to cover her face, and gently to withdraw. This is the *waning Moon*, growing smaller and smaller in the night sky. In our Moon practice, we women as well can begin to withdraw into a quieter and quieter place, becoming less outward and social. We move toward an inward place that has more to do with "being" than "doing." As the dark of the Moon comes, we are at our most inward place. If we are in cycle with the Moon, this will be the time our menses begin—a time referred to as our "Moon time."

In the *dark of the Moon*, as we begin our bleeding, is the time when the veil between us and the Great Mystery is the thinnest. It is the most feminine, receptive time for women, and its function is exactly that: to be receptive. This Moon time then becomes a time of retreat and calling for vision. . . . When we are in this place of being most receptive, we must never limit what we can receive by focusing only upon ourselves.

Grandmother Moon has completely covered her face, and so can we. At this time, then, a traditional woman goes to a Moon Lodge, a place of quiet and beauty separate from the activity of daily life. This becomes her questing place, a place of protection and nurturing. . . . During the days of her bleeding, she has the joy of doing nothing. She is not required to cook, to clean, to take care of others, to go to a job, or any other activity. Her sole purpose is to call vision for her people: to open herself to whatever the Great Spirit wishes to send through her to serve her family, her community, her world. . . .

Coming out of this dark Moon time, she has cleansed her body, nurtured herself with quiet and beauty, and received her visions. And now, Grandmother begins to uncover her face. As the tiny slice of new Moon waxes fuller and fuller, the woman comes back out into the world, carrying her vision.

Menstrual blood is a symbol of the life/death/rebirth cycle, in which dissolution and decay are inevitably followed by renewal and regeneration. Every month when a woman bleeds, she is given the opportunity to shed her inner skin and in the process renew and revive her spirit. By letting go of the old, she is able to embrace the new. As the lining of her uterus builds up and sloughs off, she is in touch with the possibility of birth, the reality of death, and the ever-changing nature of life.

If a young woman is not guided to a deeper understanding of her monthly cycle and the power of her blood, she may learn to fear and detest this seemingly pointless and interminable cycle. Linking blood with pain and physical discomfort, she may lose a sense of the healing properties of menstrual blood. Imagining her blood as foul and offensive, she dreads its inevitable arrival. Having no knowledge of the moon's phases as they work in concert with her own, she will miss this opportunity to develop a sense of kinship with the natural world.

Healing comes through knowledge, for women can be taught how to alter the nature of their experience by changing what that experience means to them. When an adolescent learns to view her menstrual blood as purifying, the experience of menstruation can be honored as a cleansing ritual of renewal. When she perceives her blood as powerful and life giving, she will feel the pride of being a woman who bleeds. When her symptoms of pain and discomfort are reinterpreted as predictable fluctuations in the pulse of power, her monthly cycle becomes a special time to focus inward in order to direct her energies in creative, life-sustaining ways.

AMY

Amy's first period, which arrived a few months after her twelfth birthday, came and went with little notice. She showed her mother her bloody underwear, and her mother showed her where the menstrual pads were stored. "Are you okay?" Amy's mother asked, tentatively placing her hand on her daughter's shoulder. "I'm just fine," Amy answered.

But as the months went by, Amy began to refer to her period as "the plague." One period would last three days while the next would go on for five days; one period would arrive six weeks after the previous period, while the next would come just four weeks later. She never knew when to expect it or how to prepare for it, and there were times—like the day she bled through her jeans and soaked the sofa cushion—when she thought she would die of shame.

Mild cramping and intermittent spotting were part of the nuisance, but those were just minor annoyances when compared to the acne. At first, just a few blemishes dotted the landscape of her cheeks, nose, and chin, but as the months went by, the pimples started cropping up everywhere. She tried Noxzema, Clearasil, steam facials, medicated soaps, and sponges as wiry and coarse as SOS pads, but nothing worked. The pimples seemed only to spread and become more inflamed, a symbol of the irritation and annoyance of the whole menstrual cycle.

"I can't stand this anymore," Amy finally confessed to her mother. "I want to take Retin A like some of my friends."

Her mother suggested that they try a gentler approach first. "Acupuncture and herbal therapy helped me with my hormonal fluctuations," she said. "Maybe these techniques would solve your problems, too."

"I'll try anything," Amy said.

When I first met Amy, I was struck by the intensity of her pent-up energy. She stared at the floor, hands clenched in her lap, shoulders hunched, neck muscles tensed, feet nervously tap-tap-tapping the floor. Watching her, I had the feeling that something exceedingly powerful was threatening to burst forth, and from fear of exposure and ridicule, she was struggling to keep it locked inside. Her voice was so soft and unvarying in tone that I had trouble hearing her; when I asked her to speak a little louder, she agreed but refused to look at me when she talked.

Before I asked Amy to give me the details of her physical and emotional history, I shared with her my philosophy of healing, emphasizing three central and indispensable concepts: responsibility, intuition, and hope. "From the very beginning, I will give you the responsibility in the healing process," I explained. "I will work with you more as an educator than a healer in the sense that I cannot wave a magic wand and make all your problems go away. But what I can do is give you the information you need to heal yourself, and offer your body the necessary support in the healing process.

"If something I do or say feels wrong to you," I continued, "if you get a gut feeling or intuition that it doesn't make sense, then it is wrong. You know best what will work for you. I have experience and expertise, and sometimes I can see or feel something that you may not be able to detect, but I am not omnipotent. Trust your own intuition, and please tell me if I make a statement or diagnosis that does not feel right to you. Taking responsibility and trusting your intuition will help us to work together as a team."

I also emphasized to Amy, as I do in every session, no matter how young or old the patient, the words *hope* and *optimism*. So many women come to me feeling defeated and hopeless; they have "been through the wringer," as they put it. I try to reframe their experiences, using the images and metaphors of nature.

Because Wood is the element of spring (the season associated with adolescence) and because Amy appeared to have a natural affinity to Wood—her well-proportioned body, soft voice, muscle tension, and restless energy all supported this first impression—I suggested that she think about the powerful impact the season of spring has on all living things. "In winter, the trees are gray and lifeless, but with the warm days and gentle breezes of spring, the limbs stretch and branch out, colors brighten, and the buds begin to swell," I said. "The sap is rising within, and all of nature is under incredible pressure, experiencing an intense need to burst forth and express itself. A similar process is taking place inside your body, for you are also part of nature. As the sap begins to rise, your energy will feel bottled up, for it is seeking a direction to flow outward into the world. The pressure creates feelings of irritability, anger, and confusion. But these uncomfortable sensations will not last forever, for once the sap reaches its peak, the stress will be released, and the buds will flower."

I asked Amy many questions, and her answers gave me information that I assembled into a pattern of imbalances and disharmonies, which guided me to a treatment plan. In addition to taking a standard medical history, I asked if she had experienced any physical or emotional traumas in her life. Where did she hold her tension? Did she ever have trouble falling asleep or waking up in the morning? Were her dreams troubling or unsettling? When was her energy level highest and when did it feel most depleted? What were her favorite colors, seasons, climates, and tastes?

Amy tended to speak in a flat monotone; her voice had no flare or "shout," a quality of dynamic energy that signals the presence of Wood energy. When this characteristic is noticeably absent, I suspect an imbalance in Wood. Around her mouth and eyes I detected a dark, greenish hue, another clear indication of deficient Wood energy. When I inspected her tongue, the redness and swelling on the sides suggested an irritation or disturbance of energy in the Liver, the yin organ associated with Wood. Her pulses were rather fast (86 beats per minute), and they were also tight and wiry, like a metal guitar string vibrating under my finger. This bounding, surging quality confirmed that her energy was constrained, which in turn signaled that her Liver was working overtime to keep up with the tumultuous changes taking place throughout her body/mind/spirit.

At this point in the examination, I asked the most critical question of all. "What are you hoping for in treatment? What would you like to change in your life?"

"I want all of this to go away," Amy said, using her hands to make a sweeping gesture over her body. "I want to be thin again, I want all these pimples to disappear. I want to feel good. I want to be normal."

"There are many safe and effective techniques that we can use to stabilize your weight, clear up your complexion, and help you feel good about yourself," I reassured her, for she was close to tears. "If one approach doesn't work, we'll simply look in another direction."

Acupuncture treatments, herbal therapy, nutritional advice, and recommendations for lifestyle changes are the basic treatments offered by Traditional Chinese Medicine. Because every person is unique, the treatments are individually tailored to the individual's specific deficiencies and imbalances.

Amy's examination revealed an excess of Wood energy and a stagnation of energy in the Liver (the organ associated with Wood). The Chinese believe that during any time of change or transformation—either physical, emotional or spiritual—the Liver orb is stressed and thrown off balance. During adolescence, hormonal fluctuations naturally stress the Liver, and the typical American high-fat, high-protein diet intensifies the problem. Dieting, fasting, binging, or purging creates further strain on the Liver. Careful attention to nutrition and stress-reduction techniques support the body's ability to heal itself, while acupuncture and herbal treatments get the energy flowing again, invigorating and nourishing the stressed organ functions.

Amy wondered how sticking a needle into her skin could strengthen her Liver.

"Your body, according to the Chinese way of thinking, is filled with a vital energy called *chi*," I explained. "*Chi* literally gives you life, but in order to give you health and happiness, it must be balanced throughout the body, with neither too much nor too little in any one place. Stress, hormonal changes, rapid growth, and nutritional deficiencies can create an increase or decrease in *chi*, and sometimes the energy gets stuck."

"Stuck?" Amy looked perplexed.

"Imagine a clear, free-flowing stream running steadily and continuously down the side of a mountain," I said. "A violent storm arises, and a huge tree is uprooted, falling into the river to create a temporary dam. If the obstacle isn't removed, the water backs up and will eventually become stagnant. That's similar to what happens in the body when the *chi* energy gets dammed up, or stuck. We use the acupuncture needles to remove the obstacle so that the energy can flow freely again."

I explained that there are 365 major acupoints in the body, 40 to 50 of which are useful for gynecological problems. (These same points have different effects for men.) Each acupoint is located on a particular meridian or channel; fourteen major channels traverse the body, running from the tips of the fingers and toes to the top of the head. Just as the earth is covered with many rivers that flow and empty into each other, drawing from numerous underground springs, so is the human body covered with a matrix of invisible channels that circulate blood and *chi* energy. Small depressions in the skin that are called gates, can be opened or closed through the technique of acupuncture, which accesses the surface channels as well as the deeper meridians leading to the various organ systems. By sticking needles in these gates, acupuncturists can alter the body's circulation, change the rhythms of the heart, raise or lower the blood pressure, reduce sensitivity to pain, increase or decrease the secretion of body fluids and the production of red and white blood cells, and even diminish the craving for addictive substances like alcohol, cocaine, and tobacco.

"Will it hurt?" Amy asked.

"Acupuncture needles are so thin and fine that they don't actually cause pain but rather create a dull throbbing sensation or even a pleasant flow of energy," I explained. "Some people describe a sense of radiating energy along the pathway of the meridian or a sensation like an electric current, while others don't feel anything specific but report an overall feeling of relaxation and gentle stimulation."

When I showed Amy one of the delicate stainless steel needles, she seemed greatly relieved, as if she had been imagining a hypodermic needle. "Okay," she said. "I guess I'm ready."

To support Amy's Liver imbalance, relax her spirits, and dispel the heat from the blood, I selected four acupoints, three of which were bilateral. I inserted the first two needles in Spleen 6, a bilateral point located approximately three inches above the ankle bone on the lower leg. "We call this point Three Yin Meeting," I explained, "and it supports the blood and yin, or fluid energy, helping your body to adapt to hormonal changes."

Next I needled Spleen 10 (Sea of Blood), a sensitive point located about two and a half inches above the kneecap on the bulge on the inner side of the leg. When the Liver has to struggle to get its work done, stagnation often ensues; over time, this congealed energy creates a condition of heat in the blood. By stimulating the Sea of Blood, we encourage the movement of the blood, dispelling the stagnant energy.

When I felt that the first four needles were inserted correctly—acupuncturists can actually feel the energy through their fingers when the needle penetrates into the meridians and suddenly becomes charged with energy—I asked Amy if she had experienced any change in her energy. The Chinese call the sensation of energy flowing through the system *de chi*, which means "obtaining the chi." In China, the acupuncturist would ask, *"De chi le mei you?"* which means "Do you feel the energy?" If the point is correctly stimulated, the patient responds, *"De le, De le,"* meaning "I feel it, I feel it."

"I feel kind of tingly," Amy said, "all the way from my feet up to here," she said, pointing to her breastbone. I took out my book *The Essentials of Chinese Acupuncture* and showed Amy a diagram of the Liver meridian, which runs precisely along the pathway she had just described.

"That's amazing," she said.

The fifth and sixth needles were placed in Liver 3 (Great Rushing), a bilateral point located in the depression between the big toe and the second toe. "Try to picture a clear mountain stream winding down the side of the mountain, easily moving around the rocks and boulders," I said as I inserted the needles. "By stimulating this point, we make sure that the flow of energy is uninterrupted so that the blood and *chi* do not pool up and become stagnant. Some acupuncturists think of this point as a kind of Roto-Rooter, or plumber's tool, that 'unplugs' the body, mind, and spirit."

The seventh and final needle was inserted approximately three inches below the navel in the acupoint known as Conception Vessel 3, (Central Pole). "Imagine the needle sinking into a hollow pole that extends deep into the earth until it reaches a clear, cool underground spring," I said. "This is the source of your life energy, and it supports and nourishes the uterus, balancing the menstrual cycle and filling the body with yin energy."

A typical acupuncture session lasts approximately thirty minutes. Inserting the needles takes less than five minutes, and then for twenty or thirty minutes the patient rests on the table. Some patients doze while others are wide awake; some are quiet and introspective, while others are talkative and playful. Amy seemed very relaxed and full of questions, so I stayed in the room to talk.

"What do the Chinese have to say about pimples?" Amy asked.

"Acne is interpreted by the Chinese as a constrainment in the Liver, which causes heat to build up in the blood. The strategy is to relieve the heat, cool the blood, and keep the *chi* energy flowing in the Liver."

"My family doctor told my mother I got pimples because I ate too many chips and french fries," Amy said.

"The Chinese would agree with your doctor that diet is an important part of treatment for acne," I said, "but Chinese doctors are more interested in the underlying nature of the problem. Because acne is viewed as a symptom of Liver constrainment and heat rising, it's best to drink lots of water and eat cooling foods like fresh fruits and vegetables, particularly if they are raw or gently steamed. Because meat and dairy foods tend to create heat in the body, as do greasy, fried, and fatty foods, these foods should be restricted. Carbonated soft drinks, coffee, tea, and chewing gum should also be avoided because caffeine and sugar drain the yin, which is already being consumed by the excess heat in the system. For some people, the nightshade family of vegetables—tomatoes, peppers, eggplants, and potatoes—aggravate an acne condition."

"Oh, darn," Amy said with a giggle, "I guess I'll have to give up my daily eggplant."

"Don't worry," I said, laughing with her, "an eggplant every now and then won't hurt you." I always try to emphasize moderation as the key to any diet. I told Amy about a recent conference I attended where an herbalist confessed her own experience with fanatical dieting. When she became a vegan (a vegetarian who follows a completely animal-free diet), she became so obsessed with eating the right foods that she became anorexic. Her menstrual periods stopped, her hair started falling out, she felt dizzy all the time, and her weight dropped to ninety-six pounds. A fellow herbalist took one look at her and said, "Well, for heaven's sake, eat a decent meal, and you'll be fine!" From that time on, hoping to maintain a sense of balance, she deliberately ate something "bad" for her every week. Her health and weight returned to normal. Now she always tells her patients, as I do mine, to eat well, but to relax and not get too hung up on the details.

Amy wanted to know what foods she could eat that would help clear up her complexion. My first suggestion was to cut down on meats and dairy products, because they are loaded with artificial estrogens, used by commercial farmers to "beef up" the meat and increase milk and egg production. Antibiotics are also pumped into farm animals—more than half of the antibiotics sold in this country are fed to animals—and when we eat meat, poultry, or dairy products, we ingest those chemicals, too. Experts estimate that every man, woman, and child in this country ingests two to three *pounds* of chemicals every year. Because the Liver is responsible for detoxifying the different chemicals, synthetic estrogens, and environmental pollutants that we ingest with the food we eat, the liquids we drink, and the air we breathe, most of my patients (both male and female) suffer from an imbalance or deficiency in Liver function.

ACNE
(ADOLESCENT AND MENOPAUSAL)

WESTERN INTERPRETATION AND TREATMENT

Hormonal changes are affecting liver function and fat metabolism; treatment includes antibiotics, topical procedures (soaps, dermatological ointments, and peels), and/or dietary changes.

CHINESE INTERPRETATION

The Chinese offer two explanations for acne conditions: (1) Abrupt hormonal changes or overconsumption of alcohol or rich, greasy foods agitate and irritate the blood, causing "heat in the blood," which generates acne. (2) Constrained Liver *chi* invades the Stomach and Spleen, interfering with the ability to assimilate and absorb foods and fats, which are then released through the skin.

COMPLEMENTARY TREATMENTS

SUPPLEMENTS

- **Zinc** (15–30 mg/day)
- **Beta carotene** (an excellent, safe source of vitamin A; 25,000 iu/day)
- **Vitamin B$_6$** (100 mg, taken with a B-complex 100*)
- **Vitamin C** (500–1,000 mg/day)
- **Vitamin E**, alpha tocopherol (400 iu/day)

EXERCISE

Movement and exercise are considered essential to oxygenate the cells and promote lymphatic drainage. Cardiovascular exercises such as brisk walking, jogging, and bicycling will help the blood to move and eliminate toxins.

---

*The B-100 designation indicates that the product contains 100 mg each of the B vitamins. Recommended dosage is one tablet per day, or as directed.

DIET

See diet box (page 176). Choose "cooling" foods such as fruits and vegetables (raw or gently cooked). Avoid animal protein and foods that create heat in the system (greasy, oily, fried, and fatty foods); refined carbohydrates, especially sugar; and alcohol. Be aware that for some people shellfish and the nightshade family of vegetables (tomatoes, peppers, eggplants, and potatoes) can exacerbate acne.

HERBAL ALLIES

- **Yellow dock** *(Rumex crispus)*, **burdock root** *(Arctium lappa)*, and **echinacea,** blood cleansers and lymphatic drainers (Take them together in equal parts as a wonderful tonic for acne.)
- **False unicorn root** or **chasteberry** to help even out the hormonal shifts and reestablish balance

CHINESE PATENT REMEDIES

- **Margarite Acne Pills** or **Armadillo Counter Poison Pills** to take the heat out of the blood (Because these are cooling herbs, they may lead to loose stools; cut back on the amount if you develop diarrhea.)

TOPICAL TREATMENTS

Yarrow steam facial (see page 177). Wash face at least twice daily with a good hypoallergenic soap; avoid using makeup; and change your pillowcase daily.

ACUPOINTS

Spleen 6, Spleen 9, Liver 3, Large Intestine 4

MIND/BODY/SPIRIT CONNECTION

The symptoms might be expressing these questions:

- "How am I not accepting myself?"
- "What is getting under my skin?"
- "What am I afraid to look at?"

A DIET FOR ALL SEASONS

In sickness and in health and in all seasons of your life, follow these general guidelines for a healthy, balanced diet:

- *Eat with awareness.* Sit down while eating, chew your food slowly, and swallow before you take a second bite. Stop eating when you are satisfied rather than waiting until you are stuffed full.
- *Drink six to eight (8-ounce) glasses of water every day.* Water diminishes appetite, dilutes waste materials, and eases the burden on your liver and kidneys.
- *Increase whole grains, fresh vegetables, fruits, nuts, and seeds,* which provide abundant sources of vitamins, minerals, and natural fiber. Add herbs and edible plants from your garden whenever possible.
- *Restrict sugars and refined carbohydrates* (white, Italian, or French breads, white flour pastas, cakes, pastries, sugary snacks, and soft drinks). These foods lack vitamins and minerals, contain little or no fiber (thus contributing to constipation), and can play havoc with your blood sugar.
- *Choose your fats carefully.* Avoid saturated fats (from animal sources) and trans-fatty acids (chemically altered fats used in margarines and many processed foods). Monosaturated fats and polyunsaturated fats can be used in moderation. Essential fatty acids such as fish oils (omega 3) and GLA oils are beneficial supplements to your diet.
- *Avoid processed cheeses and meats* (salami, bologna, hot dogs). Read labels carefully and avoid foods with artificial ingredients.
- *Restrict meat, poultry, and dairy foods.* Buy organic or free-range meats and poultry to avoid antibiotics and artificial estrogens; use nonfat dairy products such as skim milk, nonfat yogurt, and nondairy cheeses.

We heartily recommend John Robbins's book *Diet for a New America: How Your Food Choices Affect Your Health, Happiness, and the Future of Life on Earth* (Walpole, NH: Stillpoint, 1987)—one of those rare books that can actually change your life.

In addition to cutting back on meat, poultry, and dairy products and increasing her intake of fresh fruits and vegetables, I recommended that Amy take vitamin supplements. Various studies show that vitamin A reduces sebum production in high doses, but because it is a fat soluble vitamin, toxic levels can accumulate in the body. A safer way to take this vitamin is in the form of Beta carotene, a water-soluble vitamin that the body converts into vitamin A as needed. I recommended 25,000 iu/day, a standard dosage used for skin problems. Zinc (15–30 mg/day) helps with wound healing and controls inflammation. Vitamin B$_6$ (50–100 mg/day, taken with a high-potency B-complex vitamin) balances the hormones; and vitamin C (1,000 mg/day) and vitamin E alpha tocopherol (400 iu/day) are both antioxidants that work to prevent and treat acne.

For herbal remedies, I recommended the Liver-supporting herbs dandelion root and yellow dock, which help the Liver cleanse and renew itself, and burdock, which cleanses and detoxifies the blood and lymph system. Because the toxins released by the herbs should be eliminated through the bowels rather than through the skin, I instructed Amy to drink plenty of water and take fiber in the form of psyllium powder or other natural dietary fibers available at health food stores. I also recommended echinacea and goldenseal for their antimicrobial properties, and helonias root to balance her hormones.

In Chinese thought, acne always involves stagnation of blood and *chi* energy, so regular exercise is considered essential to stimulate the circulation and provide the cells with necessary oxygen. Vigorous exercise also supports the lymphatic system in its function of eliminating toxins from the body. Daily cleansing with a good hypoallergenic soap, avoiding all commercial makeups, and changing her pillowcase every night would also help improve Amy's complexion. Herbalist Susun Weed suggests a simple yarrow facial for acne and other skin problems:

Yarrow Facial

Put a handful of yarrow flowers in a quart of boiling water,
turn off the flame, cover the pot, and let the flowers steep
for ten minutes. Take off the lid, put a towel over your head,
and allow the steam to gently cleanse the pores of your skin.

Two weeks later, when Amy arrived for her second acupuncture session, the improvement in her complexion was obvious, and she excitedly told me that she had lost three pounds ("And I'm not even dieting!"). After three months, Amy's periods became more predictable, and the spotting between periods disappeared. Our sessions continued for five months, and just after summer vacation began, Amy pronounced herself cured.

That summer, Amy's mother called me several times to report on her daughter's progress and express her frustrations with adolescent behavior. One day, toward the end of August, she called to announce her own "cure." "I've been having trouble letting go," she admitted. "For so many years I was in control, and I've had a hard time watching Amy struggle with the physical and emotional changes of adolescence. I kept jumping in and interfering with her life, hoping to make things easier for her. But Amy, of course, resented my meddling. Then a few days ago my mother sent me a poem that she found in a magazine. Suddenly I understood what this whole stage means, and why it's so important for Amy to do this on her own."

Over the phone, she read me the poem:

Struggle

A man found a cocoon of the Emperor moth
and took it home to watch it emerge. One
day a small opening appeared, and for
several hours the moth struggled but couldn't
seem to force its body past a certain point.

Deciding something was wrong, the man
took scissors and snipped the remaining bit of
cocoon. The moth emerged easily, its body
large and swollen, the wings small and
shriveled.

He expected that in a few hours the wings
would spread out in their natural beauty, but
they did not. Instead of developing into a creature
free to fly, the moth spent its life
dragging around a swollen body and
shriveled wings.

The constricting cocoon and the struggle
necessary to pass through the tiny opening
are God's way of forcing fluid from the body

into the wings. The "merciful" snip was, in
reality, cruel. Sometimes the struggle is
exactly what we need.

POWER DISTURBANCES
(Otherwise Known as "Symptoms")

In adolescence, "raging" hormones are blamed for a myriad of menstrual symptoms including acne, mood swings, depression, anxiety, visual disturbances, headaches, and food cravings. The word *raging* calls to mind hostile forces that suddenly invade, wreak havoc, and just as suddenly depart, leaving a dreadful mess behind. Many young women learn to fear their hormones, as if these internal glandular secretions were somehow not part of themselves.

When, however, menstruation is viewed in the context of female power, as the time when women are most receptive to the world of intuition and spirit, then menstrual symptoms can be understood as power surges, or ebbs and flows in the energy cycle. Rather than feeling attacked and wiped out by their hormones, women can learn how to harness their wild, undomesticated power, riding them to a deeper understanding of their body/mind/spirit.

In the ancient Goddess societies, the Great Goddess was sometimes referred to as "The Lady of the Wild Things." In one artist's depiction, the Goddess stands with arms outstretched, huge birds perched on her forearms, nuzzling her wild, unruly hair, snakes crawling up the walls, wild beasts howling at her side, wheels and circles revolving around her. "The epiphany of the goddess," writes Marija Gimbutas, "is inseparable from the noise of howling and clashing, and the whirling dances."

With these ancient images as guides, perhaps young women can learn to reframe the meaning and significance of their raging hormones. While adolescent hormones are unmistakably intense and uncomfortable, at least they aren't bland and insipid. They have no manners, they refuse to be housebroken, and when they speak, they roar.

Every month the wildness courses through the female, enriching her blood and compelling her to follow down the overgrown pathway into

the depths of the psyche. The wolf stalks, the hawk circles, the mad dog
bares its teeth. Many women try to tame these beasts and control their
fury because they don't understand their meaning or their message. But
one might as well tell the moon not to rise or the high tide to control
its surge and swell. Understand them or not, make time for them or not,
like them or not, the hormones will rage, for they are part of the blood's
power.

Open the door and invite them in. Howl with them. Use their presence
to speak of the disappointments and fears that have accumulated since
they last spent time with you. Confess your fears, let go of your anger,
surrender your control. Then, when the raging is dying down, release your
emotions on the tailwinds of their departing energy. The hormonally
regulated reminder to release your emotions every month, letting go of
the old in preparation for the new, is one of the gifts of the monthly
cycle—cherish its dependability and wild grace.

The grand orchestrator of the menstrual cycle resides in a lower part
of the brain called the hypothalamus, which regulates a multitude of
functions including the releasing of hormones responsible for regulating
menstruation, metabolism, appetite, moods, and circadian (day/night)
rhythms. An imbalance in one function necessarily has an effect on other
areas; thus, even a minor fluctuation in hormonal balance will impact
metabolism, mood, and sleep patterns, while stress or emotional upset
directly affects the production and utilization of the reproductive hormones.

When the hypothalamus signals that the time is right, the pituitary
gland produces the menstrual-regulating hormones, follicle-stimulating
hormone (FSH) and luteinising hormone (LH). When released into the
bloodstream, FSH tells the ovaries that it is time to begin the cycle by
stimulating one of the eggs to ripen while creating an encasement (the
follicle) round the egg. As the follicle grows, it stimulates the ovary to
release estrogen into the body in preparation for ovulation. Estrogen is a
powerful hormone responsible for creating an atmosphere conducive to
the fertilization of the egg, including rebuilding the lining of the uterus
(the endometrium), thinning the cervical mucus to allow sperm entry into
the cervix, and creating nutrient-rich "fertile" mucus in which healthy
sperm can survive for up to five days.

Rising levels of estrogen prompt the pituitary gland to secrete LH,
which enables the ripened follicle to burst out of the ovary, releasing the

egg into the fallopian tube in the process known as ovulation. When the egg leaves the ruptured follicle behind, the follicle is transformed into a temporary endocrine gland called the corpus luteum (yellow body), which begins to produce the hormone progesterone. As its name implies, progesterone works *pro gestation* (for gestation) by creating the ideal environment in the uterus for the implantation and nourishment of the delicate egg, in the event that fertilization occurs. A heat-producing hormone, progesterone raises the body temperature and increases the viscosity of the cervical mucus, throwing up a roadblock of thick, sticky mucus to keep the sperm trapped in the cervix while also sealing off the cervix with a dense mucus plug that prevents bacteria or sperm from entering the uterus.

If fertilization does not occur, the ovum (egg) disintegrates within the uterus, the corpus luteum breaks down, progesterone production drops precipitously, and the lining of the uterus, so rich with blood and nutrients, is shed in the process of menstruation. When the shedding process is nearing completion several days later, a signal is sent to the hypothalamus to start the entire process all over again.

All these delicate, interdependent hormonal changes create noticeable physical changes and emotional fluctuations. Estrogen is responsible for the appearance of the "secondary sex characteristics," which in adolescent girls includes the growth of pubic and body hair, development of milk ducts and fat tissue in the breasts, and extra stores of fat tissue on the hips, thighs, and buttocks. In its role as a nervous system stimulant, estrogen creates a state of increased excitation and genital arousal. Progesterone is more calming and soothing, for its purpose is to create the warm, nurturing environment essential for the implantation and nourishment of the fertilized egg.

These ebbs and flows of excitation and relaxation are repeated every month, but in adolescence, the hormonal shifts are accompanied by rapid and extreme physical changes, one of the most noticeable of which is an increase in body fat. A young woman's body weight must be composed of approximately 17 percent body fat for menstruation to occur; for ovulation to take place regularly (which usually occurs two to three years after the first period), the body-fat level must be around 22 percent. Estrogen and progesterone are stored in the body's fatty tissues; when the fat level falls below a certain threshold, the necessary stores of estrogen are also depleted, and the menstrual cycle falters or stops altogether. Because estrogen works to prevent bone loss while progesterone stimulates the formation of new bone, decreased fat levels (and the resultant decrease in reproductive hormones) may also lead to premature bone loss. When we understand the delicate relationship between body fat, estrogen levels, and bone loss and consider the fact that 80 percent of adolescent girls are on diets at any given time, we can make sense of the statistic showing that 18 percent of women between twenty-five and thirty-four have abnormally low bone density.

Excessive exercise also directly influences the menstrual cycle. Studies have shown that female athletes who don't consume enough calories to replace the energy expended in exercise have abnormally low body-fat levels, causing irregular periods or cessation of periods (amenorrhea), which in turn can lead to premature bone loss. According to one study, young women who engage in strenuous exercise to the point of becoming amenorrheic have the bone density of fifty-year-old women.

Eating disorders are a major problem in our fat-obsessed society, but adolescents are at special risk. Most prepubescent and pubescent girls worry about their weight and feel uncomfortable with their new curving body. "My body is too big for me—too old—too mature—too voluptuous. I don't fit it yet," explained one fifteen-year-old girl. The voluptuous curves are only part of the problem. Another adolescent claims that she "just wasn't ready" for the changes of puberty. "I remember when I first saw that my pubic hairs were growing. I thought, 'Oh, no, I don't want this to start happening to me yet.' Then I got breasts and it was like I suddenly started having this grown-up body, but I still felt like a kid inside."

For several years the adolescent is caught in an awkward body/mind/ spirit split, when her body is developing so fast that her emotions can't quite match the pace. Extra fat stores typically result in a chubby look, creating serious body-image problems for young women who spent their childhood inside a "boy's" body and enter puberty with the desire to look like a fashion model. (In fact, only 1 in 40,000 women meets the so-called ideal requirements of a model's size and shape.) According to Naomi Wolf, author of *The Beauty Myth*, 53 percent of thirteen-year-old girls are unhappy with their bodies; by the time they are eighteen, 78 percent are dissatisfied with their body size and shape. Problems with body image often begin before adolescence; a California study showed that 80 percent of fourth-grade girls were already dieting.

Time is sometimes an effective antidote to the adolescent's need to feel at home in her new body, but the transition would be smoother if we were able to shed our culture obsession with fat. When we look at an adolescent's flat, bony body and see the dilution of her rich, crimson blood and the progressive loss of bone mass and strength, then perhaps thin will begin to look less attractive. When we look at a well-rounded, curving, womanly body, perhaps we can learn to appreciate why nature endowed women with extra fat reserves, which are essential for creating rich, nourishing, life-creating blood.

While dieting can directly affect the strength and regularity of the menstrual cycle, it should be remembered that irregular menstrual periods are normal in adolescence. During the first twelve months after menarche, the average adolescent will have only four periods. Bleeding may be heavier in one month than another, and spotting often occurs between periods. These fluctuations are absolutely normal and will stabilize when the body becomes more experienced at regulating hormone levels.

Mild cramping—see the box "Cramping (spasmodic dysmenorrhea")" on page 184—is also common among adolescent girls, although cramps generally don't become a problem until ovulation begins, approximately two years after menarche. Sixty percent of all women experience menstrual cramping, which has been connected with high levels of the hormone prostaglandin F2 alpha (PGF2 alpha). When the endometrial lining breaks down and menstruation begins, PGF2 alpha is released into the bloodstream, causing uterine spasms and cramping pain. High stress levels and a high-fat, high-protein diet (which includes the typical adolescent intake of burgers, fries, and milkshakes) tends to increase production of PGF2 alpha; dietary changes and vitamin supplements can help decrease the intensity and duration of menstrual cramps.

While cramps are definitely not "in your head," you can use your mind to focus and disperse the pain. Many women report that when their life is balanced and relatively stress-free, they don't experience the cramping sensations. "When I become too busy or stressed out, I'll have a few hours of cramps on the first day of my period," writes Dr. Christiane Northrup. "They slow me right down and are a good reminder that I need to make some adjustments and to tune in to the wisdom of my body."

Once again, a symptom can be reframed as a temporary disturbance in the energy system, when the power is revved up a bit too high. While various herbal remedies or over-the-counter pain medications can help relieve the associated pain, cramps are a reminder to slow down, breathe deep, relax, adjust, and take time out to listen to the messages emanating from the womb—the fertile, creative, life-sustaining center of the female experience.

CRAMPING

(SPASMODIC DYSMENORRHEA)

WESTERN INTERPRETATION AND TREATMENT

Approximately 60 percent of women suffer from menstrual cramps, which have traditionally been considered psychosomatic. Recent research indicates that high levels of the hormone prostaglandin F2 alpha create uterine spasms and cramping sensations. Treatments include nonsteroidal anti-inflammatory drugs (Advil, Nuprin, Motrin, Annaprox), taken before the onset of symptoms to prevent the synthesis of prostaglandin F2. Oral contraceptives are sometimes used to prevent ovulation and reduce cramping.

CHINESE INTERPRETATION

The Chinese offer two interpretations of cramping. (1) Constrained Liver *chi* with congealed blood (especially if pain precedes menstruation). (2) "Cold in the uterus," a condition that indicates a deficiency in Spleen *chi*, allowing cold to invade the uterus. If warmth on your lower belly feels good, your symptoms probably indicate a "cold" condition.

COMPLEMENTARY TREATMENTS

SUPPLEMENTS

- **Gamma linoleic acid**, found in oil of evening primrose, borage oil, or black currant seed oil (1,000–3,000 mg/day, depending on severity of symptoms)
- **Vitamin B$_6$** (100 mg twice daily—always take with a B-complex 100 vitamin*)
- **Magnesium** (1,000–1,500 mg/day)

*The B-100 designation indicates that the product contains 100 mg each of the B vitamins. Recommended dosage is one tablet per day, or as directed.

HERBAL ALLIES

- **Motherwort,** to relax and support uterus, harmonize emotions
- **Valerian,** a nervous system tonic, tranquilizer
- **Black haw,** to relax muscles of the womb
- **Ginger,** to warm and support uterus

CHINESE PATENT REMEDIES

- **Dan Shen Tablet** (Salvia Root Tablet) for relief of "stagnant pain" (sharp, stabbing pains)
- **Wu Chi Pai Feng Wan** (Black Cock, White Phoenix Pills) for cramping and general PMS symptoms

ACUPOINTS

Conception Vessel 4, Spleen 6, Spleen 10, Liver 3. Massage the lower back and sacral area, paying special attention to the tender spots (*ashi* points).

MIND/BODY/SPIRIT CONNECTION

The symptoms might be expressing these questions:

- "How am I not allowing myself to connect with my softer, more feminine qualities?"
- "Are the cramping sensations actually birthing pains—what is asking to be born within me?"
- "How can I use the pain as a signal to nurture and take care of myself?"

MOON-TIME RITUALS
(For Women of Any Age)

The word *ritual* comes from *rtu*, Sanskrit for menses. The earliest rituals were connected to the woman's monthly bleeding. The blood from the womb that nourished the unborn child was believed to have mana, magical power. Women's periodic bleeding was a cosmic event, like the cycles of the moon and the waxing and waning of the tides. We have forgotten that women were the conduit to the sacred mystery of life and death.

—*Elinor Gadon*

Rituals transform one experience into another, investing an ordinary event with extraordinary meaning. Moon-time rituals celebrating the monthly cycle of menstruation help women of any age remember and reconnect to the power of their blood. A ritual can be as simple and routine as sitting in the moonlight every night during your bleeding, writing in a daily moon-time journal, wearing a favorite necklace or pair of earrings to pick up your spirits, or stopping for a moment on your evening walk to drink in the fragrance of a rose garden.

The difference between a routine (like brushing your teeth or going to bed at night) and a ritual is the mindfulness that you bring to the act. If you are paying attention to the meaning and the message of a particular experience and using it to learn more about yourself, then the routine aspects of life become ritual acts of celebration.

"The secret of beginning a life of deep awareness and sensitivity lies in our willingness to pay attention," write Christina Feldman and Jack Kornfield in their book *Stories of the Spirit, Stories of the Heart*. "Our growth as conscious, awake human beings is marked not so much by grand gestures and visible renunciations as by extending loving attention to the minutest particulars of our lives. Every relationship, every thought, every gesture is blessed with meaning through the wholehearted attention we bring to it."

In his book *Another Roadside Attraction*, Tom Robbins describes a woman as she stands at her kitchen sink "ripping the lettuce as gently as if she feared it might cry 'ouch.'" With such tender care and focused attention, even the methodical routine of making a salad is transformed into a meaningful ritual. The following rituals, which focus on the menstrual cycle as a time for renewal and regeneration, are intended for women of all ages. While adolescents may not feel wholly comfortable participating in some of these rituals, just knowing that women from time immemorial have created both simple and elaborate traditions to honor their menstrual cycle may provide some comfort and reassurance in this season of change.

* * *

Be still. In the days before your menstrual cycle begins, imagine your blood pooling up inside, pulling on your body with its physical weight and calling your mind and spirit to attention. Heed the messages from your body/mind/spirit, and take the time to be still. Picture a deep pond at dusk, when the light is dying and day is merging into night. Focus on being still and silent like the dark water, drawing in the cooling energy of the night air and pulling it down into the warmth at your center. Feel the water moving inside you, collecting its energies until it is ready to overflow.

Menstrual blood is the water of life. Be still and feel its energy coursing through you as a river runs along the path of least resistance to its outlet in the sea.

Look at the moon. In her predictable variability, the moon reminds us of the ever-changing nature of life and the yearning for a deeper relationship with the self. When Shakespeare's Romeo professes his love to Juliet, he swears his fidelity on the moon. "O, swear not by the moon," Juliet protests, "th' inconstant moon, that monthly changes in her circle orb. Lest that thy love prove likewise variable." The moon sets the lovers' mood, but its luminous surface pulls us inward toward solitude and reflection; in her shadows, at once sheer and substantive, we see the reflected light of our own souls.

Keep a moon journal. When you bleed, think of your blood as "moon drops"—gifts from the moon, pulling on your inner tides. Buy a journal or create your own lunar diary to record your physical, emotional, and spiritual needs as they change with the phases of the moon. When the moon is full, do you find that your energy is more outgoing and other-centered? With the new moon, do you feel a stronger pull inward, away from the mundane and the everyday and into the shadow places where mind and instinct merge and the spirit comes alive? Do you bleed with the new moon or the full moon? When your cycle shifts, how does the experience of your bleeding change?

Watch the moon, note her cycles, allow her wisdom to penetrate deep into your heart and soul.

Seek out visions. In many traditional cultures, young women were taught to view the changes in their bodies as a signal to begin the process of discovering their identity and purpose in life. Adolescents were sent into the wilderness alone and without food or clothing to undergo a ritual feat of endurance. When they returned to the tribe several days later, their dreams and visions were interpreted by the Wise Ones, and a naming ceremony was held, with much feasting and celebration.

A Shoshone adolescent ritual is described by Native American medicine man Rolling Thunder:

> When our young people are twelve or thirteen years old, they go out and pray on the high mountain at certain sacred places while an older person waits at the foot of the mountain. They go up there with no clothes, just a blanket, no food or water, for as long as three days. If they drop off to sleep, they wake up praying. Then there comes a time when they have a vision showing them what they're supposed to do. They won't know the meaning of it, most likely, so they come on down to the base of the mountain and tell the older person; then they go together to the medicine man and tell of the vision again, and the medicine man looks into it. Next they have the name ceremonies and decide what the meaning of this dream is and how it's interpreted. That person then gets a feeling and a name, and they know their purpose in life.

In our culture we have no such rituals in place, so we must create our own. When you start your bleeding, watch for the dreams and visions that will give you insights into your basic nature. Ally yourself with the natural world and seek the answers to your questions—Who am I? What is my purpose in life?—in the colors, textures, sounds, and shapes of nature. Do you feel a strong kinship with a particular animal? (Common female animal allies are bears, bees, birds, cats, cows, hares, owls, snakes, spiders, toads or frogs, and wolves.) Are you a collector of pinecones, seashells, snakeskins, rocks, or fossils? Is your spirit moved by the sight of the stately oak, the wide-spreading sycamore, or the slender, fragile birch? What images recur in your dreams? Do open spaces attract you more than caves or caverns, mountains more than valleys, lakes and streams more than oceans, cities more than rural villages? Do the shadows of the night whisper to you, or do the voices speak to you at sunrise or when the sun is at its zenith?

When you understand the deepest yearnings of your heart and soul, give yourself a name that celebrates your individual spirit and your kinship with the natural world. As the seasons pass and your purpose veers off in a different direction, do not hesitate to mark the change with a new name. Celebrate in your own private way, by taking a walk in the moonlight, climbing a tree, sitting by a stream, standing on the roof of a high-rise building to look at the stars, or whispering to a spider as she spins her web.

Discover your affinity. Are you Wood, Fire, Earth, Metal, or Water? (See chapters 6 through 11.) The energy of adolescence is primarily fueled by the power of Wood, which is defined by the need for action, movement, and personal fulfillment. While every adolescent feels this driving force, each individual will experience the energy in a unique way depending on her own nature and disposition. If your basic nature is Wood, you may find that you deal with the problems and frustrations of adolescence by becoming passive or expressing intolerance for others. If you are Fire, you may become excitable and hypersensitive in times of stress and upheaval. Earth types tend to cling, Metal becomes hypercritical, and Water retreats into a detached, somber solitude. Recognizing your constitutional tendency and affinity with a particular power, you will gain a sense of your strengths and weaknesses and a vision of how to direct your energies most creatively.

Talk to yourself. Whenever you are alone for a moment and feel the need, speak your thoughts out loud, giving voice to your fears, doubts, misgivings, and disappointments. Perhaps you feel anger or resentment at the physical and emotional upheavals you are experiencing. Vent your fury and frustration, give words to your imagination, let your feelings speak their anguish without fear of judgment or censure.

For a more elaborate ritual, you might try speaking your negative thoughts to the earth. When Lara Owen, author of *Her Blood Is Gold*, could find no conventional help for her cervical dysplasia (abnormal cervical cells, often considered in Western medicine a precursor to cancer), she asked a teacher trained in Native American healing for advice. After questioning her closely, he concluded that her problem was rooted in fear and anger, for she had expressed many conflicting feelings about being a woman. He suggested that she dig a hole in her garden, put her mouth to the hole, speak her negative thoughts, and then cover up the hole with dirt. Just as the earth transforms waste material into compost, the healer assured her, so would it take these negative thoughts and convert them into positive, life-giving energy.

"When I went home, I tried this technique," Owen recalls. "I felt pretty silly, and I was glad that no one could see into my tiny garden. I didn't know that I had so many bad feelings about being a woman lurking in my highly educated feminist mind until I did this exercise. It was painful, and it was very effective."

Give your blood back to the earth. Since ancient times, menstrual blood has been used as a fertilizer. In Native American cultures, menstruating women walked into the fields or forests, squatted on soft beds of moss, and gave their nourishing, life-giving blood back to the earth. Brooke Medicine Eagle, author of *Buffalo Woman Comes Singing*, explains how she honors this ancient tradition with her own modern-day ritual:

> Something I found more wonderful and fulfilling than I could have imagined ahead of time is to actually sit upon the ground and give Moon blood directly back to the Earth. Wearing a full skirt with nothing under it, I go out and find a quiet place on the land. Then I make a pad of soft grasses or moss, upon which to sit with my wide skirt spread out around me.

Bleeding onto the earth requires time and space, precious commodities that many modern women do not enjoy. Young women may also feel a bit self-conscious walking into their backyards, naked under a flowing skirt, to squat over plants and give their blood to the earth. A less conspicuous and less time-consuming ritual involves using reusable flannel menstrual pads, washing out the pads in a special bowl filled with clean water, and then emptying the water mixed with menstrual blood onto the earth. (If you life in a city, perhaps you could give your potted plants a monthly treat!) Lara Owen describes the significance of this step-by-step ritual in her life:

> Getting my pads out marks the beginning of my period. I keep them in a pretty bag in a closet. Soaking them and washing them emphasize for me the cleansing, clearing up aspect of my period. Giving the soaking water to my plants and to nearby trees reminds me of my connection to nature, to the earth and her cycles. And then folding them up and putting them away

when my bleeding has finished marks the end of the sacred pause in the month that is my moon-time."

For a list of cloth menstrual pad suppliers and manufacturers, see page 359.

Take a bath or swim in the moonlight. Bathing rituals celebrate the cleansing and purifying qualities of menstrual blood. Before your period, when you are feeling heavy and saturated with the weight of your blood, take a long, hot bath and imagine your uterus releasing its clenched muscles and letting out a long, contented sigh. When you wash your face at night or shower in the morning, think of your blood working in a similar way to cleanse your internal spaces, removing the old, dead cells to make room for the fresh and new. On warm, summer nights, when the moon is full, swim in a lake or mountain stream. During the cold winter months, enjoy a steam bath or sauna. Let the water purify, cleanse, and renew you, just as your menstrual blood revives your womb.

Many Native American cultures honored water as the medium in which a young girl proved that she was a woman. In Anne Cameron's book *Copper Woman*, a grandmother of an unnamed Pacific Northwest tribe describes the ritual feat of endurance young women were expected to undergo after their first blood:

> They'd take you in a special dugout, all decorated up with water-bird down, the finest feathers off the breast of the bird, and you'd have on all your best clothes and all your crests, and you'd stand up there so proud and happy. And they'd chant a special chant, and the old woman would lead them, and they'd take you a certain distance. When the chant ended the old woman would sing a special prayer, and take off all your clothes and you'd dive into the water, and the dugout would go home. And you'd be out there in the water all by yourself, and you had to swim back to the village. The people would watch for you, and they'd light fires on the beach, and when they finally saw you they'd start to sing a victory song about how a girl went for a swim and a woman came home.

Celebrate the power of your blood. Blood is synonymous with power. In the Asante tribes of Ghana, priests painted a special broom with menstrual blood to ensure that they would be safe from magical charms and spells. When women of the Kwakiutl tribe traveled, they stored menstrual blood in a piece of shredded bark to protect themselves from evil. The Imperial Romans used menstrual blood to fertilize wheat fields. Moroccans used menstrual blood in dressings for open sores and wounds. In many cultures men drank red wine mixed with menstrual blood to make themselves spiritually powerful. Egyptian pharaohs drank a fluid named *Sa*—"the blood of Isis"—to give them sacred, holy powers.

In the ancient Greek festival of Thesmophoria, women mixed their menstrual blood with the seed corn before planting.

> The women, who according to some authorities invented agriculture, did so because only they had the secret of the strong fertility of the seed corn. The reason for this was that originally the women mixed the seed corn with menstrual blood, which was the best possible fertilizer, before planting it. Since the man had no magic blood of this kind, they could not grow corn as well as the women could, any more than they could grow babies.

Celebrate your blood, as it has been celebrated for thousands of years, for now, as then, it is imbued with the power of life, the inevitability of death, and the miracle of rebirth.

MOTHER GIFTS

I love my daughter. She and I have shared my body. There is a part of her mind that is a part of mine. But when she was born, she sprang from me like a slippery fish, and has been swimming away ever since.

—Amy Tan

My mother is my mirror, and I am hers.
What do we see? Our face grown young again.

—Marge Piercy

If you are the mother (or grandmother, relative, or friend) of an adolescent, with her permission you can participate in her moon-time rituals or create rituals of your own to honor the life-giving, life-sustaining nature of the female experience. Here are just a few ideas:

Celebrate the darkness. Teach your daughter not to fear the dark but to appreciate its beauty and power, for darkness teaches us how to go inward, listening to our intuitive voice and finding the courage to follow its wisdom. Tell your daughter about insights and experiences that have come to you in the dark. Take walks with her on moonless nights. Teach her how to "see" in the dark—to look with her inner eye and trust her intuitive visions.

Offer small gifts. Remind your daughter of your affection and respect by bestowing small, inexpensive gifts. If she asks, "What is this for?" respond with a simple statement such as "I was thinking about you" or "I thought you might like this." This list of suggestions will get you thinking:

- A moon journal or lunar diary
- A photograph or graphic representation of the moon
- A poster showing the phases of the moon
- A hand-painted frame for a favorite photograph
- A small hand-crafted box to hold her favorite trinkets
- A candle for her room
- A lavender sache for her clothing drawers (The sweet, tranquil smell of lavender is said to ease the mind and soothe the spirit.)
- A snakeskin (Not every adolescent will appreciate this gift, but remember that snakes were revered by the ancient Goddess societies as symbols of immortality; their presence guaranteed, in Marija Gimbutas's words, "that nature's enigmatic cycle would be maintained and its life-giving powers not diminished.")

Tell her stories. Become a collector of stories featuring your intelligent, powerful, and resourceful female ancestors. Tell your daughter about the time you won the school spelling bee, your mother fought off a life-threatening disease, or your grandmother walked ten miles to buy a dozen eggs. Remind her that she is the descendant of strong, powerful women. At night, when she is sleepy, tell her stories about spirited women like

Mary Magdalen, Joan of Arc, Florence Nightingale, Amelia Earhart, and Anne Morrow Lindbergh. Talk about the goddesses, witches, and wise women of the past. Read stories to her from *Women Who Run with the Wolves* or *Tatterhood*, a collection of folktales featuring young, intrepid heroines. Encourage her to write and tell stories of her own.

Buy her flowers. To celebrate your daughter's first blood, give her red roses, one for each year of her life. Leave the flowers in her room so that she can discover them on her own. If she chooses to acknowledge the gift, that is fine; if she decides to keep the secret of the roses to herself, respect her need for privacy on this special day. (To celebrate the new moon, which represents the first stages of becoming, or to remind yourself of the power of your blood, give yourself the gift of a red rose.)

Give her a backrub. We learned this simple bedtime ritual from a mother of three children, whose oldest child is now twelve. Every night after her children brush their teeth and settle into bed, she asks if they would like a backrub. While her younger children enjoy the physical contact and time alone with their mother, her adolescent daughter frequently uses this time to talk about the events of her day, sharing her thoughts, concerns, and problems with her mother. "I don't ask her questions," this mother explains. "I just massage her back and listen."

An important part of this ritual is to let your child guide you: if she wants you to scratch rather than massage, or concentrate in a specific area, follow her directions. Perhaps she has a growing pain in her leg; ask her where it hurts and gently knead the affected muscles. If she wants to talk, listen carefully and respectfully. If she wants to be quiet, try not to disturb her need for silence. In these ways, you are acknowledging that it hurts to grow, that life can be stressful, that rest and relaxation are an essential part of the day, and that you are available to offer physical comfort and emotional support when she asks for your assistance.

Brew her a cup of herbal tea or hot cider. At the end of a long day, or to warm up on a cold, snowy afternoon, make your daughter a cup of tea using raspberry leaves and motherwort, both supportive, relaxing, and nourishing herbs. Raspberry, which contains rich concentrations of vitamins A, B complex, and C, numerous minerals, including phosphorus and potassium, and easily assimilated calcium and iron, tones and nourishes the reproductive organs and reduces the pain of cramping. Motherwort, a common weed, invigorates circulation, calms the nerves, relieves anxiety, strengthens the heart, improves digestion, eases cramps, and reduces water retention.

To make the brew more flavorful, add cinnamon (a blood invigorator and regulator of the menstrual cycle) and/or honey, which is used by the Chinese to dissipate frustration and was revered by the ancients as a healing food that contributes to health and longevity. Although the tea could be considered a medicine, think of it as a gift to be shared and savored.

Share your power places. Where do you feel most comfortable, most at ease, most at home, most yourself? Is there a room, a chair, a special place in your yard or garden where you feel particularly peaceful or powerful? Talk to your daughter about the distinctive energies associated with different spaces: How a grove of trees makes you feel secure and protected, or a mound in the earth reminds you of a female's rounded breast or belly. Crossroads offer a place to reflect on important life decisions, meadows celebrate openness and honesty, plateaus give us a chance to catch our breath, and cliffs show us how high we can go and how far we can fall. By sharing your power places and your sense of the different energies available in the natural world, you will help your daughter discover the meaning of different spaces and how, by temporarily limiting her vision, they expand her world.

These rituals and others that you will discover on your own attest to the sacredness of the ordinary—the pure, untouched beauty that can be discovered in the most ordinary acts of everyday living. When we move too fast and forget to pay attention, we lose a sense of the "now"; always looking to the past or the future, we neglect the opportunity to appreciate life as it is happening, right now, in this very moment. The ability to be utterly and intensely absorbed in the unfolding moment has been equated with the childlike state of awe and wonder called innocence. "Innocence is the spirit's unself-conscious state at any moment of pure devotion to any object," writes Annie Dillard.

The object itself isn't important—what matters is the spirit of devotion, which is apparent in the simple pleasure of "doing" something just for the sake of doing it. Devotion means that we do not have to find a reason why we embark on a certain task or enjoy a particular activity; we do it because, in the most basic sense, we are it. As Lao-tzu noted, "The way to do is to be."

The Zen teacher stood at the gates of the monastery, waiting for five of his students to return from a bicycle ride to the marketplace.

"Why do you ride your bicycles?" he asked when they had returned and were gathered around him.

"This sack of potatoes is heavy and cumbersome," said the first student, "and I am grateful that my bicycle was able to carry the load."

"What a smart boy you are!" marveled the teacher. "When you grow old, you will stand straight and tall rather than hunched over as I am."

"I enjoy the scenery as the wheels turn beneath me," said the second student, and the teacher praised him for keeping his eyes open to the beauty of the world.

The third student explained that the wheels, which symbolize a circle with no beginning or end, put his mind at peace, allowing him to meditate and chant as he rode serenely along.

"Your mind rolls with absolute ease, like the perfectly balanced wheel," the teacher said approvingly.

"When I ride my bicycle, I am in harmony with all earth's creatures," said the fourth student.

"The path of peace and tranquillity opens up before you," the teacher commended him.

"And you?" The teacher turned to the fifth and final student. "Tell me—why do you ride?"

"I ride my bicycle to ride my bicycle," the student answered.

The teacher kneeled down before the fifth student and said, "I am your student."

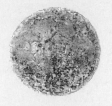

CHAPTER 14

SUMMER: FROM LOVER TO MOTHER

The Tao is called the Great Mother:
empty yet inexhaustible,
it gives birth to infinite worlds.

It is always present within you.
You can use it any way you want.
—**Tao te Ching**

American Indian women valued their role as vitalizers. Through their own bodies they could bring vital beings into the world. . . . They were mothers, and that word did not imply slaves, drudges, or drones who are required to live only for others rather than for themselves. . . . The ancient ones were empowered by their certain knowledge that the power to make life is the source of all power and that no other power can gainsay it.
—*Paula Gunn Allen*

In the gilded days of the summer of life, when the light's liquid fire spills out of solar cells and human pores, a woman discovers the depths of her passion, devotion, trust, and sacrifice. Memories of innocent childhood days fade, bleached by the hot white light of desire, which swells and bursts, only to swell and burst again, delirious with its own resurging energy. A woman in love is infused with the energy of Fire; like black asphalt absorbing and holding the heat of the sun even after night falls, she burns hot.

Although not a traditional story, the following section from William Goldman's *The Princess Bride* conveys the anguished intensity that accompanies "true love." Buttercup has just spent a sleepless night thrashing in her bed, sick with longing for the farm boy Westley. Before dawn she knocks on the door of his hut, and when he appears, she has to look away, nearly blinded with desire. Beyond fear, beyond hope, beyond any attempt at self-control, she confesses her love.

> *"I love you," Buttercup said. "I have loved you for several hours now, and every second, more. I thought an hour ago that I loved you more than any woman has ever loved a man, but a half hour after that I knew that what I felt before was nothing compared to what I felt then. But ten minutes after that, I understood that my previous love was a puddle compared to the high seas before a storm. Your eyes are like that, did you know? Well they are. How many minutes ago was I? Twenty? Had I brought my feelings up to then? It doesn't matter." Buttercup still could not look at him. The sun was rising behind her now; she could feel the heat on her back, and it gave her courage. "I love you so much more now than twenty minutes ago that there cannot be comparison. I love you so much more now than when you opened your hovel door, there cannot be comparison. There is no room in my body for anything but you. My arms love you, my ears adore you, my knees shake with blind affection. My mind begs you to ask it something so it can obey. Do you want me to follow you for the rest of your days? I will do that. Do you want me to crawl? I will crawl. I will be quiet for you or sing for you, or if you are hungry, let me bring you food, or if you have thirst and nothing will quench it but Arabian wine, I will go to Araby, even though it is across the world, and bring a bottle back for your lunch. Anything there is that I can do for you, I will do for you; anything there is that I cannot do, I will learn to do. . . . Westley, Westley, Westley, Westley, Westley,—*

darling Westley, adored Westley, sweet perfect Westley, whisper that
I have a chance to win your love." And with that, she dared the bravest
thing she'd ever done: she looked right into his eyes.

The savage, desperate nature of true love is all-consuming; it cannot
blaze so bright for long, or it will exhaust itself. As the season passes,
and Fire's flame burns down, the energy of Earth builds up, nourishing
the longing for an enduring attachment, a passionate devotion, a love that
knows no bounds. The intensity of Fire consumes; the stability of Earth
preserves. As Earth exerts its steady, calming influence, the firestorm is
contained and transformed into the controlled blaze of mature love. The
hearth fires cook up food for the body, mind, and spirit, nourishing the
creative life, kindling the desire for relationships of depth and substance,
igniting ideas, brewing up courage.

The Fire/Lover–Earth/Mother knows the value of patience and the
meaning of self-sacrifice. As her wisdom grows, she understands that even
true love dies and must be reborn again, many, many times in a single
relationship. For love, if it is genuine, is never perfect, and for all the joy
we experience within its embrace, we must also accept a measure of pain
and suffering. To truly love another person means to give your heart to
that person, and when you hand over your heart, you risk having it broken.
Brokenness, however, is the human way to wholeness. "No one is as whole
as he who has a broken heart," said Rabbi Moshe Leib.

Love that embraces brokenness calls for a fearless spirit and a willingness
to endure pain and loss. The challenge to stay with love through all its
stages is explored in an old Inuit story titled "Skeleton Woman," which
Clarissa Pinkola Estés relates in her book *Women Who Run with the Wolves*.
This is a story about a fisherman who one day brings in an unexpected
catch from the sea—the skeleton of a young woman. The fisherman labors
mightily to reel in his line, but once he discovers the exact nature of his
catch, he recoils in terror and futilely attempts to escape it. But he cannot
run away from Skeleton Woman, who is hopelessly tangled in his fishing
line. Eventually he takes pity on the heap of bones pulled from the sea,
and with great tenderness he begins to untangle them, trying to make
the skeleton whole again.

The story then tells how the fisherman falls asleep, and as he dreams
he sheds a tear. The salty tear revives Skeleton Woman, who borrows
the sleeping man's heart, using its power to put flesh on her bones.
Fully restored, she returns the heart to the fisherman's body and falls

fast asleep. When the two awake, they are in each other's arms, linked forever.

This strange but wonderful tale has much to teach us about the cycles of love, life, and death. Estés uses the story as a teaching tool to describe the "seven tasks that teach one soul to love another deeply and well." The first task, Estés writes, is the discovery of another human being as a "spiritual treasure, even though one may not at first realize what one has found." A ferocious struggle ensues as the fisherman brings in the line, unaware that he is about to come face to face with death. When the bones break through the surface of the water, he cries in terror, for this is not the trophy fish he was expecting. Worse, no matter what he does to untangle his line, Skeleton Woman will not let go.

But her tenacious spirit is precisely what is required in the first stages of love, providing the fisherman with the opportunity to prove his mettle. "This is the premier time when there is a real opportunity to show courage and to know love," Estés writes. "To love means to stay with. It means to emerge from a fantasy world into a world where sustainable love is possible, face to face, bones to bones, a love of devotion. To love means to stay when every cell says 'run!' "

Terror rules the day in the second task, when the fisherman runs for his life. But he cannot escape Skeleton Woman, who is always right on his heels. In love relationships, this is the stage when one of the lovers, having glimpsed the not-so-pretty aspects of the other, begins to fear the claustrophobic clutch of a long-term relationship. Thoughts of being trapped, consumed, and engulfed by the labor involved in loving another human being drive the fear. This temporary loss of courage signals the dawning awareness that love is more than simple pleasure and that to love truly and deeply requires hard work. "Without a task that challenges, there can be no transformation," writes Estés. "Without a task there is no real sense of satisfaction. To love pleasure takes little. To love truly takes a hero who can manage his own fear."

In the arduous process of untangling the bones, the fisherman proves that he is capable of completing the third task. With great courage and compassion, he comes face to face with what Estés calls "the not-beautiful," or as she notes in a footnote, "the not-yet beautiful." "What is the not-beautiful?" Estés asks. "Our own secret hunger to be loved is the not-beautiful. Our disuse and misuse of love is the not-beautiful. Our dereliction in loyalty and devotion is unlovely, our sense of soul-separateness is homely, our psychological warts, inadequacies, misunderstandings, and infantile fantasies are the not-beautiful."

The bones of death, the fisherman is beginning to intuit, are also the bones of life, for "when Death moves, the bones of Life begin to turn too." The fourth stage is marked by sleep and the return to innocence, when the fisherman surrenders to the mysterious longings that have been awakened in his soul. As the fisherman sleeps, he sheds a tear (the fifth task), a symbol of his desire for union and communion with another. "When the man cries the tear, he has come upon his pain," Estés writes, "and he knows it when he touches it . . . the fisherman is letting his heart break—not break down, but break open."

In the sixth task he offers his heart—"the only thing that really matters, the only thing capable of creating pure and innocent feeling"—to Skeleton Woman, who uses it to sing life into her body and flesh onto her bones. From death emerges life, and from life, love. Flesh and spirit merge in the final stage as the fisherman and Skeleton Woman share their strength and their power, transformed by love into soul mates who will be "nourished to the end of their days."

From the story of Skeleton Woman, we learn that the work of love (for love is nothing if it is not work) begins with discovery (which is not always pleasant to behold) and cycles through the stages of fear, hope, compassion, surrender, and trust to the final stages when the heart breaks open, allowing flesh and spirit to merge and become one. Sometimes— often, it seems, in the modern world—we get the stages mixed up, and love is consummated before it is created. Because we are afraid of the work involved or uncertain how to accomplish it, the cycle runs backward, the bones get even more tangled in the line, and fear and confusion reign.

If love teaches us anything, though, it is the knowledge that what dies will be reborn. If we are willing to commit the time, take the responsibility, and heal the wounds, love will return again and again and again, growing stronger and more vital with each passing stage. Estés describes the cyclical nature of love:

> Love in its fullest form is a series of deaths and rebirths. We let go of one phase, one aspect of love, and enter another. Passion dies and is brought back. Pain is chased away and surfaces another time. To love means to embrace and at the same time

to withstand many many endings, and many many beginnings—
all in the same relationship.

LAURIE

Laurie, a twenty-four-year-old graduate student, was referred for acupuncture treatments by her gynecologist, who described the significant details
of her medical history over the phone. As a child, Laurie had chronic strep
infections, which were treated with heavy doses of antibiotics; when she
was ten years old, she became seriously ill with scarlet fever and was
treated with antibiotics; and in her teenage years, she took the antibiotic
tetracycline for acne.

"I'm convinced those repeated courses of antibiotics have contributed
to a chronic condition of excessive vaginal yeast," Laurie's doctor concluded.
"The antiyeast treatments we've been using work for a short time, but
then the infections return with a vengeance."

The incidence of yeast vaginitis—the proliferation of yeast bacteria
in the vagina—has increased dramatically since the introduction of
antibiotics in the 1940s and 1950s. Antibiotics are exceedingly powerful
drugs, but they aren't particularly discriminating about which bacteria
they kill; their firepower resembles a machine-gun spray more than it
does a sharpshooter's bullet capable of singling out the bad guy. When
antibiotics are used to fight bacterial infections anywhere in the female
body, one of the good guys killed off is the vagina's Döderlein bacillus,
which is responsible for maintaining the proper vaginal pH level. As
the Döderlein bacilli die off in massive numbers, the pH level in the
vagina drops, resulting in reduced acidity—the perfect environment
for yeast to thrive. According to gynecologist Neils Lauersen, M.D.,
author of *It's Your Body*, one of every two women visiting a gynecologist's
office is suffering from vaginitis; while vaginal bacteria like chlamydia,
gardnerella, and trichomona can also rage out of control and cause
vaginitis, half of all vaginal infections are caused by excessive yeast,
particularly candida albicans.

"Do you think you could work your magic on this patient?" asked
Laurie's doctor, who knew firsthand about the "magic" of acupuncture
and herbal therapy. Three years earlier, he had suffered from the pain and
discomfort of an enlarged prostate; his doctor recommended exploratory

surgery, but his wife, a former patient of mine, suggested that he try an alternative approach before submitting to the knife. After two months of acupuncture and herbal treatments, his inflamed prostate tissue had returned to normal, and his doctor canceled surgery.

"Yeast infections respond very well to acupuncture and herbal therapy," I said. "I'd be happy to meet with your patient. By the way, how is your prostate these days?"

"Good as new," he said.

The first thing I noticed about Laurie was a deep yellow/orange hue around her eyes and temples, alerting me to an excess of Earth energy and potential problems with the Spleen and Stomach, the yin and yang organs associated with the power of Earth. Complaints of bloating and swelling, metabolic problems ("I think I must have a slow metabolism," she confided, "because I don't eat very much, and I'm always on the run, but I can't seem to lose weight"), general lack of energy, heaviness of spirit, and PMS-type symptoms of lethargy and fatigue also pointed to an imbalance in Earth energies.

Laurie's pulses were "slippery," a term that indicates a feeling of excess fluid in the body. When I put my fingers in the middle position on her right hand (the Earth pulse), I noted the thick, heavy quality of the energy, which felt somewhat like grease when it begins to congeal into lard. Earth's function is to assimilate food, fluids, and emotional nutrients and break them down into energy, blood, and waste products; when Earth's energy is out of balance, it cannot fully break down and assimilate the substances we ingest. Fluids in the body stagnate, jelling into a substance the Chinese call tan, and a quality of dampness begins to invade the body/mind/spirit. One external manifestation of that dampness is a yeast infection; other external signs of dampness include headaches, stomach rumblings or gurglings, and aching joints that become more painful in damp weather. Internally, dampness manifests itself as lethargy, foggy thinking, and a heavy feeling in the limbs—all symptoms that Laurie reported feeling.

I also noticed an irregularity to the rhythm of the pulse beat. As the Heart pumps the blood through the vessels, it establishes a steady, predictable beat; the irregular rhythm indicated that Laurie might be experiencing an excess of Fire, the energy that rules the Heart. The Liver pulses felt thin and thready to the touch, indicating that the excess Fire energy in the Heart was consuming the Liver's Wood energy. The power of Wood has two basic controlling functions: to feed Fire and to regulate Earth. When Wood is unable to keep the Earth energies in check, digestive disturbances can ensue, leading to excess dampness throughout the system. (See the chart detailing the generation and control cycles, page 95.)

Laurie's tongue was pale and a bit flabby or swollen; the tip and sides were red, and a thick white coating covered the lower aspect of the tongue, near the root. The paleness and swelling supported a diagnosis of deficient Spleen energy, while the inflamed tips and sides indicated a constrainment of Liver energy and heat in the Heart or Pericardium. The coating pointed to a damp condition in the Lower Heater, the functional organ system governing the pelvic region.

As we discussed her symptoms, Laurie appeared to be extremely anxious and was often close to tears. Her voice had a singsong, overly melodious quality, confirming a diagnosis of excess Earth energy. What surprised me was her tendency to laugh out loud when she seemed most distressed or frustrated—further evidence that her Fire energy was also out of control.

"Whenever I become involved in a new relationship, I get a yeast infection," Laurie said. "I've taken every medicine under the sun, and nothing works. Do you suppose these infections are trying to tell me something?"

"What do you think they might be trying to tell you?" I asked.

"This is silly, I know, but I find myself wondering if anyone will be able to love me, really love me, if I'm so obviously imperfect," Laurie said. "Every time I get an infection, I ask myself—will this man stay with me when my body is so obviously malfunctioning?"

"Your questions are very important, because they reveal the emotional impact of your illness," I said. "The Chinese believe that we must look at all the potential factors—physical, emotional, and spiritual—contributing to an imbalance. Because stress can contribute to the development of yeast infections, we have to look carefully at the principal stressors in your life. One of the most valuable questions to ask yourself is, How is this problem preventing me from expressing myself? What am I sitting on?"

"What aren't I sitting on?" Laurie laughed. "Anger, disappointment, grief, fear—you name it, I'm sitting on it!"

As Laurie talked about the various relationships in her life, she revealed a tendency to mother her friends and lovers, always making herself available to listen, offer advice or support, deliver a home-cooked meal or a bouquet of flowers from her garden. But when she was feeling low in energy and needed help, her friends didn't seem to have time to listen to her complaints, and she found herself fretting over numerous real or imagined insults.

In lovemaking Laurie's main objective was to satisfy her partner; she had never had an orgasm because, she surmised, she feared losing control. "I'm too intense," she explained. "I come on too strong, so I purposely hold myself back. I know that my intensity scares other people, and to tell the truth, it scares me, too. I feel so needy, so anxious to please, but I don't seem to know how to take care of my own needs."

"Do you like to be praised and win approval from others?" This is the classic question I ask when I suspect an imbalance in Earth energy.

"Yes, of course," Laurie said.

"And can you take that praise in, assimilate it, and say to yourself, 'I deserve that compliment'?"

Laurie shook her head and began to cry. "What's wrong with me?" she asked, wiping at her tears.

"Your energies are just slightly out of balance," I reassured her. "In Chinese terminology, you have an imbalance in your Earth and Fire energies. Earth's energy is receptive and nourishing, while Fire's energy is joyful and extroverted. Both of these elements, which are basic to your nature, are beginning to build up and get out of control. An imbalance in Earth energy is connected with blurred boundaries, meaning that you have problems knowing where you end and others begin, while disharmonies in the power of Fire lead to a state of hyperexcitability, which is frequently connected with problems in relationships. With acupuncture and herbal therapy, we'll attempt to balance your Earth energies and drain the excess heat from the Heart and the Liver."

Because Laurie's problems stemmed from both a Fire and Earth imbalance, with stagnant *chi* building up throughout her system and most noticeably in the Lower Heater (vagina), my treatment strategy involved needling seven different points. Spleen 6 (Three Yin Meeting), located just behind the tibia, three thumb-widths above the interior ankle bone, helps to nourish the blood, supports and balances the menstrual cycles, and reinforces the yin energy, which in turn helps to subdue excess Fire. This acupoint is also universally used to support digestion and promote the proper assimilation and distribution of food.

To bring the *chi* energy to the pelvic area, I stimulated Conception Vessel (CV) 2 (Crooked Bone) and CV3 (Central Pole). The Conception Vessel is the archetypical yin meridian and thus the original source of water and fluid energy. CV2, located just above the pubic bone on the midline of the abdomen, is traditionally used to support and nourish the uterus and other sexual organs, helping to move the *chi* and blood through the lower pelvis to resolve and disperse any obstructions. CV3, located on the midline of the belly just a thumb-width below the midpoint between the umbilicus and the top of the pubic bone, plays a vital role in sexual function, balancing the menstrual cycles and supporting Kidney functions.

To harmonize Laurie's Heart energies and calm her spirit, I needled acupoints Heart 7 (Spirit Gate) and Pericardium 6 (Inner Frontier Gate). Spirit Gate, located about half an inch in from the pinky side of the wrist crease, is perhaps the most commonly used acupoint for settling a troubled or anxious spirit; needling or pressing this point also helps to regulate and stabilize the Heart *chi* by supporting the yin (cooling) energy in the Heart. Inner Frontier Gate, located approximately two inches above the crease of the wrist on the midline of the inner arm between two tendons, has a similar calming effect but is typically used when Liver agitation is suspected. I showed Laurie how to locate the point, also known as Gate to the Heart, so that she could open and close the doors to her Heart as the situation demanded.

Stomach 36 (Walks Three Miles) is a very important point for supporting metabolism, as it nourishes the Earth functions of digestion, assimilation, and elimination. Located on the outer aspect of the lower leg, about three inches below the knee and a finger's width lateral to the tibia bone, this point reminds us to slow down, digest, and receive. A delightful story explains the origin of the name Walks Three Miles. In the old days, monks traversed the continent by foot, walking many miles each day to visit various monasteries. When they reached the point of exhaustion and felt they could go no further, they would needle or press this acupoint and experience a resurgence of energy that would allow them to continue for several more miles.

The archetypical point for excessive dampness and problems of conges-tion throughout the body is Stomach 40 (Abundant Splendor or Bountiful Bulge). "This point," I said as I inserted the needle in the side of the calf muscle halfway between the lateral ankle bone and lower knee, "clears away the dampness in your system. Imagine that a thick fog bank is enveloping you when a sudden, brisk wind disperses the fog, allowing the sun to shine through for the first time in weeks. To help this point do its work, you might ask yourself if there is anything preventing you from allowing the warmth of the sun to penetrate deep into your life."

"It must be fear," Laurie said after reflecting for a moment. "It seems that every time I open myself up, I get hurt. It's easier to have this cushion around me, because then I don't feel so much pain. But if the fear acts as a kind of fog that prevents me from seeing clearly, then it doesn't protect me, does it?"

"Not if it prevents you from being yourself," I agreed.

After that first acupuncture session, Laurie and I talked at length about exercise, diet, and stress management. Although she jogged every other day and appeared to be in good physical shape, her back and neck muscles were knotted and thick with tension. I recommended yoga stretching exercises, daily breathing techniques, and hot baths before she went to bed to help relieve the muscle tension.

Laurie's diet was far from ideal, for like many graduate students, she studied late at night, drinking cup after cup of coffee to stay awake and frequently snacking on candy bars and donuts. Sweets gave her the feeling that she was being nourished and the stimulating effects of caffeine provided her with an energy rush, temporarily lifting the weight of fog and lethargy. But soon after the rush, the physical lethargy and emotional apathy returned. I recommended that Laurie eliminate sugar and refined carbohydrates from her diet and avoid dairy products, especially milk and ice cream, because of the high lactose (milk sugar) content, which stimulates yeast growth in the vagina and bowel. Raw foods were temporarily off limits because they are difficult to digest and they stress the Spleen; therefore, I recommended that she gently steam or stir fry her vegetables as the Chinese do. ("Have you ever tried to get a fresh green salad at a Chinese restaurant?" I asked, and she laughed.) Warming spices like ginger and garlic would help mobilize the Earth energies and dissipate excess dampness.

For supplements, I suggested vitamin B_6 (50–100 mg/day), which tends to calm the spirit, nourish the Heart, regulate the hormones, and balance the fluid levels in the body (as with any recommended B vitamin, B_6 should be combined with a well-balanced B-complex vitamin). Acidophilus bifidus capsules would help rebalance and recolonize the healthy intestinal flora, which had been systematically destroyed by the regular use of antibiotics.

For herbs, I suggested those with a bitter taste on the tongue, for bitterness promotes the production of bile, helps the Liver detoxify and eliminate unhealthy substances, and improves appetite and digestion. The main ingredient in Laurie's formula was the mildly bitter herb dandelion root, which cools down the Fire energy and supports the Liver. To warm up Laurie's internal organs, I relied on ginger, which nourishes the entire pelvis, eases menstrual cramps, and relieves indigestion and gas pains; hawthorn berries, which work to support the Heart both physically and spiritually; lady's mantle, a natural astringent that would help dry up the vaginal discharge; and echinacea, an antimicrobial, antifungal herb that supports the immune system.

I also recommended that Laurie douche three to four times a week with a special decoction (an herbal brew in which the plant substance, including the roots and bark, is boiled for ten minutes or more) consisting of echinacea (the purple coneflower) and calendula (marigolds). The recipe: Boil the echinacea root in water for ten minutes, turn down the heat, add the calendula, and let simmer for thirty minutes. Add a few drops of tincture of myrrh (or tea tree oil if myrrh is not available). A tampon can be saturated in the tea and then inserted in the vagina for no more than an hour or two. Many women follow this ritual with a yogurt douche to replenish the vaginal membranes. (Regular douching can disrupt the normal pH levels of the vaginal membranes, but when the body needs help cleansing or ridding itself of bacteria, a medicinal douche like this one can be extremely helpful.)

Laurie's yeast infections responded immediately to these treatments, and within a month, her vaginal yeast flora was back to normal. For nearly a year, she had no recurrence of symptoms; when she became involved in a new relationship, the yeast cropped up again, but with careful attention to diet and supplements, we quickly brought it under control. Laurie continued with seasonal acupuncture sessions ("It's like having an oil change every three thousand miles," she said with a laugh), and in a recent session, she talked about the new man in her life.

"He listens to me, he really seems to care about my needs," she said. "Oddly enough, although he likes my intensity, I don't feel so intense anymore. It's as if I was always chasing after these relationships, hoping to make them work, and suddenly I got tired and decided to sit down and wait for something to catch up with me. I feel patient. I don't want to rush through this relationship, to push things faster than they should go."

Lying on the table with her eyes closed, acupuncture needles in her calves, wrists, and abdomen, Laurie was silent for a few moments. "You know, when I came to you, I had almost given up hope," she said finally. "My family doctor referred me to a gynecologist, who did what he could for me and then passed me along to you. Even though both my doctors were kind and understanding, I felt as if I had run out of options, and you were the last straw. I know my condition isn't life threatening, but I felt as if I was a lost cause."

She started to cry. "I'm fine, just a little emotional," she assured me when I asked if she was all right. "Lying here with these little needles poking in me, I can feel the energy flowing through me, cleaning out the passageways of my body. Sometimes in these sessions, I feel as if the needles penetrate my soul."

"I think that's exactly what they do," I said. "I like to think of the needles as little pinpricks that open up a space for the light to shine through. But in order for the light to penetrate, you have to be awake and aware. Remember, you didn't ignore your symptoms—you listened to them, and when help was offered, you took it. Some people, from fear or pride, or hoping that a better or easier answer will come along, never reach out for help."

I told Laurie one of my favorite stories (some might call it a joke) about the priest and the flood.

The forecasters were predicting a severe storm, with torrential downpours and very high winds. City officials advised that everyone in the area be evacuated until the storm had passed. When the news reached the priest, he declared that his faith in God was strong; he would ride out the storm in his church, for God would save him.

The storm came as predicted, and its force was even more severe than anticipated. When the waters flooded the streets, a group of emergency workers offered to help the priest to safety. "My trust in the Lord is complete! He will save me," said the priest, refusing their help.

When the waters covered the entrance to the church, more rescuers appeared, pleading with the priest to come with them or he would surely drown. "God will protect me, my faith will save me!" cried the priest.

In no time at all, the church was flooded, and the priest was forced up into the steeple. A helicopter hovered overhead, and someone shouted through a megaphone at the priest: "Father, grab the rope and save yourself!"

"God will save me!" the priest called back.

CHRONIC YEAST INFECTIONS

WESTERN INTERPRETATION AND TREATMENT

Yeast live normally (and happily) in the vagina, but infections, emotional or physical stress, and use of antibiotics can deplete friendly bacteria that control the yeast, creating an imbalance of pH levels and contributing to chronic yeast infections. Diagnosis is confirmed microscopically in the laboratory. Yeast infections are treated topically with prescription or over-the-counter antiyeast medications; in extreme cases, stronger prescription drugs are used.

CHINESE INTERPRETATION

The Chinese view yeast infections as either chronic or acute, and either hot or cold: (1) Hot/acute is sudden onset, with more dramatic, acute symptoms, such as intense itching, burning, and thick yellow discharge. (2) Cold/acute is sudden onset with intense itching but less burning and a profuse white discharge. Over time, these acute symptoms can become more chronic and insidious, leading to (3) Hot/chronic, which is similar to the hot/acute condition but with less-dramatic symptoms, or (4) Cold/chronic, which is similar to cold/acute but with less-dramatic symptoms. With both chronic conditions, deficiency symptoms such as lethargy, fatigue, and sluggishness often occur.

COMPLEMENTARY TREATMENTS

SUPPLEMENTS

- The friendly bacteria **Acidophilus**, which helps to reinstate a healthy bacterial environment in the digestive system, is available in two common forms: *Lactobacillus acidophilus* and *Lactobacillus bifidus*. I have a slight preference for the *bifidus* variety, which works quickly and efficiently to stem the proliferation of yeast. Tablets or liquids are usually taken with each meal; follow directions on the product label.

- **Yeast-free multivitamin and mineral tablets** (ask your health food store for recommendations or consult the list of recommended nutritional supplements in Appendix 3).

Dosages for these and other recommended supplements may vary according to the product; when amounts aren't clearly specified, ask a professional for advice.

TOPICAL STRATEGIES

- Avoid pantyhose, tight clothing, and tampons.
- Try a yogurt vaginal rinse to help rebalance the vaginal pH levels. Use plain yogurt (no sugar or flavorings). Place in the vagina with a vaginal (spermacide) applicator; repeat every other day until symptoms abate. To absorb the leakage, use a sanitary napkin or a tampon. Combine the rinse with *one* of the following methods:
  1. Australian tea tree oil vaginal rinse (Mix the oil with water according to instructions on package; dip a tampon into the mixture and insert vaginally; remove after one hour.)
  2. Garlic suppository (Wrap a peeled clove in gauze, insert vaginally, and leave overnight.)
  3. Boric acid suppository (Insert vaginally. Capsules are available in health food stores, or ask your pharmacy to make this for you, using 600 mg boric acid powder in "0" gelatin capsules.)

DIET

Avoid yeasty or moldy foods such as cheese, dried fruits, peanuts, alcohol, milk and dairy products (except for nonfat yogurt). Avoid whenever possible antibiotics, birth-control pills, and steroids.

HERBAL ALLIES

Each of the following herbs can be beneficial. Combined in equal parts, they make a wonderfully effective tonic:

- **Echinacea**, an excellent immune tonic with antimicrobial actions
- **Lady's mantle**, an astringent and uterine toner
- **Pau d'arco** (*Tabecuia Impetiginosa*), a South American herb with strong antifungal properties

CHINESE PATENT REMEDIES

- **Chien Chin Chih Tai Wan** (Thousand Pieces of Gold, Stop Leukorrhea Pills) for cold (acute or chronic) conditions with white discharges (support the kidneys and dry out discharges)
- **Lung Dan Xie Gan Wan** (Gentiana Purge Liver Pills) for hot (acute or chronic) conditions with itchy discharges that have a burning quality
- **Yudai Wan** (Vaginal Discharge Curing Pills) for acute/hot conditions with hot, yellow, smelly discharges (not to be used with cases of deficiency)

ACUPOINTS

Spleen 6, Spleen 9, Kidney 3, Kidney 7, Conception Vessel 4

MIND/BODY/SPIRIT CONNECTION

The symptoms might be expressing these questions:

- "How is this symptom preventing me from expressing myself, sexually or otherwise?"
- "How do I feel conflicted about my sexuality?"
- "How am I bogged down with repetitive or excessive thoughts?"
- "What am I worried about?"

Moments later the church was engulfed by the flood, and the priest drowned. When he arrived in heaven, he was met by St. Peter, who was astonished to see him. "Why, Father, you're not due here for another twenty years!" said St. Peter.

"I trusted in God," the priest said, shaking his head sadly, "but it was a terrible flood and even God couldn't save me."

"That doesn't sound quite right," said St. Peter. "Let me go speak to God and find out what happened."

St. Peter returned a few moments later, a distressed look on his wise old face. "I'm sorry, Father," he said, putting his hand on the priest's shoulder, "but God said he came three times to help you, and you refused him each time."

"I didn't refuse help, did I?" Laurie asked with a smile. "I could still be standing up on that roof waiting for help, but I chose to come back to earth."

"You are Earth," I reminded her.

"Earth *and* Fire." She laughed. "Remember—I may be grounded, but I'm full of spark and flare."

"You are indeed," I said.

As love matures, questions of life and death arise as naturally as vapor lifting up from a lake at nightfall. At first, these questions concern the health and longevity of the relationship itself: Will it last? What must I let go, and what must I keep? What needs to die within me in order to give birth to love? For many women, these questions eventually focus on the desire to have a child. The decision to create a new life requires profound courage and trust, for this is uncharted territory, and although much can go right, much can also go wrong. Stripped of her defenses and forced to wander unarmed and unprotected, a woman embarking on this pathway must learn to trust that love itself will take her where she needs to go, that if she loves deeply enough, miracles can happen.

But even miracles (especially those that are human made) require hard work and careful planning. One in every six to ten couples experiences problems with fertility, and many women seek out the advice and support of complementary medical treatments such as acupuncture, herbal and nutritional therapies, body work, and psychotherapy. If no clear structural factors prevent conception, approximately 50 percent of these clients will conceive and carry a fetus to term when treated by a qualified acupuncturist and herbalist. When a woman is taking fertility drugs such as Clomid or Pergonal, acupuncture and herbal and nutritional therapies will increase the likelihood of conception. If miscarriage has been a problem in the past, numerous alternative treatment options can reduce the risk.

"When a father's sperm and the mother's blood contact each other, they unite and congeal to become the fetus in the womb," wrote Chang Huang in the sixteenth century. The entire diagnosis and treatment of infertility in Traditional Chinese Medicine is an extension of this basic tenet, for anything that might block, obstruct, or weaken the blood (or in males, the sperm) is considered a potential cause of infertility— even if the blockage occurs in such seemingly unrelated organs as the

Heart, the Kidneys, or the Liver. Whenever I see a patient who is having difficulty conceiving or who has a history of miscarriage, I consider the mind/body connection and ask myself these questions: How has the natural rhythm of ovulation and conception been disrupted? What parts of the mind/body/spirit need to be nourished before conception can take place? Are there relationship conflicts that need to be addressed? Where is the energy blocked?

ANNA

Anna, thirty-two years old, and her husband, John, finally conceived after nearly two years of faithful effort; but ten weeks into her pregnancy, the fetus spontaneously aborted. Deeply depressed by the miscarriage and fearing that she was running out of time, Anna agreed to try a fertility drug. Six months later she was pregnant, but once again, just eight weeks into her pregnancy, she miscarried.

Afraid to take more drugs and desperate for an answer to her questions about her ability to carry a child to term, she decided to try acupuncture treatments. "Let's just give it five or six months," she begged her husband, who was skeptical about the alternative therapy. "If I don't get pregnant, we'll take the gynecologist's advice and go back on fertility drugs."

When I first spotted Anna in the waiting room of my office, her body was slumped over in the chair, her head buried in a book. I approached her to introduce myself, but she was so shut off from the world around her that I had to speak before she noticed my presence. Stammering hello, she gathered up her belongings and followed me into my office.

"I don't feel very hopeful," she began, and indeed she seemed apathetic and lifeless, as if her energy was slowly draining out. Her voice was totally without animation, and I detected a distinct moaning quality, a clear indication that her Water energy was calling out for attention. Her complexion was pale, and she had a bluish hue around the temples and dark circles underneath her eyes. I suspected a Kidney (Water) imbalance, and the medical history and physical examination confirmed my preliminary diagnosis. As a child, Anna suffered from numerous urinary tract infections, and from infancy to age four or five, she had persistent ear infections. "Even today whenever I get a cold or the flu, I inevitably get an earache. I just seem to lose my equilibrium and balance," she explained.

In Chinese theory, urinary tract infections are caused by a deficiency of Kidney energy, which allows heat and humidity to invade the Lower Heater, where the Bladder is located. Anna's earaches also suggested a Kidney imbalance, for the ear is the sense organ governed by the Water element, and symptoms involving pain, vertigo, dizziness, loss of equilibrium, and problems with hearing are linked to the Kidneys.

I asked Anna about her sleeping patterns. Sleep is directly affected by energy imbalances, and problems with sleeping—difficulty falling asleep, restlessness during the night, a tendency to startle and wake up suddenly, nightmares, or grogginess in the morning—provide important clues about the nature of the underlying imbalance. Although Anna slept well at night and enjoyed regular naps during the day, she said she never really felt rested. Every day around 4:00 or 5:00 P.M., she would begin to get sleepy and irritable; her energy was typically depleted until about 8:00 P.M., when she began to feel more active and energetic.

When I asked about her sleeping habits, Anna described a recent dream that deeply disturbed her. She and her husband were on vacation, taking a cruise around the Caribbean, and she was trying to find her way back to their room. Following the narrow corridors, she descended deeper and deeper into the bowels of the ship and, with all the twists and turns, became lost. Overwhelmed with feelings of terror, she approached a corridor with two doors, one of which looked familiar. Opening the door, she walked into a room where a baby, who appeared to be abandoned, was lying on the floor crying. Panicked, Anna cried out for her husband, but he was far away and couldn't hear her. When she woke up, she was sweating and her heart was racing.

Anna gave me a beseeching look. "Do you have any idea what it means?" she asked.

Dreams are taken very seriously in Traditional Chinese Medicine, and the symbols are interpreted as indications of imbalance (excesses or deficiencies) in the Five Transforming Powers of Wood, Fire, Earth, Metal, and Water. Anna's dream included symbols of Water (the ocean and the corridors or channels deep within the ship) and Metal (the ship itself and, because grief is the emotion associated with Metal, the tears she cried when she found the baby). Because the interpretation of a dream must always involve the dreamer's analysis of the relative importance and personal meaning of its symbols, I asked Anna if there were any images in the dream that particularly affected her.

"The tears seem important," she said. "I feel as if I spent half my childhood crying for attention, but my mother never listened to me, never really heard me—she always told me to grow up and stop acting like a child." As Anna continued to explore her feelings about her dream, she began to focus on the crying baby. "Why didn't I pick up the baby and comfort it?" she asked. "Why did I feel so afraid when I saw the baby that I cried out for my husband?"

"Do you know why?" I asked, gently tossing the question back at her.

Anna was silent for a moment. "Maybe I'm afraid I won't be able to be there for my child, the way my mother wasn't there for me," she said, a troubled look on her face. "But in the dream, my husband wasn't available, either. Before I miscarried, I was worried about my husband's work schedule and wondered if he would be able to spend enough time with me and the baby. He works in the city and has to commute an hour each way. I'm just afraid he won't have time for a child."

I told Anna a story about Joleen, another patient with fertility problems who had a dream about swimming in the ocean with a porpoise. As they swam and played together, they became fast friends, and at one point, the porpoise turned to her and asked, "How can I help you? What do you need to know?" In the dream, Joleen started to cry and explained that she couldn't get pregnant even though she desperately wanted children.

"If you were able to have a child," the porpoise asked her, "what would you like to give it?"

"I would give my child unconditional love, self-confidence, and the freedom to express his or her feelings without shame or guilt," Joleen answered.

"As soon as you are able to give these gifts to yourself, you will be ready to conceive a child," the porpoise said.

"Did Joleen ever get pregnant?" Anna asked.

"Not yet," I said, "but she is filled with hope and working hard to give herself the gifts she mentioned in the dream."

"Do you think I can get pregnant and carry a child to term?" Anna asked.

"Based on your medical tests and your previous pregnancies, I have no doubt that you can conceive," I said, "but to help your body nourish a growing fetus, we need to treat the imbalance in your Water energy. Water is the element of the Kidney, and when a woman conceives, she gives a gift of *jing*, or Kidney essence, to her baby. This gift is taken from her own supply of Kidney energy, and so to conceive and carry a child to term, a woman needs an abundance of *jing* energy. Acupuncture treatments, herbal remedies, and good nutrition can all contribute to this vital, essential energy."

I briefly explained the Chinese theory of the Five Transforming Powers and then discussed Anna's specific energy imbalances. The pulses, tongue examination, and medical history revealed a deficiency of Kidney energy and stagnation of blood and *chi* energy in the uterus. Using acupuncture and herbal treatments, we would support and replenish the Kidneys and promote the movement of energy and blood through the Lower Heater, paying specific attention to the Liver's role in promoting the free and easy flow of energy, blood, and emotions.

On the examining table, I gently palpated Anna's abdomen, searching for any particularly sensitive spots that might indicate blockage or obstruction in a specific meridian. Then I checked her muscles, limbs, joints, and vertebrae for firmness and signs of tension.

I also assessed the energy in the Three Chou, or the Triple Heater, to get a sense of her body's temperature-regulating ability. The Triple Heater should have a relatively consistent temperature, with the upper body as warm or cool to the touch as the lower body. If one area is significantly cooler or warmer than another, this difference in temperature indicates an imbalance of energy that requires attention. Because Anna's lower belly felt cold to the touch, I decided to warm her uterus with a technique called moxabustion, or simply, moxa. Moxa involves burning the herb mugwort *(Artemisia vulgaris)* over the part of the body that needs to be warmed, in this case the acupoints CV3 (Central Pole) and CV4 (Gate at the Source), located on the midline of the abdomen just an inch apart. While both points relate to Kidney function, CV3 is more concerned with strengthening the yin, while CV4 sustains the *chi*.

When an acupuncturist decides which points to needle, he or she follows the Law of Least Action. If I tried to treat every one of Anna's presenting symptoms, I would have to use several dozen needles and acupoints, thus confusing the messages and diffusing the energy available to the body/mind/spirit. The art of acupuncture is to select those specific points that give a clear message to the individual and her unique problem, using the points as a kind of poetry in which a few carefully selected needles, like a few well-chosen words, express the inexpressible.

The acupoints I selected for Anna were Kidney 3 (Great Stream), a powerful point that nourishes and replenishes Kidney energy; Kidney 10 (Yin Valley, or the Master Point), the Water point on the Water channel of the Kidney meridian, which strongly supports the yin qualities of the Kidney; and Spleen 10 (Sea of Blood), which sweeps aside the debris and clutter in the pelvic basin, building the blood and ensuring an even and smooth flow of energy. To direct the energy to the pelvis, support the yin and *chi* of the Kidneys, and directly nourish the uterus, I needled acupoints CV3 (Central Pole) and CV4 (Gate at the Source).

When I needled the final bilateral points *Zi Gong* (Baby Palace), located approximately three inches above the pubic bone and three inches to either side of the midline of the belly, I asked Anna to imagine the cool, fresh waters of a mountain stream flowing steadily toward the ocean. "You are part of this stream, caught up in its flow," I said, "and as you move with the water, bending and flowing around the rocks and other obstacles confronting you, you are filled up with vital energy. When you feel that you are about to overflow, direct your energy to your womb, filling it with light and power."

After I removed the needles, we discussed a natural fertility awareness technique known as "conscious fertility," which would help Anna to pinpoint her most fertile time. This method relies on three critical signs of fertility: mucous changes, alterations in the cervix itself, and basal body temperature changes. The cervical and mucous changes are caused by increased estrogen production; approximately six days prior to ovulation, rising levels of estrogen create E-type mucus. This "fertile" mucus contains microscopic channels that allow the sperm to swim up through the cervix and stay healthy and viable in the woman's reproduction system for up to five days. Fertile mucus is wet and slippery, somewhat like raw egg white, and can be stretched between two fingers; many women notice this wetter mucus as a thin discharge on their underwear in midcycle.

Rising estrogen levels also cause the cervix to soften up and move farther away from the vaginal opening (tucking up closer to the uterus), and the os, or cervical opening, begins to enlarge. All these changes favor conception. After ovulation, when estrogen levels are decreasing and progesterone levels are increasing, the cervical mucus gradually dries out, becoming pasty, sticky, and crumbly. (In remembering their fertile and infertile periods, many women find it helpful to imagine sperm as rain-forest creatures who dislike dry, desertlike conditions and prefer wet climates with many rivers to swim in.) This dense, thick, "infertile" G-type mucus destroys sperm and blocks entry to the uterus. Rising progesterone levels also cause the cervix to drop deeper into the vaginal canal, the os closes up, and the cervix feels firmer to the touch (more like the tip of your nose than the softness of your lips).

The third fertility sign is a rising basal body temperature (BBT). Shortly before, during, or after ovulation, the BBT rises between 0.3 and 1.0 degree Fahrenheit, signaling the increased production of progesterone, a heat-producing hormone. Since progesterone is released immediately after ovulation by the corpus luteum, rising BBTs indicate that the ideal time for fertilization of the egg has arrived. (Subtle changes in BBT can be easily detected with a basal thermometer, available in most drugstores or pharmacies.)

Dr. Serafina Corsello suggests a unique method for taking the BBT. As soon as you wake up in the morning, urinate in a styrofoam cup ("the only good use of a styrofoam cup," says Dr. Corsello), place the BBT thermometer in the cup for five minutes, and then record the temperature. Be sure, however, to use this or any other temperature-taking method (oral, rectal, or vaginal) consistently, as variations in temperature will occur depending on which method is used.

"By periodically testing your cervical mucus to determine its consistency and texture, feeling the position and firmness of the cervix, and carefully recording your basal body temperature changes, you will know when you are most fertile and therefore most likely to conceive," I told Anna. When she left my office, I gave her a basal thermometer, a fertility awareness chart, and a copy of *The Fertility Awareness Handbook*, which clearly describes the techniques of conscious fertility. (This technique is also 98 percent effective as a contraceptive method; the only potential drawback for both contraception and conception is the need for active participation and continuous monitoring.)

For supplements, I recommended a natural, high-potency multi-vitamin and-mineral with iron and 400 mg/day of folic acid. A component of the vitamin B complex, folic acid aids in the growth and reproduction of blood cells and provides essential support to a developing fetus; studies have shown that a folic acid deficiency increases the risk of birth defects. A healthy diet rich in green vegetables and high-quality fats such as olive, canola, and flaxseed oils was essential.

For herbal allies I suggested the following: helonias root (false unicorn root) to promote fertility; black cohosh to nourish the uterus; black haw to relax and support the uterus; verbena (or vervain) and St. John's wort to calm and restore the nerves, support the yin, and dispel anxiety and irritability; the Chinese herb *Dong Quai* (also spelled *Dong Kwai*, *Dong Gway*, *Dang Gui*, *Tang Gwei*, or *Tang Kuei*), a superior herb for numerous reproductive and hormonal problems; and garden sage (*Salvia officinalis*) to keep the blood flowing freely, relieve stagnation, and regulate hormonal changes to increase fertility.

Anna returned for ten more acupuncture sessions; five months after her first session, she called to tell me that she was pregnant. After we whooped and hollered over the phone, I suggested that she drink a daily infusion of red raspberry leaves and nettles (see recipe below), a lovely, uterus-nourishing pregnancy tonic; increase her folic acid to 800 mg/day; continue with the multi-vitamin and -mineral supplement; and take 400 iu/day of vitamin E alpha tocopherol. Although herbs and acupuncture can be very helpful in pregnancy, fear of lawsuits and litigation lead most acupuncturists and herbalists to abstain from using these methods when treating pregnant women. I continued to advise Anna during her pregnancy, but we decided to wait until after she delivered before continuing with acupuncture and herbs.

Pregnancy Tonic

Red raspberry leaves
Nettles

Buy or pick the fresh herbs, put an equal amount of each herb in hot water (not boiling), and let them steep for a few hours.

Herbalist Susun Weed suggests putting half an ounce of each herb in a quart thermos filled with hot water at bedtime; the concoction will be ready to drink in the morning and throughout the day.

In her third month, Anna complained of morning sickness, and I suggested that she try a small amount of ginger, either by preparing a weak tea with a teaspoon of the powdered root mixed with a cup of boiling water (taking little sips until the symptoms dissipate), or putting a drop of ginger tincture (available in health food stores) on her tongue whenever she felt nauseous. (Ginger, like many other dietary spices, can overstimulate the womb if used in large amounts, although small doses are completely safe.) The Chinese often recommend that pregnant women chew dried tangerine peel as an antidote for morning sickness. Pressing acupoint Pericardium 6 (Inner Gate), located two inches above the crease of the wrist, is also surprisingly effective for relieving nausea. (A recent study demonstrates that this acupoint is effective for preventing postsurgery nausea.)

Toward the end of Anna's pregnancy, we spent several hours discussing breathing techniques to prepare her for labor and delivery; after the session, she asked if I would like to be present at the birth. "I wouldn't miss it for the world," I said. Anna called me five days after her due date, and I met her at the hospital, where she labored in a birthing center, attended by a midwife. During her labor, she sipped raspberry leaf tea, and when her contractions intensified, I added black cohosh, which works to relax the uterine muscles and simultaneously intensify the contractions.

Ten hours after her labor began, Anna delivered a beautiful, healthy, eight-pound baby boy. To aid the uterus in expelling the placenta, Anna drank a mixture of black and blue cohosh, Native American gynecological herbs that have been used for centuries to support the uterus and help the muscles contract more efficiently.

I continue to see Anna four times a year, once every season, for acupuncture sessions and herbal therapy. In her last session, she brought her eighteen-month-old baby with her, and while she lay on the table with needles poking out of her abdomen, arms, and legs, he played happily on the floor with his toys. Listening to her child squealing with delight at a red, blue, and yellow clown that jumped up and down on a spring, Anna smiled from ear to ear.

"I just feel so full of life, so full of love," she said. "My marriage is so much stronger now, even though we have less time together. John cut back on his work hours to spend more time with me and the baby. He's happier than I've ever seen him, and we both feel so much more flexible and adaptable. Tell me—in Chinese theory, what accounts for this infusion of energy in our lives when it would seem that we should have less energy?"

I remembered when I first saw Anna, her head buried in her book, her expression forlorn, her voice sad and hopeless. Looking at her face now, so radiant with love and happiness, I was struck by the remarkable changes in her life.

DIFFICULTY CONCEIVING

WESTERN INTERPRETATION AND TREATMENT

Most physicians accept the general formula that 40 percent of all infertility problems are related to deficiency in the number or quality of sperm; 40 percent can be traced to anovulation (lack of ovulation) or structural blockages; and for 20 percent, no obvious reason can be found. Structural causes of infertility include tubal blockage, endometriosis, and scarring from recurrent pelvic inflammatory disease (PID). Functional causes include irregular ovulation due to pituitary, adrenal, or thyroid imbalances and ovarian cysts or tumors. For problems connected with anovulation, fertility drugs or high-tech conception techniques such as in-vitro fertilization are common treatments. For some structural blockages, surgery can be helpful.

CHINESE INTERPRETATION

The Chinese offer three different explanations for infertility or difficulty with conception: (1) Deficiency in Kidney *chi* and *jing*, which, over time, creates general weakness, lack of vitality, and the inability to produce a healthy egg; (2) Stagnant Liver *chi* (the energy is not circulating properly), which can lead to "congealed blood" (structural blockage); (3) Deficiency in Spleen *chi*, which causes improper digestion of fluids, leading to buildup of phlegm (*tan*), which can obstruct the pelvic area and prevent conception.

COMPLEMENTARY TREATMENTS

SUPPLEMENTS

- **B-complex vitamin** (choose the high-potency B-100 formula*)
- **Folic acid** (included in B-complex but add 100 mg/day)
- **Calcium** (500 mg/day)
- **Magnesium** (1,000 mg/day)

*The B-100 designation indicates that the product contains 100 mg each of the B vitamins. Recommended dosage is one tablet per day, or as directed.

- **Zinc** (15–30 mg/day)
- **Vitamin C** (1,000 mg/day)

EXERCISE

If conception difficulties are caused by an obstruction, gentle cardiovascular exercises can be extremely helpful; however, if the problem is caused by a deficiency condition, make sure that the exercise is nonstrenuous (walking or swimming). Natural light and sunlight may increase fertility, so whenever possible, exercise outdoors. Neuromuscular skeletal imbalances may be involved, blocking circulation to the pelvic organs; consult with an acupuncturist, massage therapist, or chiropractor.

DIET

Avoid caffeine, alcohol, nicotine, and over-the-counter, prescription, and recreational drugs.

HERBAL ALLIES

The following herbs are gentle enough to be combined. Use false unicorn root as the main herb and add other herbs as needed.

- **False unicorn root**, a fertility tonic and hormone balancer
- **Red clover** (*Trifolium pratense*), rich in vital nutrients, to restore and balance hormonal functioning (Make a tea with the flowers.)
- **Red raspberry** leaf tea, a general uterine tonic
- **Nettles,** high in iron and nutrients
- **Dong Quai,** to build the blood

CHINESE PATENT REMEDIES

- **Chai Pai Di Huang Wan** (Eight Flavor Rehmannia Pills) to nourish the Kidney *chi* and dispel heat from the pelvis
- **Lung Dan Xie Gan Wan** (Gentiana Purge Liver Pills) for Liver constrainment or buildup or phlegm in the pelvic area (a draining formula, not to be used for deficient conditions)

ACUPOINTS

For Kidney deficiency: **Conception Vessel 4, Spleen 6,** and **Stomach 36**

For Liver constrainment and phlegm: **Conception Vessel 3, Conception Vessel 4, Liver 3, Pericardium 6,** and **Stomach 40**

MIND/BODY/SPIRIT CONNECTION

The symptoms might be expressing these questions:

- "What unfinished business do I need to address before I can conceive a child?"
- "How can I nourish myself so that I have the strength and resilience needed to nourish a child?"
- "Are there problems in my marriage (or partnership)? Can we as a couple work together to support each other and offer support and nourishment to our child?"

"The Chinese would ask you to look outside at nature and recognize the processes of change that are going on at all times in your life," I said. "Life energy is produced from the constant interaction of yin and yang, and love is just one of the energies essential to a successful union. A strong marriage, like a healthy and happy life, requires the delicate balancing of all the powers of nature."

I told Anna one of my favorite stories, called "The Lesson."

In ancient times, a young couple approached an old master and asked, "Please, Master, speak to us of marriage and the place of love in our union."

And the Master said, "See that marriage is a union manifesting the five energies of nature held within us and that love is only but one of the energies."

"Then please, Master, speak to us of the energies in nature that are held within us."

And the Master said, "The first energy, the Fire energy, is like the Sun, always warming the body/mind/spirit, bathing your relationship with love. Experience this manifestation of nature within you as the urge to love, and express that love to your partner.

"The Earth energy is like the soil, always giving to the body/mind/ spirit, providing your relationship with nourishment. Experience this manifestation of nature within you as the urge to nurture, and express that nurturing to your partner.

"The Metal energy is like the gem, always sustaining to the body/mind/spirit, endowing your relationship with strength. Experience this manifestation of nature within you as the urge to be strong, and express that strength to your partner.

"The Water energy is like the spring, always refreshing to the body/mind/spirit, forming your relationship in change. Experience this manifestation of nature within you as the urge to change, and express that change to your partner.

"The Wood energy is like the tree, always supportive of the body/mind/spirit, seeding your relationship in growth. Experience this manifestation of nature within you as the urge to grow, and express that growth to your partner.

"You are the laws of nature—you are love, you are nourishment, you are strength, you are change, you are growth. Know that these energies will move and be moved, seeking their balance between the forces of control and creativity, and so your relationship will seek those balances also."

And with that the Master turned and gently walked away.

Every woman's life contains a thousand deaths—eggs that were not fertilized, love that was not consummated, dreams that were never realized, hopes that never materialized. When a piece of the self dies, we sometimes forget to mourn. Life goes on, and we march on with it; in our haste to keep moving, we do not take the time to stop and pay our respects to those parts of the self that died before they had a chance to live. But grief is always just a step behind, part of the shadow self, and when we are forced to rest for a time, waylaid by illness, fatigue, or a heavy heart, a sense of loss rises up unbidden. At those undefended moments, we mourn silently for the casualties of our past.

For millions of women—an estimated 50 to 60 percent of all women between the ages of eighteen and fifty—a time of grief and mourning returns every month. When their hormones are switching gears and their defenses are low, a crack of sorts develops between the world of action and the world of reflection, and they feel the pull to go inward, to dream, to imagine, to confront the deeper mysteries. If they resist this natural inclination to retreat into the recesses of their being, feelings of anxiety and irritability build, moods grow dark, and confusion reigns. The pressure gradually intensifies until the blood is released, and then the gloom is washed away, the heavy air is dispelled, and everything is washed clean.

This cyclic recurrence of grief, anxiety, and heightened sensibility in the second half of the menstrual cycle is called premenstrual syndrome, or PMS. During the luteal phase of the menstrual cycle—from ovulation through the onset of menstruation—many women feel a compelling, even overwhelming need to acknowledge the thickening energy and gathering storm clouds of emotion. This is the time, in Dr. Christiane Northrup's words, when women prepare to "develop or give birth to something that comes from within ourselves"; it is the phase when women are "most in tune with their inner knowing and with what isn't working in their lives."

The luteal phase calls out for solitude, silence, and introspection. In Native American cultures, women prepared at this time to enter the Moon Lodge, where they were shut off from the noise and activity of the outside world, their household and child care duties assumed by other members of the tribe. No space or time has been created in our culture to respect and honor the moon cycle, and so women must create their own House of the Moon, asking friends and family to give them the time and space to retreat into a dark, silent place to meditate, read, reflect, and gather wisdom.

In the Skeleton Woman story, Skeleton Woman gave birth to herself by reaching into the fisherman's body and removing his heart. Holding the secret of life and love in her bloody hands, listening to its pulse and putting her soul in touch with its rhythms, she drummed flesh onto her bones and gave herself new life. From the bones of death, life was created. Love is like that, too, for the flesh of love is created from the bones of longing and desire. The only requirement for this process of renewal and regeneration is that we honor and act on the need for change. If we don't take the time or can't find the courage to reach in and grab the heart, creating ourselves anew, we suffer deeply, haunted by thoughts of what might have been, grieving for the dead and the dying parts of the undeveloped self.

KATE

"I love my children, I adore them, nothing in my life matters more than them, but I feel like I'm not a very good mother, because at least two weeks out of the month I lose control and start ranting and raving." Kate took a deep breath, let out a sigh, and continued.

"My friends keep telling me I should get a job, do something creative. I *was* creative before I got married and had children, but now I feel like I'm not doing anything productive, just spending all day with my kids, and I love that, I really do, I don't want to be doing anything else. But I just feel like something is missing, and I don't know what it is. To be truthful, I only have one good week out of the whole month. The rest of the time I'm edgy, moody, and out of control. The silliest thing sets me off, and after I blow up at the kids for some stupid reason or another, I feel so guilty that I want to die from shame."

Kate was sitting on the edge of her chair, her dark eyes searching mine ("Do you understand?"), her hands beating the air like a conductor's baton, keeping time to the music of her frenzied beat. Thin and delicately boned, with graceful hands and slender feet, she wore her long dark hair pulled back in a ponytail that waved in the air behind her as she talked. With her flushed complexion, manic speech patterns, restlessness, and hyperexcitability, Kate clearly demonstrated an imbalance in Fire energy.

"So I was complaining to one of my friends that I was out of options. I had already tried"—she started counting off on her fingers—"macrobiotic diets, megavitamins, estrogen pills, progesterone pills, and my doctor was trying to talk me into tranquilizers. I cried on my friend's shoulder, telling her that I didn't want to be tranquilized, I wanted to figure out what was going on, and she suggested I come to you. She said hormones are your specialty." Kate leaned toward me and put her hand on my arm. "I have to tell you I'm not a believer in this alternative therapy stuff. Getting stuck with needles is not my idea of fun. But I'm out of options. If I don't do something fast, my husband and children are going to throw me out of the house, and I'll have to check myself into a loony bin."

In that first session, Kate and I talked for almost an hour. She told me about her life before marriage, when she was a lead singer in a female rock band. "We partied and played all night." She sighed, remembering. "Looking back, I have this distorted sense that I was happy all the time, full of life, energy, optimism. I can't remember ever being moody or depressed back then—at least not like this. I didn't just suddenly blow up at my friends and family for no reason whatsoever. What has happened to me? Is it PMS—or is it all in my head?"

"Your symptoms are not in your head," I assured Kate, briefly relating the most recent theories about the causes of PMS. For many years, obstetricians and gynecologists thought the symptoms of PMS—the emotional ups and downs, moodiness, irritability, panic attacks, insomnia, confusion, depression, explosions of anger, even the headaches, fatigue, fainting spells, heart palpitations, cramping, and bloating—were psychological, or "in the head." But careful research and clinical experience have conclusively proven that PMS is related to hormonal imbalances, which are often subtle and difficult to detect through laboratory tests.

PMS appears to be a "luteal phase defect," which means that something goes awry after ovulation, when the corpus luteum begins to break down, and progesterone, a calming, relaxing hormone, is slowly released into the bloodstream. The corpus luteum normally disintegrates slowly, releasing a steady influx of progesterone into the bloodstream; but in women who suffer from PMS, the corpus luteum appears to deteriorate too rapidly, causing several bursts of progesterone rather than a steady, regulated flow. Rather than experiencing the soothing, calming effects of progesterone, a woman with a luteal phase defect is overexcited and overstimulated by an excess of estrogen.

"What exactly goes wrong?" Kate asked.

"No one really knows for sure," I said, "although there are dozens of different theories. Diet, stress, overstimulation, lack of sunlight, any number of different factors working alone or in concert are capable of upsetting the body's delicate endocrine balance."

One disturbing explanation for the increased numbers of women suffering from PMS, as well as the increased intensity of their symptoms, focuses on the exogenous, or "unopposed," estrogens that proliferate in our modern-day society. Our entire food supply is high in synthetic (man-made) estrogens, which are directly injected into farm animals or added to feed to make the animals grow faster and produce more milk or eggs. These synthetic hormones are stored in the animal's fat reserves, and when we eat beef, chicken, eggs, and cheese, we also ingest the hormones. Another potential cause of adrenal and endocrine malfunction is overstimulation in the form of violence and explicit sex scenes in movies, television, and video games. When the nervous system is subjected to excessive stress or stimulation, certain hormones (such as estrogen) are overproduced, while other hormones (such as progesterone) are rapidly depleted.

A growing reliance on toxic chemicals also contributes to an overly estrogenic environment. Hundreds of chemicals used in our modern society—PCBs used to make electronics; polycarbonite plastics found in water jugs and baby bottles; chlorine compounds used to bleach paper; surfactants used in dishwashing liquids, toilet paper, and various pesticides—have molecular structures similar to the hormone estrogen. Scientists theorize that these "xeno-estrogens" fit into the body's estrogen receptor sites, tricking the body into switching off or turning on certain biological pathways. As a result, men and women alike are being pumped up with excess estrogen and are "overfeminized." In 1940, an average milliliter of human semen contained 113 million sperm, while in 1990 the number had dropped to 66 million. Animals are also affected; a Florida researcher recently discovered that male alligators' penises were only one-quarter their normal size, while their testosterone levels were low enough to make the animals sterile.

"What's the effect of extra estrogen on women?" Kate asked.

"Many experts believe that the profusion of gynecological problems that we are dealing with today—including infertility, PMS, endometriosis, estrogenic cancers (breast, uterine, endometrial, ovarian, bone), and various menopausal complaints—can be traced to the unopposed estrogens cycling and recycling throughout our bodies. Women can't produce enough progesterone on their own to counteract the effects of our highly estrogenic environment, and so the necessary support must come through dietary changes, stress reduction techniques, herbal remedies, and if necessary, a natural progesterone supplement."

"I don't get it," Kate said, a confused look on her face. "I thought estrogen was the good hormone and progesterone was the bad one. I have friends who gave up hormone replacement therapy because of the effects of the progesterone. And when my doctor gave me Provera to help with my mood swings and irritability, it only made things worse. My heart was thumping out of my chest, and I became even more of a crank."

I explained to Kate that because the hormones used by most physicians are synthetic (like Provera), their molecular structure is subtly different from natural hormones. Synthetic hormonal compounds are basically foreign substances that alter normal functioning, creating unpleasant side effects such as irritability, migraines, bloating, breast tenderness, and in more severe cases, blood clots and cancer. Studies show that taking progestins (synthetic progesterone) actually decreases the body's natural progesterone levels, thus intensifying and extending the symptoms of PMS.

A natural source of progesterone is available, however, which is derived from the wild yam, an herb that grows in Southern Mexico. The wild yam contains a chemical called diosgenin (also found in soya products), which is virtually identical to the progesterone naturally produced by women and mimics the natural actions of the hormone (rather than altering normal functioning as synthetic progestins do). The herb can be taken orally, transdermally (through the skin), or as a rectal or vaginal suppository, and it is extremely effective for relieving symptoms of irritability, anxiety, mood swings, insomnia, bloating, and tenderness. Completely safe and relatively inexpensive (approximately thirty dollars for a two-month supply), natural progesterone stimulates the growth of new bone, helping to heal and prevent osteoporosis.

"If a woman's symptoms are severe, and she requires immediate results," I told Kate, "I have no hesitation recommending natural progesterone."

"My symptoms are severe," Kate said, putting her hand over her forehead as if she felt faint. "Give me some of that stuff right now!"

"Let's see what else is going on," I laughed, "and then we'll make a complete diagnosis and treatment plan."

Kate's pulses were wiry and tight, feeling like a taut, thick string vibrating under my fingers in the Liver, Kidney, and Heart positions; this quality indicated a constrainment of energy in those organ systems. The Lower Heater (Kidney) seemed weaker, while the Upper Heater (Heart) and the Middle Heater (Liver) were literally bounding under my fingers. From this examination, I learned that Kate's energy was trapped and constrained above the diaphragm, creating the symptoms of a tight chest, heart palpitations, and insomnia. In Chinese terminology, Kate's Liver was consuming the Water of the Kidney, causing excess Heat and Fire to irritate the Heart, which in turn disturbed the Spirit (shen), creating anxiety and restlessness. She was clearly a combination of Wood (Liver) and Fire (Heart) energies.

I described my recommendations for treatment. We would begin with weekly acupuncture treatments; when she felt better, we would switch to bimonthly and then monthly treatments. Dietary changes, vitamin and mineral supplements, herbal remedies, and the natural progesterone cream would support her Liver and Kidney functions, draining the excess Fire and stabilizing the Heart and Spirit. (See appendix 3 for information on obtaining natural progesterone.)

For her diet, I recommended plenty of fresh fruits, vegetables, and fiber. A bulking fiber such as psyllium would help to eliminate circulating estrogens more efficiently through the bowels. (I prefer this natural fiber to Metamucil and other synthetic fibers that contain sugar and artificial coloring and flavoring.) To help create bulk and flush out her system, she should drink a minimum of six glasses of water each day. I strongly recommended that she cut back on highly estrogenic foods such as beef, poultry, and dairy products: I also urged that she eliminate from her diet alcohol, caffeine, and tobacco, all of which increase blood acidity, deplete calcium, and burden the Liver, the organ responsible for metabolizing hormones.

To help her Liver break down the circulating hormones, I recommended oil of evening primrose (500 mg, three or four times a day), which contains the essential fatty acid gamma linoleic acid (GLA); flaxseed, borage oil, and black currant seed oil are also good sources of GLA, which appears to "oil the hormonal machinery," in Dr. Serafina Corsello's words, and promote a healthy menstrual cycle. Vitamin B_6 (200 to 400 mg/day, taken with a high-potency B-complex vitamin) helps eliminate excess water and swelling, and magnesium (500 mg/day) diminishes uterine contractions and relieves cramping.

As for herbs, I recommended a tincture of chasteberry, dandelion root, motherwort, and black haw, but when Kate couldn't tolerate the alcohol in the formula, I suggested two prepared Chinese remedies: *Wu Chi Pai Feng Wan* (Black Cock, White Phoenix pills), an excellent female tonic for stuck energy, especially in the Lower Heater (the pelvic region), containing herbs that warm the uterus, support the yin, and build and move the blood; and *Hsiao Yao Wan* (Free and Easy Wanderer pills), the archetypical remedy in Chinese herbology for constrained Liver *chi*, helping to move the energy and blood in a relaxed way throughout the body/mind/spirit.

I chose six acupoints for Kate. Liver 3 (Great Rushing), located in the depression between the big toe and the second toe, is the source point on the Liver channel and the archetypical point to instigate the flow of *chi* and blood when obstruction has occurred. When we stimulate this point, the energy gently flows through the system, breaking down barriers and obstructions and clearing out the clogged channels. Liver 14 (Gate of Hope), located on the nipple line two ribs below the nipple on both sides, directly supports the Liver's function of flowing and spreading, helping to break up stagnating energy and renew feelings of hope and optimism.

Spleen 6 (Three Yin Meeting), located three thumb-widths above the interior ankle bone, just behind the tibia, nourishes the blood, balances

PREMENSTRUAL SYNDROME (PMS)

WESTERN INTERPRETATION AND TREATMENT

Until recently, PMS was considered a form of hysteria and often labeled psychosomatic, but studies convincingly demonstrate that the symptoms are caused by deficient progesterone production, most likely due to a "luteal phase defect" involving the corpus luteum (see page 228). The emotional instability so often associated with PMS is created by relative imbalances in estrogen and progesterone levels. The syndrome tends to intensify with age but resolves with menopause. Western treatments include progesterone therapy (Provera) for general symptoms, diuretics for bloating, painkillers for headaches, tranquilizers for anxiety, and antidepressants or psychotherapy for depression.

CHINESE INTERPRETATION

The Chinese offer two interpretations of PMS, which can occur independently but often coexist: (1) Constrained Liver *chi* creates blockage and stagnation, which leads to symptoms such as irritability, breast pain, headaches, bloating (especially in breasts). (2) Deficient Spleen and Kidney *chi* creates the symptoms of general bloating, chronic depression, fatigue, lassitude, aches and pains throughout the body, and intensified sugar cravings.

COMPLEMENTARY TREATMENTS

SUPPLEMENTS

- **Gamma linoleic acid,** or GLA, an essential fatty acid, found in oil of evening primrose, borage, and black currant seed oil (1,000–3,000 mg/day, depending on severity of symptoms)
- **Vitamin B$_6$** (100 mg twice daily; always take any single B vitamin with a B-complex 100 vitamin*)

*The B-100 designation indicates that the product contains 100 mg each of the B vitamins. Recommended dosage is one tablet per day, or as directed.

- **Vitamin E**, alpha tocopherol (400 iu/day)
- **Magnesium** and **calcium** (Take two units of magnesium for every unit of calcium. Try 500 mg/day of calcium and 1,000 mg/day of magnesium; increase magnesium to 1,500 mg/day with onset of menses until symptoms abate.)

EXERCISE

Because PMS is considered a form of stagnation, exercise is essential to keep the energy and blood flowing. Walk, jog, work out gently on exercise machines at least three times every week. Whenever possible, exercise outdoors as fresh air and natural light appear to reduce the intensity of the symptoms.

HERBAL ALLIES

For General Symptoms

- **Chasteberry**, to support progesterone production
- **Motherwort**, to balance hormones and calm irritability
- **False unicorn root**, to balance hormonal cycles
- **Dandelion root**, a liver cleanser

For Specific Symptoms

- Bloating: **Dandelion** leaves
- Cystic breasts and breast tenderness: **Cleavers** (a lymphatic draining herb). Increase **vitamin E** to 800 iu/day. (Be sure to eliminate *all* caffeine products.) Also, try a poultice of cabbage leaves to relieve tenderness: soak cabbage leaves in hot water; bruise the leaves to allow the natural oils to escape; place over breasts while still hot; cover with cheesecloth.
- Irritability: **St. John's wort, valerian root,** or **vervain**
- Depression: **St. John's wort** or **damiana** (*Turnera diffusa* or *Damiana aphrodisica*)
- Headaches: **Common garden sage**

CHINESE PATENT REMEDIES

- **Woman's Precious Pills** and/or **Wu Chi Pai Feng Wan** (Black Cock, White Phoenix Pills) for PMS with signs of deficiency (pale, bloated tongue and chronic symptoms such as lethargy and weak pulses)

- **Hsiao Yao Wan** (Relaxed Wanderer Pills) or **Ji Xue Teng Qin Gao Pian** (Milletia Reticulata Liquid Extract, excellent for more severe PMS symptoms) for stagnant Liver or stagnant blood signs (red or purplish tongue and more acute symptoms such as stabbing pains, chronic depression, hopelessness)

ACUPOINTS

Spleen 6, Spleen 8, Spleen 10, Conception Vessel 4, Conception Vessel 6, Liver 3. For mood swings, press **Heart 7** and **Pericardium 6**: For sweet cravings or digestive problems, add **Stomach 36**.

MIND/BODY/SPIRIT CONNECTIONS

The symptoms might be expressing these questions:

- "How am I blocking my creativity from expressing itself?"
- "How do I prevent myself from receiving warmth and nourishment from others?"
- "I need time and space to rest, reflect, and dream—how am I neglecting to take care of myself?"

the menstrual cycle, supports the yin energy, and subdues excess Fire. Spleen 8 (Earth's Crux), located in a depression three inches below the bump on the inner knee, regulates Earth energies, specifically targeting Earth disharmonies below the umbilicus. This point also nourishes the Spleen, regulates the blood, and relieves symptoms of PMS, cramping, lower back pain, abnormal uterine bleeding, water retention, and pain and distention in the lower belly or sides of the body.

Pericardium 6 (Inner Frontier Gate), located on the inner arm two inches above the wrist crease, relaxes the spirit and calms the Heart; this crucial point is often used in conjunction with Liver 3 to treat and subdue the symptoms of constrained Liver *chi*, which include uncontrollable anger, irritability, insomnia, headaches, and hot flashes.

The most symbolic point for Kate was Heart 7 (Gate of Spirit), which is the most commonly used acupoint for settling the spirit. "The Spirit Gate is a very stabilizing point," I told Kate as I inserted the needle in a depression on the crease of each wrist, "calming and pacifying the spirit, easing anxiety, nervousness, and agitation, relieving insomnia, and dissipating the heat of the Heart."

"What's wrong with my heart?" Kate asked.

"The Spirit Gate is more concerned with emotional and spiritual problems," I said. "The Heart in this sense signifies home, and this point will help you discover where you feel most at home, where your Heart yearns to be. If you meditate on this point, you might ask yourself what you love most in the world. What means the most to you? How do you choose to express that love? How might that love be blocked or prevented from going where it needs to go?"

"I love being with my kids," Kate said without a moment's hesitation. "That's where my heart is, because when I'm with them, I'm totally content. But when I talk to my friends and they discuss their jobs, the money they make, all the people they meet, and the places they go, I feel jealous and inadequate. They're out there in the real world becoming rich and famous, or at least having lots of fun, and here I am sitting at home, drawing with crayons and baking cookies with my kids. I spend my whole day answering my kids' questions, feeding and cleaning up after them, and wiping the tears off their faces."

"But are you happy?"

"At times I'm totally content," Kate said. "I love my children more than anything in the whole world. It's just when I start to think about what I could be doing, how much more creative I could be, or how much money I could make—that's when I start to go crazy."

"I wonder if we all don't go a little crazy at different times in our lives," I said. "Perhaps women are wiser, more adaptable, and live longer than men because they learn through their menstrual cycles that the craziness is cyclical—it comes, and it goes, over and over again. Women intuitively know how to go crazy and then be sane again, how to be patient and when to run out of patience, how to give and how to take, how to let part of themselves die so that other, more essential parts might live."

"The craziness gets even worse when you become a parent," Kate said. "I can't tell you how many times I've said to myself, 'This too shall pass.' It's my current theme song."

"The nature of a parent's work is sacrifice," I agreed with Kate, "for you must necessarily take away from yourself in order to give your children what they need. Let me tell you a story."

One of the old men had just finished putting handles on his baskets when he overheard a brother voicing concern about his own unfinished work.

"The marketplace is about to open," said the brother, "and I have no handles for my baskets. What shall I do?"

The old man quietly removed the handles from his baskets and gave them to his neighbor. "Please accept these handles," he said, "for I have no need of them."

In his benevolence the old man left his own work unfinished so that his brother's needs would be met.

"Just as the old man willingly gave his brother the handles from his baskets, so does a mother offer the gift of her time, energy, and love to her children," I said.

"Handles on the baskets," Kate mused. "That's a nice way of thinking about it."

The herbs, acupuncture treatments, dietary changes, vitamin and mineral supplements, and natural progesterone cream worked wonders for Kate, and her symptoms gradually resolved over a period of three to four months. After six months, she decided to stop using the natural progesterone cream ("Let's see how strong I am by myself," she said) and discovered that her body was able to maintain its hormonal equilibrium without external assistance. For preventative purposes, she comes in for acupuncture treatments five times a year, once during each season, and an extra session in spring, to help support her Wood energy and prepare her for the approaching season of Fire (summer).

"My Liver's been acting up," Kate announced in a recent visit, throwing her backpack on the floor and grinning from ear to ear. "Let's poke a few holes in it, shall we?"

In summer, the season of passion, devotion, and self-sacrifice, women learn how to sing the songs that put flesh on the bones. Through their boundless, limitless love, they move the wheel of life along, acknowledging the presence of death but refusing to let it drown out the song of life. Life and death form the alternating spokes on the wheel; as one spoke sings "Life," the other groans "Death." The wheel turns, and the separate sounds merge into a humming song of renewal and regeneration. Love drives the wheel.

A story is told about this kind of love—the love that knows no bounds. The story takes place a long time ago when, it is said, men first wrested control from women and began to build up their power. Life was filled with anger and fear, for the men did not yet understand the responsibility that comes with power, and they spent their time punishing and restricting the women and children, giving orders, telling their daughters whom they should marry, and forcing their wives into submission. One of the women in the tribe rebelled. Her name is Tem Eyos Ki, and this is her story.

> *Tem Eyos Ki went to the waiting house to pass her sacred time in a sacred place, sitting on moss and giving her inner blood to the Earth Mother. Men were not allowed near the waiting house, it was too sacred for them to understand or approach. And Tem Eyos Ki stayed in the waiting house with some of the other women whose time it was, and she was there for more than four days.*
>
> *When she came from the waiting house she was a woman hit by lightning, a woman struck by wonder, a woman shaked with power, a woman filled with love. She walked from the waiting house with a look on her face more potent than magic. Seeds of life glittered in her hair.*
>
> *She smiled, and sang a song that told of love that knew no limits, of love that knew no bounds, of love that demanded nothing and expected nothing but fulfilled everything. She sang of a place so wondrous the minds of people could not even begin to imagine it. A place without anger or fear, a place without loneliness or incompletion.*
>
> *She walked through the village singing her song, and the women followed her. They collected their children, boys and girls alike, and followed Tem Eyos Ki, leaving behind the cooking pots and weaving looms, leaving behind the husbands and fathers.*
>
> *Tem Eyos Ki walked past the village, along the beach, toward the forest, singing her song of love and wonder. And the women followed.*
>
> *The men found the village empty, the meals uncooked, the work unfinished. They followed the women, angry and threatening. They followed the women into the forest. Followed the women who followed Tem Eyos Ki, who followed the song she learned in the waiting house when she found love.*
>
> *Storm wind tried to stop the men with gales and rain. The forest tried to stop them. Even the sky tried to stop them with thunder and lightning and the sea smashed herself against the rocks to warn the women.*
>
> *The women wept and said they did not want to return home. The*

men threatened to kill Tem Eyos Ki. To silence her song so that she would never again tempt their women from their hearth fires. They went after Tem Eyos Ki to kill her.

But Qolus, who is a female figure and was father of the four sons who fathered all ordinary people, sent a magic dugout, and Tem Eyos Ki leaped into it, still singing her song. She flew above the heads of the shouting men and the weeping women and sang of things people had forgotten. The storm stopped, the wind calmed, the rain stopped falling, and the sea became still. All creation listened to the song of Tem Eyos Ki. And then she flew away.

The men stopped arguing and began to talk. The women said why they had wanted to leave. The men listened. The women listened. They went home together, to try to live properly again.

But sometimes a woman will think she hears a song, or think she remembers beautiful words, and she will weep a little for the beauty that she almost knew. Sometimes she will dream of a place that is not like this one. Sometimes she almost thinks she knows what it was Tem Eyos Ki was singing in her song. And she weeps for the beauty she never knew.

—**The Daughters of Copper Woman** *(1981)*

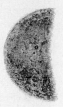

CHAPTER 15

AUTUMN: FROM MATRIARCH TO WISE WOMAN

Whoever is soft and yielding
is a disciple of life.

The hard and stiff will be broken.
The soft and supple will prevail.
        —Tao te Ching

The power of woman is great, and the more discipline and devotion she
renders, the greater her power grows.

        —*Paula Gunn Allen*

As a woman moves beyond her childbearing years into the autumn of her
life, she begins to harvest the essential materials that will sustain and
nurture her for the rest of her journey. Autumn is the season of ripening
and maturity, when fruits fall plump and sweet to the ground, and paper-

thin seeds delicate as spiderwebs are borne off on the stiffening wind to await the season of rebirth and renewal. The season sings "Surrender," and all of nature listens, letting go of the old in preparation for the new. Trees fling off their colorful headdresses with a few mighty shakes to stand shorn but proud, knot-muscled limbs extended upward and outward in a show of strength and endurance. Life-giving sap retreats, pulling back into the core to nourish and sustain the roots. Flowers drop their petals one by one, broken limbs litter the ground, leaves crumble to the touch, and the soil blankets itself with death and decay, laying the groundwork for the creation of new life.

The symbol of autumn is the seed, where future life lies compressed and perfectly ordered within a tender, flexible space. Dry and lifeless on the outside, filled with the delicate potential of growth and animation on the inside, the seed enfolds life within the arms of death. "Here, in the seed," notes *The I Ching*, "in the deep hidden stillness, the end of everything is joined to a new beginning."

"From such small beginnings—a mere grain of dust, as it were—do mighty trees take their rise," wrote Henry David Thoreau in *The Dispersion of Seeds*, his final manuscript, written in the years before his death at the age of forty-five. Drawn to the core, the inner substance and deeper meaning of life, Thoreau wandered through the woods and fields of his native Massachusetts, carefully observing how seeds were scattered by the wind or transported by birds, squirrels, foxes, and other forest creatures. In the seed, Thoreau found his metaphor for death and rebirth. "We find ourselves in a world that is already planted but is also still being planted as at first," he wrote. In the tiny, frail seeds of autumn, the wholeness and holiness of the world were revealed to him. "The very earth itself is a granary and a seminary, so that to some minds, its surface is regarded as the cuticle of one living creature."

To the unconcerned, seed cases may appear useless and barren, dried out and weather worn. But for those who would look deeper, who would stoop to peel away the outer core in order to contemplate the inner substance, untold treasures are revealed, for, as Thoreau notes, "that which seemed a mere brown and worn-out side of the summer, sinking into the earth of the roadside, turns out to be a precious casket."

Life whispers its meaning in such "little things." In a lovely passage introducing his manuscript on wild fruits, Thoreau bemoans the fact that so few appreciate "the little things" in life, for most of us are forever chasing after the big things. "The Wellingtonia gigantea, the famous California tree, is a great thing, the seed from which it sprang a little thing," he wrote. "Scarcely one traveller has noticed the seed at all, and so with all the seeds or origins of things."

It was to the little things that Thoreau devoted his life, and his precise, finely drawn observations take us down and inward to the core. With the same tender care that nature bestows on even its lowly weeds to ensure their survival, we must treat our own seeds. With focused attention to the little things, we move ever closer to an understanding of the meaning of life.

In human life, the tender seeds of autumn are the seeds of heart and soul. In the autumn of a woman's life, she collects the grains, bulbs, tubers, and roots that will sustain her for the rest of her days. Using her powers of discipline and devotion, she searches for the essentials that will carry her through the winter. She is a collector of wisdom, a harvester of experience, a preserver of the little things, and she knows that for everything she keeps, she must give something away. *What is essential?* she asks herself with each step. *What can I do without?*

In Native American lore, the woman who has moved beyond her childbearing years is viewed as a *gatherer*. A thoughtful, solitary, somewhat eccentric character, she walks the woods with a penetrating eye, marveling at the patience and devotion nature bestows on all her handiwork. Searching for the essential truths, the gatherer is said to *"walk in a sacred manner," "to walk in beauty,"* and *"to walk in balance."* Symmetry and correspondences attract her eye; paradox pleases her; nature's intricate, overlapping patterns engage her spirit. Over time, she comes to understand the value of her own "perfectly dry and bristly" exterior, for her inner ripening and maturity could not proceed without a sacrifice of vital energy from the outer shell. As time goes by, all her energies become focused on the interior, where the seeds of heart and soul are steadily nurtured.

The Chinese refer to autumn as the season of Metal, the time when a woman learns to draw on her inner stores of discipline, order, and perseverance. The power of Metal prepares her for whatever situation might present itself; while her body may be weakening, her heart and soul cannot afford to be frail. "There are great obstacles to be overcome," notes *The I Ching*, and "it is necessary to be hard as metal and straight as an arrow to surmount the difficulties." Muscles of perception, intuition, and inner knowing must be developed and continually strengthened, for just as the body grows stronger through exercise, so does the soul become more powerful through self-discipline and focused attention. The season of autumn signals the time to develop the muscles of the soul.

* * *

The transition between the seasons of life is not always smooth and orderly. Profound transformations are taking place, and the body/mind/spirit may be ill prepared to cope with the sudden shifts of energy. Caught off guard, a woman may struggle for balance, only to discover in her deepest fears the very source of her strength and resilience. Forced to acknowledge that part of the self is dying, grieving for what is gone and can never be recovered, she turns her focus inward, where she works over the seeds, picking and choosing, taking stock, continually asking the same questions over and over again—*Who am I now? What am I yet to become?* With each repetition of these questions, she sinks deeper into the meaning of her own existence, moving steadily through the shadows in order to come fully into the light.

CLAIRE

The bleeding began on a Sunday; by Wednesday, Claire knew that something was terribly wrong. In less than three days, she had used up a box of forty super Tampax and two dozen menstrual pads, and the thick, clotted blood showed no sign of weakening. When she woke up early Saturday morning in a pool of blood, her husband rushed her to the emergency room, where she spent a harrowing day hooked up to IVs, afraid that her life, poised at its midpoint, was coming to a violent, bloody end. The emergency room doctor assured her that the bleeding was not life threatening but emphasized the need for more tests to determine the precise cause of the hemorrhage. Claire was released from the hospital with an iron supplement and instructions to make an appointment with her gynecologist for a D & C (dilation and curettage).

Just the mention of surgery sent Claire into a panic; her father died at age fifty-three—just eight years older than she was now—from complications arising from minor surgery. "I can't go to a doctor," Claire told her husband, nearly hysterical with fear. "I'm too scared. I don't want to die." Desperate to help his wife, he spent hours on the phone, asking friends and relatives for ideas about alternative treatments; realizing how frightened her husband was, Claire agreed to try acupuncture.

The day after she was released from the hospital, Claire was sitting in my office, her eyes red and swollen from crying, her face pale and ashen. Her voice was weak and the vocal quality was monotonous, revealing a potential imbalance in Wood and/or Earth energies. The subtle greenish hue around her eyes and her naturally dark-skinned complexion also spoke to an affinity to Wood, but Claire was in so much distress that I couldn't trust my first impressions. When the hemorrhaging was under control and her fears had abated, we could proceed more slowly, working to understand the inherent strengths and weaknesses of her basic constitution.

Claire's pulses were thin and feeble, exerting little force against my fingers; the weakness of her pulses indicated a deficiency of *chi* and blood, a diagnosis that was supported by the pale, bloated quality of her tongue. Her menstrual history was relatively straightforward and uneventful: She began menstruating when she was thirteen, and her cycles ran predictably, twenty-eight to thirty days. She had no significant premenstrual tension, cramping, clotting, or emotional lability. At age thirty-five she married, and two years later her husband had a vasectomy; the decision not to have children was mutual. Around the age of forty-one or forty-two, Claire's periods became more erratic, with heavier flows lasting three or four days, but nothing in her past history could have prepared her for the violent, unrelieved hemorrhaging she had just experienced.

"What does the bleeding mean?" she asked me. "Is a D and C absolutely necessary? Do you think I might have cancer?"

Whenever a patient asks me questions about her condition, and particularly when those questions are so clearly rooted in anxiety and fear, I respond with practical information and constant reassurances in an effort to keep her spirits up and her hope alive. "Heavy bleeding is a common problem associated with perimenopause, the transition period between normal periods and the cessation of menstruation," I said.

Then I briefly explained the Chinese theory of "reckless bleeding." When the physical and emotional stresses of life become overly burdensome, the Liver has to work harder to keep the energy, blood, and emotions flowing smoothly; over time, the Liver's reserves are drained. If the Liver reaches a point of exhaustion, it can no longer perform its yin function of cooling the blood and keeping the body/mind/spirit calm and well lubricated. Friction and stagnation result, generating heat in the blood and causing it to "run recklessly." Because the deficient yin cannot contain the heat, the blood boils over, escaping its pathways and creating signs and symptoms such as hot flashes, night sweats, and hemorrhaging. Heavy, abnormal bleeding is also viewed by the Chinese as a deficient *chi* condition, for one of the functions of *chi* is to keep the blood contained within its vessels.

If the *chi* becomes depleted, the blood is said to leak from the vessels, indicating a problem in the Spleen/Pancreas orb.

The symptoms associated with reckless bleeding are often transitional, indicating a temporary condition that will eventually correct itself. Because Claire was still bleeding heavily, however, the first priority of treatment was to slow down the flow of blood and restore her strength through the use of acupuncture techniques and herbal remedies. After we had accomplished those goals, we could begin to explore the root of the problem.

Because Claire had expressed fears about a D & C and the possibility of cancer, I addressed those concerns, explaining that factors other than hormonal shifts can also cause heavy bleeding, including uterine fibroids, cysts, hyperplasia of the endometrial tissues, vaginitis, and in rare cases, cancer. Although the odds were slim that Claire suffered from any of these more serious disorders, it was essential that we rule them out through a pap smear and various blood analyses. Claire immediately balked, insisting that she would have nothing to do with conventional medicine; only when I offered to refer her to a gynecologist who I knew would proceed slowly and cautiously, did she agree to make an appointment. In the meantime, I reassured her, we would treat the bleeding as a hormonal imbalance, using several strategies to get the bleeding under control.

Acupuncture and herbal remedies are remarkably effective in controlling bleeding; when used together they complement each other, supporting and energizing the entire system. While acupuncture tends to focus more on the Five Transforming Powers, restoring balance in subtle ways to the energetic networks that ebb and flow throughout the body, herbal medicine directly affects the balance of yin and yang, and the interchange between blood, fluid, and *chi*. Herbalists use dozens (even hundreds) of herbs, changing the combinations of herbal ingredients to suit the individual disorder, for each herb has a distinct effect on specific bodily functions. Different herbs work in different ways to expel toxins, induce sweating, dry up excess dampness or humidity, warm the blood, build up fluids, subdue Fire, and nourish the yin, while acupuncture works in indirect ways to restore balance and recreate a healthy energy flow throughout the body/mind/spirit.

In that first session, I needled eight points. Spleen 6 (Three Yin Meeting), located on the lower leg just behind the tibia bone, supports the three yin meridians (the Spleen, Liver, and Kidneys), which join up at this point. Conception Vessel 3 (CV3) (Central Pole), located on the midline of the belly, nourishes the yin energy at the root (the Kidneys). Conception Vessel 4 (Gate at the Source), located an inch above CV3, supports the digestive and assimilative functions of the Stomach and Spleen and strengthens the "source *chi*," nourishing the Kidneys and thus invigorating the entire system. Liver 3 (Great Rushing), located between the big toe and second toe, is the source point on the Liver meridian and works to renew and reinforce Liver functions by resolving the stagnation of blood and *chi*. Liver 1 (Great Sincerity) and Spleen 1 (Hidden Clarity) are the archetypical points used to stop heavy bleeding (the Liver and the Spleen are considered the two orbs most responsible for heavy bleeding).

The herbal remedies were critically important in Claire's treatment. Certain herbs work quickly and efficiently to stop hemorrhaging in the body, and for gynecological purposes the most effective is a remarkable Chinese patent (ready-made) formula called Yunnan Pai Yao (Yunnan White Powder). A life-saving remedy for acute problems such as hemorrhages, shock, and infections, Yunnan Pai Yao is also a wonderful antidote for the pain and inflammation associated with menstrual cramps, ulcers, sprains, and hemorrhoids.

I also recommended an herbal formula consisting of dandelion, a rich source of iron and plant hormones that nourishes the Kidneys and Liver; nettles, a nourishing and strengthening herb that works to strengthen blood vessels and provides an abundant source of vitamins A, C, D, and K, calcium, potassium, phosphorus, iron, and sulfur; yellow dock, a gentle source of iron and replenisher of hemoglobin; lady's mantle, an excellent blood coagulant; and agrimony or shepherd's purse, both excellent astringents and well-known remedies for uterine hemorrhaging.

For as long as Claire continued to bleed heavily, I advised her to avoid any foods or drinks with caffeine (tea, coffee, chocolate, colas), because they inhibit the absorption of iron. Alcohol and aspirin thin the blood and should also be avoided. Hot baths or showers were off limits because heat dilates the blood vessels, aggravating and intensifying bleeding. Claire was a vegetarian, so as a substitute for my usual recommendation of calf's liver (an excellent source of iron, B vitamins, and vitamin A) in cases of iron deficiency, I suggested that she eat plenty of iron-rich foods such as spinach, kale, and seaweeds.

Claire left that first session feeling much more hopeful, and she called the next evening to report that the heavy bleeding had stopped. When she walked into my office a few days later for her second appointment, she looked completely transformed. Animated and playful, she held her

MENORRHAGIA

(HEAVY MENSTRUAL BLEEDING)[1]

WESTERN INTERPRETATION AND TREATMENT

Heavy bleeding during regular menses can be caused by endometriosis, fibroid tumors, or cysts. Chronic stress is sometimes considered a contributing factor. Traditional treatments include progesterone therapy or oral contraceptives, which can help stop the bleeding; dilation and curettage (D & C) for diagnostic purposes and to stop the bleeding; and hysterectomy (removal of the uterus) as a final solution. For anemia (often caused by excessive bleeding), iron supplements are prescribed.

CHINESE INTERPRETATION

The Chinese offer two interpretations of heavy menstrual bleeding: (1) Deficient Spleen and Kidney *chi* cannot hold the blood in its channels; the symptoms include pale, flabby tongue, prolonged light bleeding (blood is pinkish in color rather than bright red), fatigue, and shortness of breath. (2) Liver *chi* stagnation, which leads to heat in the blood; the symptoms include a dark-colored tongue with yellow coating, profuse bleeding with dark red blood, and irritability.

COMPLEMENTARY TREATMENTS

SUPPLEMENTS

- **Iron** (Try Liquid Floradix Iron, a European herbal formula rich in natural iron herbs, available in health food stores; and follow the directions on the bottle.)
- **Beta carotene** (25,000 iu/day)
- **Vitamin C** with bioflavonoids (1,000 to 5,000 mg/day)

[1]**Warning:** As prolonged heavy bleeding may involve serious illness, see your gynecologist before trying these complementary treatment methods; also, anemia may occur and must be treated.

TOPICAL STRATEGIES

Tampons can irritate inflamed vaginal tissues. Switch to pads, and try natural cloth pads (see appendix 3).

EXERCISE

Try to stay off your feet and allow gravity to assist in the healing process.

DIET

Choose dark green, iron-rich vegetables (kale, spinach, broccoli, and kelp) and root vegetables (carrots, radishes, turnips). Avoid spicy foods, fatty foods, dairy foods, refined carbohydrates, sugar, caffeine, nicotine, and alcohol.

HERBAL ALLIES

- **Yellow dock** (*Rumex crispus*), to replenish iron
- **Nettles**, rich in iron and other essential vitamins and minerals
- **Lady's mantle**, to stop the bleeding

Caution: do not use *Dong Quai* while experiencing heavy bleeding, for it is a blood mover and may intensify the bleeding.

CHINESE PATENT REMEDIES

- **Yunnan Pai Yao** (Yunnan White Powder); use until the bleeding stops
- **Gui Pi Wan** (Restore Spleen Pill) to support the Spleen, *or* **Bu Tiao** (Nourish Blood, Adjust Period Pill) to support Kidney and Spleen energies and relieve congestion in the pelvic area

ACUPOINTS

A special point to control bleeding is located on the knuckle of the big toe. Press hard on both toes.

For deficient Spleen and Kidney *chi*: **Spleen 4**, **Spleen 6**, **Kidney 3**, and **Conception Vessel 4**.

For Liver stagnation and heat in the blood, add **Liver 3**.

body proudly, with shoulders back and chin held high. Her color had returned, and around her temples, I detected a greenish-yellow hue, an indication of imbalances in Wood and possibly Earth energies. Her square physique, well-proportioned body, and strong voice supported the presence of wood energy, but her affinity to Earth was clear in the fleshiness of her skin, the singsong quality to her voice, and a persistent heaviness of spirit, expressed in her tendency to worry and obsess about her problems.

Most people don't fall cleanly into any one constitutional type, and when an individual is healthy, happy, and asymptomatic (experiencing no unusual pain or discomfort), she will typically display a blended mixture of the Five Transforming Powers. The particular affinities become most obvious when an imbalance or deficiency exists, and in Claire's case, both Wood and Earth were calling out for attention. As time went by and Claire's symptoms gradually resolved, her natural Wood constitution and strong connections to Earth kept shifting and changing; as her body/mind/spirit became more balanced and integrated, she became more difficult to classify as one type or another.

In this second session, I reported the good news from the gynecologist: Claire's laboratory tests revealed no pathology or abnormalities. As a result, we would continue to treat Claire's problems as symptoms of an underlying hormonal imbalance and energy blockage. "Your symptoms of flooding, clotting, lethargy, and exhaustion support a diagnosis of what the Chinese call 'stuck' energy," I said.

"That's exactly how I feel, as if I'm dammed up inside," Claire said, immediately responding to the word *stuck*. "No matter how hard I try, I can't seem to break through. I feel as if I'm beating my head against the proverbial wall."

"The bleeding was certainly a breakthrough," I said.

"Yes, it was, wasn't it?" Claire said, surprised by the sudden insight.

"When you started to bleed uncontrollably, what do you think your body was trying to say?" I asked.

Claire was thoughtful for a moment. "I think I know," she said, looking proud of herself. "I think my body was trying to say, 'I won't be held back.'"

"What have you been holding back?"

"My creativity—I've always had this deep need to express myself, but for years now I've been stuck." Claire started to cry then, and her words tumbled over each other, seeking an outlet. In her twenties and early thirties, she had committed her life to writing poetry, and after several years of devoted effort she succeeded in publishing several poems. When she met her future husband, also a struggling writer, she was working on a collection of poems and had just secured an agent. But after they were married, she immersed herself in his work, helping to research and edit his nonfiction articles; the more successful he became, the more she devoted herself to his career and neglected her own. Eventually she stopped writing altogether.

"I used to love editing my husband's work," Claire said, "but now I feel as if I'm all dried up and have no creative spark. I can't seem to drum up the energy to get my own work done and most of the time I just sit at home, trying to get interested in a book or watching a talk show and eating junk food."

In Chinese philosophy, the "creative spark" is called the *Hun*, and the Liver, which is responsible for the steady flow of energy throughout the system, is called the House of the *Hun*. If we imagine that we are each a hollow bamboo pipe, then the breath that fills the pipe and creates a unique sound is the *Hun*—the individual's creative spirit. If the bamboo pipe is occupied by another person's breath (in Claire's case, her husband's) or if it is somehow obstructed, the tone and pitch will be distorted. Because a healthy Liver allows the spirit to be expressed clearly and forcefully, the Chinese use acupuncture to support and strengthen the Liver functions, thus nourishing the *Hun* and permitting its clear, undistorted expression.

In that session and others that followed, we concentrated on acupoints that would help build the blood and yin, break up energy blockages, and allow nourishment to penetrate deep into Claire's body/mind/spirit. Pericardium 6 (Inner Frontier Gate), located on the forearm a few inches above the wrist crease, is considered the gateway to the Heart; when we stimulate this point, we oil the hinges to the Heart, permitting the gate to open and close easily and efficiently. Liver 3 (Great Rushing), located between the big toe and second toe, helps to dispel blockages and obstructions, allowing the *chi* and blood to flow freely. Liver 13 (Camphorwood Gate, or Official Gate), located on the rib cage two inches above the navel and about six inches on either side of the midline, directly supports the Spleen/Pancreas functions and would help Claire assimilate physical and emotional nourishment. Spleen 6 (Three Yin Meeting), located above the interior ankle bone just behind the tibia, builds and supports the yin, nourishing the blood and balancing the menstrual cycle.

The most important point for Claire was Spleen 4 (Ancestor and Descendant), located on the inner arch of the foot in a hollow approximately one and a half inches behind the knuckle of the big toe. This point is used to open a special channel called chong mo (penetration channel), which builds and supports the blood and, on a more basic level, allows nourishment to penetrate deep into the body/mind/spirit. The Chinese believe that only when we are well nourished, balanced, and whole can we be of any real assistance to others. When I stimulate this point, I talk about the importance of taking in and absorbing nourishment (food, water, love, creative energy) so that these live-giving forces can flow through the system, creating more blood to replenish what has been lost, breaking up areas of stagnation, and building a strong, healthy sense of the self.

As we talked about various strategies to help Claire overcome her feelings of stuckness and stagnation, I shared several stories with her. One particular story seemed to affect her deeply.

> *Abbot Mark and Abbot Arsenius were discussing the role of pleasure in the life of a monk. "I once knew a brother who noticed a wildflower growing in his cell and immediately pulled it up by the roots," said Abbot Mark. "Is it right, I wonder, to deny oneself such small pleasures?"*
>
> *"Well, yes, that is fine," said Abbot Arsenius after a moment's reflection, "for each human being must follow his own mind and heart. But if the brother realized later that he was unable to live without the flower, then he should plant it again and nurture it with tender care and devotion."*

"I uprooted my own career when I devoted my life to my husband," Claire said, immediately applying the story to her own life. "For a while,

I got along just fine without it. But times have changed, and I'm ready to plant the flower again."

Claire decided to resume her poetry writing. As she began to devote more time to her own career, her relationship with her husband became strained; eventually they decided to separate. Although her life is in transition, marked by many emotional and spiritual upheavals, Claire insists that she has never been happier. "I keep thinking about that hollow bamboo pipe," she told me in a recent session. "My goal right now is to fill it with pure, clean energy. Once I recognize the sound of my own creative voice, I won't ever again allow myself to forget it."

The seeds of creativity that burst forth in such abundance in the spring and early summer of a woman's life often lay dormant when she turns her attention to a lover, husband, or children. But during the transition period known as menopause, women instinctively turn their attention to those neglected seeds, seeking to rediscover the unique individual they were before sexuality and reproduction became the primary focus of their lives. If menopause is reframed as an opportunity to recover and recreate your "real" self—the "passionate, idealistic, energetic young individual who existed before menstruation," as Germaine Greer puts it in *The Change*—then we can begin to understand the depth and potential of this remarkable metamorphosis.

But first, a good deal of work needs to be done to clear away the prevailing conception of menopause as a dreaded event to be forestalled and pushed out of mind as long as possible. In our modern-day culture women have learned to view the onset of menopause as the beginning of the end of their life, marking an inevitable (and inevitably accelerating) descent into frailty, debility, and dependence. Subtle symptoms and signs are ignored and left untreated in the hope that life can go on as usual. Beneath the surface, however, profound changes are taking place in the body/mind/spirit, which begins to call out for additional sources of nourishment in order to deal with the increased strain.

"A good horse jumps at the shadow of the whip," states a Zen proverb, but in our culture, we have become immune to shadows. Indeed, we have to feel the full sting of the whip—the telltale hot flash, the sudden hemorrhage, the deep depression—before we agree to slow down and listen to what our body is trying to tell us.

In her book *The Silent Passage*, Gail Sheehy relates her personal experience with the "first bombshell of the battle with menopause":

It was a Sunday evening. Snug inside a remarriage not yet a year old, I was sitting utterly still, reading, in a velvet-covered armchair. A pillow's throw away my husband was doing the same, while jazz lapped at our ears and snow curtained the window. Every so often we looked up and congratulated ourselves on staying home in this cocoon of comfort and safeness and love we had created.

Then the little grenade went off in my brain. A flash, a shock, a sudden surge of electrical current that whizzed through my head and left me feeling shaken, nervous, off-balance. . . . I felt hot, then clammy. I tried lying down, but sleep could not soak up the agitation. My heart was racing, but from what? Complete repose? I felt, for perhaps the first time in my life since the age of thirteen, profoundly ill at ease in my body.

Hoping to find some relief for her distress, Sheehy made an appointment with her gynecologist, who asked her a series of questions, noted her symptoms, dutifully stuck her with a needle, and sent her blood to be analyzed. After receiving the laboratory report, he announced that yes, indeed, her estrogen levels were very low. What about hormone replacement therapy? she asked. That wasn't an option, he explained, because she was still menstruating. According to the strict medical definition of menopause, Sheehy learned, you're not really *in* it until you're "menstruation-free" for at least a year.

Hesitantly, she brought up the painful subject of her waning interest in sex. "It's nothing I can help you with," her physician responded. "Decrease in sexual response is just a natural part of aging." Sheehy left her doctor's office feeling as though she had been handed a "one-way ticket to the Dumpster." The question that haunted her restless days and sleepless nights was, "Does this mean I can't be me anymore?"

When women walk into my office after an experience like Gail Sheehy's, I know I have a lot of work to do. I notice their hunched shoulders, I listen to their expressions of hopelessness, I feel as if I could touch their despair. Their encounters with conventional Western medicine have taken their hope away; without hope, they feel powerless and out of control. The most commonly asked question is inevitably some variation of Gail Sheehy's question: *Is this normal? Am I dying? Is this the beginning of the end? What is happening to me?*

My first and most important task is to swing open the gates of hope, and I begin that process by listening, reassuring, and sharing the wisdom of ancient and modern-day healers through the vehicle of storytelling. I explain that the Western view of menopause—a view based on an obsession with youth and beauty—is not the only "frame" available. Borrowing the rich images of rebirth and regeneration offered by Native American, Chinese, and other traditional cultures, this momentous life experience can be reimagined as a time for celebration rather than mourning.

Many traditional cultures teach that when a woman stops menstruating, she leaves the purely physical world and steps up to a higher spiritual plane. The Native American culture, for example, emphasizes the power that menstrual blood confers on the "grandmothers" of the tribe, who are no longer required to give their blood away.

> When a woman stops her bleeding, she is permitted into the Grandmother Lodge. Her rich blood, which she has given away for all the years of her fertility and childbearing, is held inside now; it cleanses and renews her, giving her the strength of a powerful warrior. In the Grandmother Lodge she gathers together with the other white-haired women to see what can be done about the world and to use her great powers to nurture and protect all life: not just the lives of her children, her tribe, or her nation, but the life of the earth itself and all its living inhabitants.
>
> The great and mystical powers of the white-haired women are used for peace and to ensure the renewal of the cycle of life.

The Native Americans view menstrual blood as inestimably precious; in the process of aging and maturing, a woman gives the gift of the blood back to herself, strengthening and renewing herself to become a powerful warrior whose wisdom is treasured by all members of the tribe. Traditional Chinese Medicine shares this view of menstrual blood as powerful and life enhancing. The Chinese consider the long transition from monthly bleeding to no bleeding at all a strain on the body's energy resources, but as long as a woman lives in harmony with nature and gets sufficient rest, exercise, and nutritious foods, menopause should not cause any serious or long-lasting problems. If a woman experiences long-term pain or discomfort, a doctor schooled in Traditional Chinese Medicine would ask her to view these symptoms as distress signals alerting her to an underlying deficiency or imbalance.

The Chinese offer a lovely analysis of the aging process. During pregnancy, a woman gives to her offspring the gift of *jing*, an inherited form of vital energy that lasts thirty to forty years, depending on the health of the mother during her pregnancy. As our prenatal (inherited) *jing* is gradually depleted in the process of living, we must create our own *chi* and blood, which is transformed into postnatal *jing* and stored in the Kidneys. This acquired *jing* supplements and augments our original inheritance, and as long as we stay healthy and happy, the body/mind/spirit will continue to have access to an abundant supply of *jing*.

But by age thirty-five to forty, the reserves of prenatal *jing* have been steadily depleted, a condition that signals the beginning of the aging process. When a woman gives away her blood each month during her menstrual period, she loses a significant amount of *jing*; when the prenatal *jing* nears exhaustion, her body wisely cuts back on the monthly blood flow in order to conserve the precious *jing*. By holding on to her nourishing and life-giving blood, a woman protects her vital essence, replenishes her *chi* energy, and slows down the aging process.

The Kidneys, which store the *jing* and govern the entire life cycle of birth, maturation, and decline, are organs of mystery and magic in the Chinese system, cauldrons that bubble and teem with life. The authors of *Between Heaven and Earth* describe this organ orb in lyrical, almost mystical terms:

> The Kidney is like an island sea: on the surface languid and serene, fed by seasonal rains and crystal-pure underground rivers, with warm mineral-rich vapors bubbling up from beneath its floor, breathing renewal into salty waters that teem with primordial marine life. Submerged within us, the Kidney envelops the hidden, quintessential treasure house of life's potentiating power.

By midlife, when the initial investment of prenatal *jing* is nearly depleted, the Kidneys require continuous replenishing and support. "Tell me about your restorative lifestyle," a Chinese doctor might ask a woman who is approaching the change of life. The physician would want to hear that she is getting plenty of rest, exercising daily, managing her stress levels at work and home, meditating, eating and drinking wisely, taking various herbs and tonics to support her Kidney *chi*, and generally striving to live in harmony with her fellow human beings. If she has neglected to support her body/mind/spirit in these ways, she will begin to hear the Kidneys calling out to her with symptoms such as hot flashes, irritability, mood swings, back pain, sex drive changes, and heavier menstrual flow. If these distress signals go unheeded, they will arouse a reaction in the Liver, creating a rebellion of energy and blood, which in turn causes increasingly severe symptoms such as heavy bleeding and clotting, migraine headaches, depression, exhaustion, insomnia, and panic attacks.

Acupuncture and herbal remedies work at both the superficial and profound levels, helping to ease the symptoms and make the patient more comfortable while simultaneously working to correct the underlying cause of the problem. To reinstate balance and harmony, the Chinese doctor replenishes Kidney functions by stimulating certain acupuncture points and prescribing appropriate herbs and supplements. But equally important, the doctor sits down with the patient, listening, looking, advising, and encouraging her to discover creative ways to listen to her body/mind/spirit's cries for help. The doctor knows that once the patient understands that her symptoms point to a deeper disharmony, she must also accept the basic wisdom that the answers to her problems cannot be found outside herself but must emanate from within.

JANET

Fifty-year-old Janet walked into my office dressed in a beautiful wool suit with matching shoes and purse. Her prematurely white hair was pulled back from her finely chiseled face and fastened with a gold clip; not a strand of hair was out of place. Smoothing out her skirt, she sat down on the edge of the chair, back perfectly straight, chin high. Then she burst into tears.

"I'm a basket case," she said, reaching for a tissue and drying her tears. Ticking off her problems like a grocery list—hot flashes, mood swings, heavy periods with clotting, migraines, dry skin, depression, irritability, the blues, and the blahs—she looked me straight in the eye and said, "I'm afraid there's no hope for me."

"There's always hope," I said. "For example, your *shen* is very good."

"What is heaven's name is *shen?*" she asked, her frown indicating that she wanted straight-line answers and would not welcome unnecessary diversions.

"The Chinese believe that the quality of a person's heart or spirit can be seen in their eyes, which are considered the window to the soul," I explained. "Brilliantly clear eyes with lots of shine and sparkle indicate good, healthy *shen*; clouded eyes that emit no sparkle or glint point to an alarming weakening of the life force. Your eyes sparkle and shine, which means that your spirit is strong, and thus your prognosis is very good."

"Well, that's good, I guess," Janet said. Her mouth suddenly twisted, and she started crying again. "But then why am I so miserable?"

I talked about *jing* and *chi* and the natural stresses of menopause on the Kidney and the Liver, explaining that when Janet's body adjusted to the hormonal changes and when the underlying imbalances were corrected, she would feel herself again. Then I asked Janet to put her symptoms into the context of her life. When and how did they begin? What was happening in her life at the time—were there any unusual life stresses, career changes, emotional upheavals? Were the mood swings, irritability, and depression constant and consistent, or did they change in intensity or duration from day to day or from month to month? How did she cope with the demands of her busy life when she was experiencing these painful and debilitating symptoms? What effect did her emotions have on the more purely physical symptoms of hot flashes, heavy periods, migraines, and dry skin?

The Chinese believe that powerful emotions, especially repressed anger, grief, and frustration, can trigger hot flashes, heavy bleeding, migraines, and insomnia. Any intense emotion, even an overabundance of excitement or joy, restricts the blood vessels and creates certain autonomic nervous system symptoms.

"When you repress or stifle an emotion, the pent-up energy can cause hot flashes and other physical symptoms," I explained to Janet. "It's not necessarily the anger itself that causes the reaction but the feeling of being pent up inside and unable to express your feelings. In the Western world, we try to separate ourselves from our emotions, but in that process, we actually contribute to the disease process. When people stuff their feelings inside, they increase the pressure on an already stressed system. If we can reclaim our emotions, even (or perhaps especially) our negative emotions, and give ourselves permission to express them clearly, we will become more whole."

As Janet talked about her problems, it became clear that her major emotional symptom was an overwhelming feeling of hopelessness. She believed that something was deeply wrong with her—"I'm a monster in disguise," she said in that first session. But every doctor she had consulted (and there had been half a dozen in the last year) told her that nothing was *physically* wrong with her, everything was perfectly "normal," and if she would relax and stop working so hard, all would be well.

"All is not well," Janet told me, "and if this is normal and I'm only in the beginning of menopause, then how will I ever make it through the next week, let alone the next five or ten years?"

Accustomed to thinking logically and rationally, always looking for the shortest route from here to there, Janet wanted answers *right now*. As she discussed her situation, always taking care to be precise and meticulously detailed, I began to get a sense of her underlying strength and vitality. After college, she married, raised two children, and devoted herself to volunteer work in her community. When her children were in high school, she went back to law school and, just a few years after graduation, established a successful practice as an environmental lawyer with a large New York City legal firm. She valued discipline and order, and expressed an impatience with "superficial" people, "trite" conversations, and "meaningless" pursuits. Her immaculate appearance, precisely organized schedule, and well-developed aesthetic sense revealed a strong affinity to Metal. Wood was also an important part of her basic constitution and was apparent in the choppy, aggressive tone of her voice, the subtle greenish hue around her mouth and temples, and the solid, muscular nature of her physical constitution. Many of her symptoms, particularly the symptoms of being stuck or constrained—hot flashes, shortness of breath, muscle tension, and blood clotting—supported a diagnosis of deficient Wood energy.

The tongue and pulse examinations confirmed that imbalances existed in both Wood and Metal. Janet's tongue was relatively dry with a red tip and sides; the surface of her tongue was covered with a slight yellow film. The dryness indicated a depletion of moisture, or yin (fluid), strongly suggesting a deficiency in Kidney energy. The tip of the tongue relates to the Heart and the Lung, and the sides reveal information about health and vitality of the Liver; the redness and swelling signaled irritation in those organ functions. The slight yellow coating suggested minor digestive upsets. When I explained that her Liver functions seemed to be out of balance, apparently aggravating her digestion, Janet confirmed that she was experiencing digestive upsets.

Janet's pulse felt like a thin, tight thread against my finger. The feeble, forceless quality of her pulse supported a diagnosis of deficient Kidney yin, and the tightness suggested hyperactivity in the Liver, suggesting constrained Liver energy. In the Lung position (the pulse closest to the wrist on the radial artery of the right hand), I detected a soft, deficient quality, indicating some sadness or ongoing depression, or perhaps a chronic mucous condition in the Lungs.

When I palpated the fourteen bilateral trigger points on the Liver meridian, which begins at the big toe and runs all the way up the inside of the leg onto the torso, ending on the thoracic cage, two ribs below the nipple, Janet involuntarily flinched or shuddered. Every point along the Liver meridian appeared to be sensitive to the touch, and I could feel the muscle tension overlying the meridian itself, another indication that the energy along this pathway was blocked or constrained.

After completing the various examinations, I discussed my diagnosis and treatment plan, explaining that her Liver functions appeared to be out of balance, caused in part by a deficiency in Kidney yin, or fluid. When the Kidney yin dries up, the Liver (which is governed by Wood) becomes dry, brittle, and easily inflamed, creating the symptoms of hot flashes, irritability, and mood swings. When this occurs (and it is a common condition in menopausal women), the acupuncturist stimulates and invigorates the different meridians by inserting acupuncture needles in specific sites. Herbal therapy, dietary changes, and various stress-reduction techniques also help to correct the underlying imbalances.

"Will the acupuncture and herbs offer me any long-term protection?" Janet asked. "Several doctors have told me that my combination of symptoms—specifically the depression, insomnia, night sweats, and hot flashes—makes me a perfect candidate for hormone replacement therapy. But I'm not convinced that long-term drug therapy is the answer. What do you think I should do?"

Whenever I am asked about hormone replacement therapy (HRT), I take a deep breath and prepare to dive into troubled waters. *To take or not to take:* that is the question most women ask as they enter the menopausal years, and unfortunately there is no easy answer. A woman must learn everything she can about the risks and benefits of HRT and then make the choice for herself. My job is to offer advice about the various tests and laboratory analyses available, suggest resources and reading materials, and then step back, letting the patient make the final decision.

The benefits of HRT relate to the bones and the heart. Osteoporosis is a progressive disease in which the bones thin and become more porous, leading to a higher risk of broken arms, hip fractures, and spinal (vertebral) fractures. Estrogen appears to retard bone loss, which in women is accelerated for several years after menstrual periods cease due to a progressive loss of ovarian function and decreasing estrogen levels. At high risk for osteoporosis are thin white women who drink, smoke, and lead a sedentary lifestyle; if a woman has a family history of osteoporosis or if she had her ovaries removed before the age of forty, the risk is increased. For these high-risk patients, I recommend a bone scan to determine bone density and porosity; if the scan reveals a problem, hormone replacement therapy may be indicated for several years or even for the rest of her life (if the side effects can be tolerated).

To help reverse and retard the process of bone loss in women predisposed to osteoporosis, I recommend various lifestyle changes; a natural progesterone cream (progesterone in its natural form promotes the new growth of bone cells); a diet high in complex carbohydrates and low in fat, with severe limits on red meat and carbonated beverages (because these products are high in phosphorus, which leaches calcium from the bones); supplementation with vitamins A, C, D, magnesium, and calcium; and weight-bearing exercises such as walking, running, and weight training. With careful attention to diet, exercise, and stress management, hormone replacement therapy may not be necessary, even in high-risk patients.

While estrogen clearly prevents the loss of old bone, the hormone's protective effect against heart disease is more complicated. Estrogen supplements appear to increase levels of HDL (the "good" lipoproteins that help to lower blood cholesterol) and lower levels of LDL (the "bad" lipoproteins that raise blood cholesterol). Since LDL levels rise significantly after menopause, thereby increasing a woman's risk of heart disease, estrogen appears to reduce this risk. However, the studies showing that estrogen has a protective effect against heart disease have been accused of selective bias. In other words, it may not be the hormone that protects the heart from disease, but the fact that women who take the hormones are typically upper middle class and well educated, and thus more likely to be well nourished, to exercise regularly, have relatively low blood pressure, and follow their doctor's instructions. Their lifestyle may offer them more protection from disease than the fact that they take a daily hormone pill.

The heart-protecting benefits of hormone therapy are still theoretical and therefore controversial, but the risks are clear. Numerous studies conducted in the last two decades show that women who take estrogen are five to fourteen times more likely to develop uterine cancer; a 1986 study demonstrated that the risk of breast cancer is doubled. The risk of cancer increases the longer a woman takes the drug. By adding progestins (synthetic progesterone) to the hormone cocktail, the incidence of endometrial cancer was reduced to normal, but progestins do not appear to protect against breast cancer and may, in fact, increase the risk. The *level* of risk is currently being debated by the medical community, but no one argues that there aren't serious risks involved.

"Female reproductive hormones may someday be remembered as the most recklessly prescribed and dangerous drugs of this century," writes Sidney M. Wolfe, M.D., in his book *Women's Health Alert*. Many doctors, acupuncturists, and herbal therapists would agree, arguing the basic position that if menopause is not a disease, why use long-term drug therapy to treat it? I support Dr. Christiane Northrup's claim that "the best way to protect the heart is to live with passion and joy," and my work is dedicated to helping women look for ways in which their passion might be thwarted and suppressed. But in the end, the decision to take or not to take hormones must be left to the woman herself, who has to live with the consequences.

As we discussed the pros and cons of hormone replacement therapy, Janet admitted that she was seeking support for her decision not to use hormones. She had a deep and abiding faith in her body's ability to handle the stress of the change of life, and a natural distrust of external crutches and support. Her body, she knew, was strong and inherently sound; it had provided the firm foundation that kept her on her feet for all these years, and she felt a deep commitment to returning the favor. "I can't explain it," she told me, "but I feel as if I owe it to my body to give it everything I can, to support it as it has supported me all these years."

"Acupuncture and herbal therapy will be your allies in that decision," I said.

In that first session, I stimulated seven acupoints, six of which were bilateral. Kidney 3 (Great Mountain Stream), located between the inner ankle bone and Achilles tendon, is the source point of the Kidneys and strongly balances Kidney energies. Kidney 10 (Yin Valley), located in the back of the knee on the inner side in the depression between the tendons, is the Water point on the Water meridian and thus strongly supports the yin. Spleen 6 (Three Yin Meeting), located three inches above the inner ankle bone behind the tibia, is the classic point to nourish the yin. Liver 3 (Great Rushing), located between the big toe and the second toe, is the most important point to break through blockage and obstruction, helping to unclog constrained energy. Liver 8 (Spring at the Bend), located on the inside of the knee where the bones meet on the inside crease, is used to support the yin of the Liver.

MENOPAUSAL SYNDROME

(HOT FLASHES, ANXIETY, DEPRESSION, DIGESTIVE PROBLEMS, SEXUAL PROBLEMS)

WESTERN INTERPRETATION AND TREATMENT

A hormonal imbalance with a depletion of estrogen is identified as the cause of this syndrome, which is intensified by psychological complaints such as "empty nest syndrome" and "midlife crisis." It is generally treated with hormone replacement therapy (HRT), although symptoms are often treated individually: for depression, antidepressants are prescribed; for insomnia, sleeping pills; for bloating, diuretics; and for anxiety, tranquilizers.

CHINESE INTERPRETATION

The Chinese identify two major syndromes underlying the menopausal transition; these syndromes may or may not occur together: (1) Deficient Kidney yin leads to deficient Liver yin with rising Fire signs (anxiety, palpitations, headaches, hot flashes, night sweats). In predisposed women, the deficient Liver yin can lead to deficient Heart yin, causing such symptoms as insomnia, forgetfulness, and palpitations. (2) Deficiency in Kidney and Liver *chi* is characterized by stagnation and stuckness, which further weaken the Spleen and Kidney, creating a condition of chronic depression and hopelessness, as well as symptoms of indigestion, metabolic sluggishness, weight gain, lethargy, and fatigue.

COMPLEMENTARY TREATMENTS

SUPPLEMENTS

- **Vitamin B-complex** (best to use the high potency B-100 formula*)

*The B-100 designation indicates that the product contains 100 mg each of the B vitamins. Recommended dosage is one tablet per day, or as directed.

- **Vitamin B$_6$** (100–200 mg/day in addition to B-complex)
- **Calcium** (500 mg/day)
- **Magnesium** (1,000 mg/day)
- **Natural progesterone cream** (ProGest Cream or Wild Yam Cream), which can prevent and reverse osteoporosis, subdue hot flashes, and reduce anxiety; use ¼ to ½ teaspoon rubbed into lower belly, inner thighs, or armpits twice daily or as directed by your practitioner. If you are still menstruating, use the cream from midcycle until the onset of menses; if your periods have stopped, use it for fifteen days of each month.

EXERCISE

Exercise is extremely important during the menopausal years. General movement keeps the blood and energy flowing and prevents problems from occurring later on in life. Cardiovascular exercise keeps the heart healthy, while weight-bearing exercises help prevent osteoporosis.

HERBAL ALLIES

- **Chasteberry** and **St. John's wort** are the premier menopausal allies. For specific menopausal symptoms, see recommendations below.

CHINESE PATENT REMEDIES

- **Gia Wei Hsiao Yao Wan** (Relaxed Wanderer Pills)—a variation of **Hsiao Yao Wan** formulated specifically for the menopausal woman—for relief of the deficient yin/rising heat symptoms (hot flashes, insomnia, night sweats)
- **Ding Xin Wan** (Heart Stabilizing Tablets) for relief of anxiety, depression, insomnia, forgetfulness, hot flashes

ACUPOINTS

Conception Vessel 4, Kidney 3, Kidney 10, Liver 3, Liver 14, Pericardium 6, and **Heart 7**

SPECIFIC SYMPTOMS AND TREATMENTS

- **Mood swings:** Exercise is essential, for depression and anxiety both reflect stuckness, or stagnation, and physical exercise will assist the Liver in moving the stuck *chi* energy. **St. John's wort** stabilizes the nervous system. For chronic anxiety try **skullcap** (*Scutellaria*) and the Chinese patent formula **An Mian Pian** (Peaceful Sleep Pills). **Natural sunlight** helps to counter depression; also for depression try **Gui Pi Wan** (Restore Spleen Pills), which strengthen the Spleen, nurture the Heart and spirit, and build *chi*.

- Digestive problems (weight gain, sluggish metabolism, constipation, diarrhea, chronic nausea): To support metabolic function, try **dandelion root**. If "cold" prevails (loose bowels, chills, fear of the cold, pale tongue), try **ginger**. Add acupoints **Spleen 6** and **Stomach 36**.

- Sexual problems (lack of desire, lubrication problems): If vaginal dryness is a problem, try a lubricant such as K-Y Jelly, vitamin E oil, or cold-pressed natural oils such as sesame, safflower, almond, or coconut; use your fingers to rub the oil or jelly into the vaginal area. **Nettles** and **raspberry leaves** gently build up the *chi* energy and replenish the system. *Dong Quai* or **ginseng** support Kidney function to increase lubrication and sexual interest. **Natural progesterone cream** helps relieve dryness of vaginal tissues. **Kegel exercises** increase circulation to the pelvic area, nourishing and toning vaginal and uterine tissues and enhancing orgasms. To stimulate sexual desire, try acupoints **Kidney 3**, **Kidney 7**, **Governing Vessel 4**, and **Conception Vessel 4**. To stimulate lubrication, try **Spleen 6**, **Kidney 3**, and **Kidney 10**.

- Hot flashes: Avoid spicy foods and caffeine. Add **vitamin E** (800 iu/day alpha tocopherol). For herbal allies, try **motherwort, black cohosh, Chasteberry,** and *Dong Quai*. A specific Chinese patent remedy for hot flashes, insomnia, and night sweats is **Da Bu Yin Wan** (Major Yin Supplement Pills). **Natural progesterone** subdues hot flashes. For acupoints, add **Liver 3**. Ask yourself, What's burning me up? How have I suppressed my passion (or my pain, creativity, anger)?

- Flooding: See menorrhagia box (page 246).

MIND/BODY/SPIRIT CONNECTION

The symptoms might be expressing these questions:

- "I feel stuck—how can I move through these feelings of stagnation and stuckness?"

- "I'm being called to move on in my life, but where am I going?"
- "I'm holding on to my blood so that I can become stronger and wiser—how can I share what I've learned and move forward with strength and vigor?"
- "What is essential in my life? What can I give up? What must I keep?"

The final two points—Liver 14 (Gate of Hope), located two ribs below each nipple, and Conception Vessel 3 (Central Pole), located three inches above the pubic bone on the midline of the belly—were particularly important for revitalizing and rejuvenating Janet's body/mind/spirit. When I inserted the needles, I asked her to meditate on the poetry of these points.

"Think of the Central Pole as sinking deep into the earth and tapping an underground stream of perfectly clear and unpolluted water," I suggested. "Imagine that the needle is bringing this pure springwater up into your body to cleanse and renew your cells."

Liver 14 is the quintessential point for stagnation of stuckness. "This point will help ease your feelings of being stuck in one place and unable to proceed," I said. "From your symptoms, it seems that you feel as if you are trying to open a door that is cemented shut. No matter how hard you try, you can't get this door open; the more you work at it, the more frustrated and disheartened you become. Imagine, as I stimulate this point, that you are suddenly freed from a one-dimensional view of the world. Now you have a three hundred sixty-five–degree view, and you can see that there are other doors to open, each of which has well-oiled hinges. Practice going up to these doors, and opening and closing them whenever you wish. Become familiar with the many choices available to you."

It took only a few minutes to insert the needles; afterward, Janet and I talked about the meaning and significance of Metal, both the underlying energy supporting her body/mind/spirit, and the nature of the season she was entering. We talked about grief and loss and letting go, and I told her a popular Zen teaching story that illustrates the necessary mind-set for this stage of life.

A university professor approached a master hoping to learn about the nature of Zen. "I know a great deal about the workings of the physical world," the scholar explained, "but perhaps you could add to

*my knowledge by offering some thoughts about the nature of the spiritual
world."*

*"Let us have a cup of tea," said the master, "and then we shall
talk." The professor held out his cup as the master poured, filling the
cup to the brim and then continuing to pour while the tea spilled onto
the floor.*

"It is overflowing!" protested the professor. "No more will go in!"

*"Yes, it is so," said the master. "Just as this cup is full to overflowing,
so is your mind filled with opinions and speculations, leaving no room
to receive the teachings. Only when you empty your cup, can we begin."*

When I removed the needles and asked Janet how she was feeling, she
claimed she was "floating." "Something has changed," she said. "Everything looks calmer and brighter. I'm not sure I understand what you were
talking about, but it sounded beautiful in a strange kind of way, and
something broke through. I feel this amazing energy—it's an incredible
feeling."

Janet responded to the herbs in the same openhearted, open-minded
manner. As I discussed the different personalities and properties of the
herbal remedies, explaining that their basic purpose was to nourish the
yin energy, building up the fluid levels in her body, while supporting
and invigorating the *chi*, she listened attentively.

"Chasteberry is a very earthy, grounded herb that works differently for
each person, adapting itself to your specific imbalances and deficiencies,"
I explained. "It will help you feel more supported and balanced, physically,
emotionally, and spiritually. Dandelion root is one of my favorite herbs
and a wonderful ally for a constrained Liver. It will help support your
digestion and replenish your Liver *chi*. St. John's wort is a comforting and
soothing nervous-system restorant with very calm, waterlike qualities. It
will help smooth out your irritability, anxiety, depression, and hot flashes.
Motherwort, a Native American herb with a balancing effect on the heart,
nervous system, and uterus, will help you to relax, ease your worries, and
allow you to get a good night's sleep."

We ended that first session with some thoughts on "a restorative lifestyle." For her diet, I strongly recommended that she avoid caffeine,
alcohol, and excessively greasy or spicy foods, all of which exacerbate Liver
imbalances. I encouraged her to continue her habit of daily exercise; because
her affinity to Wood was so strong, exercise was particularly important for
overcoming a tendency to stasis, the feeling of being stuck. She enjoyed

walking, and I recommended daily brisk walks of at least two miles, suggesting that she add weights as she walked or try some easy weight-bearing exercises to build up bone strength and density, thus preventing future problems with osteoporosis. As she exercised, she could try a wonderful breathing technique that would help to relieve tension and focus her mind.

Breathing Exercise

1. Breathe in to the count of 6; as you breathe in, imagine the pure, clean air entering your lungs.
2. Hold the breath for 24 counts and imagine that your cells are using this opportunity to empty their waste products into the bloodstream.
3. Exhale to 12 counts, visualizing the waste products exiting with your breath from your body.

Over the next three months Janet's hot flashes dissipated, her emotional fluctuations evened out, and she began to sleep "like a baby." At the end of that period, she was feeling so much better that she began bimonthly sessions, which eventually became monthly and then seasonal visits. Recently Janet sent me a quotation from the book *The Wit and Wisdom of Women*, with a short note attached. "I never did understand what you were talking about with the Metal this and the Wood that, the Liver this and the Kidney that," she wrote, "but somehow the meaning got through."

The quotation was Anne Morrow Lindbergh's:

Perhaps middle age is, or should be, a period of shedding shells; the shell of ambition, the shell of material accumulations and possessions, the shell of the ego. Perhaps one can shed at this stage in life as one sheds in beach-living; one's pride, one's false ambitions, one's mask, one's armor. Was that armor not put on to protect one from the competitive world? If one ceases to compete, does one need it? Perhaps one can at least in middle age, if not earlier, be completely oneself. And what a liberation that would be!

* * *

"All healing is *bian-bao*," the Chinese are fond of saying. If a tree has a diseased branch (*bian*), it is possible to treat only the symptoms by cutting off the branch, but a sick tree will eventually sprout another diseased branch and then another and another. To understand the nature of the problem, we must look deeper, to the root (*bao*) and then beyond the root to the soil and the atmosphere that nurture and support life.

Continuing with this metaphor, we gain a different perspective on the inherent biases of conventional Western medicine, which focuses almost exclusively on the diseased branch, ignoring prevention in favor of cure. Faced with a middle-aged woman who reports a myriad of "psychosomatic" symptoms, the conventional doctor hopes to track down an illness so that he can then suggest a treatment. If no illness is found and laboratory tests indicate that a woman's hormones are within normal range, her symptoms are typically ignored or treated with hormones, tranquilizers, sleeping pills, antidepressants, or painkillers.

"Pragmatic Americans consider the very existence of problems intolerable and life with problems unacceptable," wrote Luigi Barzini in *The Europeans*. "They believe . . . that all problems not only *must* be solved, but also that they *can* be solved, and that in fact the main purpose of a man's life is the solution of problems. They also believe (or want to believe) that 'a' solution, if not 'the' solution, can always be discovered."

But what can be done with the "problem" of menopause? Where is the enemy and how can it be neutralized? Unfortunately, even tragically, when the problem is identified as menopause itself, the uterus is targeted as the enemy and automatically placed in the crosshairs of conventional medicine's impressive weaponry.

"After the last planned pregnancy, the uterus becomes a useless, bleeding, symptom-producing, potentially cancer-bearing organ and therefore should be removed," suggested Dr. Ralph C. Wright in 1969. Although Wright's position is extreme (and thus often cited), his distaste for the uterus is publicly shared by other doctors, male and female alike. "Hysterectomy fits women's present needs," asserted Dr. Eleanor B. Easley, a gynecologist, in 1971. "It is an excellent procedure for sterilization. A woman is a more reliable worker after she's had one. It is advantageous at the menopause if only to simplify estrogen therapy. For some time I've been telling women that in another twenty years I expect hysterectomy to have become almost routine at the menopause."

"Menstruation is a nuisance to most women, and if this can be abolished without impairing ovarian function, it would probably be a blessing to not only the woman but to her husband," notes the 1975 edition of the widely used *Novak's Textbook of Gynecology*.

A 1987 editorial in the British medical journal *Lancet* promoted hysterectomy as an "attractive" solution for the woman who wishes to be finished with the business of reproduction, for the operation promises "relief from her symptoms and other expected benefits—greater reliability at work, availability at all times for sexual intercourse, saving on sanitary protection, freedom from pregnancy and freedom from uterine cancer."

In the United States, hysterectomy is the second most commonly performed operation (after cesarean sections); 90 percent of these operations are performed for benign or idiopathic diseases (those with an unidentified cause), which, if left to time and the healing power of nature, might well disappear without treatment. Sixty percent of hysterectomies are performed on women under the age of forty-four; one-third of all women in the United States will have their uterus surgically removed before they reach the age of sixty.

The popularity of this operation for conditions that are not life threatening and might eventually go away on their own would seem to indicate that it is completely safe and without complication, but hysterectomy, like all major surgeries, has its risks, many of them serious. One in one thousand hysterectomy patients die. Forty of every thousand patients suffer from complications that require hospitalization. Eight to 15 percent of patients require blood transfusions. One to 3 percent will need a second operation. The risk of urinary stress incontinence is significantly higher in women who have had hysterectomies. When both the uterus and ovaries are removed in a procedure called a hysterectomy-oophorectomy, between 33 and 46 percent of women report decreased sexual response; this procedure also doubles the patient's risk of coronary heart disease.

The uterus continues to be a functioning organ even after menopause, acting as a receptor site for estrogen and progesterone, which are continuously circulated throughout the system. The ovaries produce estrogen well past menopause; although the types of estrogen change, these hormones are believed to reduce cholesterol (a benefit to the heart) and aid in calcium absorption (a benefit to the bones). The uterus also serves an important function in keeping other pelvic organs in place and affecting in numerous ways (even, perhaps, just by its presence) sexual responsiveness.

In *Women's Health Alert*, Dr. Wolfe suggests that there are only three sufficient reasons for removing this organ: cancer of the uterus, ovaries, cervix, or fallopian tubes; abnormal uterine bleeding (uterine ruptures in childbirth or during an abortion or D & C, for example); and severe infections of the uterus and fallopian tubes associated with peritonitis, abscesses, and shock. Even in these cases, whenever possible, a woman should carefully discuss the alternatives with her doctor before surgery.

Whether a woman enters menopause naturally or artificially (via hysterectomy), this stage of life should be viewed as both significant and potentially life transforming. The various symptoms of pain and discomfort are important clues to the internal process of change, for the symptoms are literally and figuratively messages signaling the presence of deficiencies or imbalances that may be preventing change from occurring. Pain and discomfort are like road signs warning us to stop, yield, or slow down for the curves ahead; these symptoms also function as reminders that some maintenance work might be necessary in order to make the going a little smoother. Through careful attention to her symptoms, a woman can learn where her energy is blocked or stagnant and help her body heal itself.

If we did not feel pain, we would put our fingers to the flame and notice the wounded tissue only after the blisters had formed. Pain teaches and instructs; its purpose is to keep us healthy and alive. We cry out because we are in pain, and we are in pain because an imbalance or deficiency is calling out for attention. When we are in pain, something is wrong; it needs to be put right. But pain also reveals an entire world that would be closed off if we had only joy and happiness to contend with.

"Most people begin to open to their life not because there is joy, but because there is pain," writes Steven Levine in *Who Dies?* And Helen Keller once said: "We could never learn to be brave and patient if there were only joy in the world."

One of the most beautiful stories ever told about pain and loss is *The Wizard of Oz*. Four eccentric characters set off on a journey to search for the one trait they believe they are missing and cannot live without. Dorothy is searching for her home, the Scarecrow needs a brain, the Tin Man wants a heart, and the Lion is hoping to build up his courage. Filled with high hopes and eager for quick solutions, they follow the Yellow Brick Road— the road well traveled, the ordinary route, the established means to an end—and wend their way to Oz, convinced that the omnipotent Wizard will restore them to health and wholeness. But tricks of fate, good and evil witches, mind-altering poppy fields, singing dwarves, and flying monkeys create numerous detours in their journey.

Eventually the foursome encounters their shadow, the symbol of their deepest fears and insecurities—the wicked witch. Forced to defy evil with only her wits to save her, Dorothy tosses a bucket of water at the witch, and the specter melts before her very eyes. But still she does not understand the nature of her power, and with her faithful companions, she completes the journey to Oz for the final encounter with the Wizard.

When the great Wizard is exposed as a fraud, Dorothy is heartbroken. "You're a very bad man!" she accuses, to which the Wizard kindly responds, "Oh no, my dear, I'm a very good man. I'm just a very bad wizard."

The Wizard knows that his talents lie in his ability to guide others to the understanding that what they need has been inside them all along— to help them understand, through sleight of hand, magic, a spectacular light show, or whatever means necessary, that what they are searching for has also been searching for them.

A story is told about a monk—one of the Desert Fathers, an unorthodox group of ascetics who lived in the deserts of Egypt in the third and fourth centuries—who asked his elder for advice.

> *The brother had traveled a long way across the desert to see Abbot Moses in Scete, and he was exceedingly tired. "Can you give me a good word, Abbot?" he asked.*
>
> *"Return home," advised Abbot Moses, "sit quietly and patiently in your cell, and you will learn everything you need to know."*

The message in Oz and in the desert (and indeed in all of life) is the same: Be alert and sensitive to the inner self, refine your spirit, use your mind, trust your inner guides, and reject the dogmatic formulas of others who would tell you how to live your life. Listen to your heart, and you will find your way back home.

ALICE

Eight years ago a surgeon cut into Alice's womb and uprooted a fibroid the size of a four-month fetus. When another growth appeared, doubling in size within a year, her gynecologist recommended removing the uterus. "I'm afraid it's a breeding ground for these tumors," he said. Feeling like a petri dish swimming with noxious bacteria, Alice consulted another specialist, who recommended even more radical surgery. "Let's take out the works, even the appendix," he said, explaining that since she was nearing menopause and had no plans to have children, "these organs are really quite useless."

Alice came to me feeling frightened and defeated, hoping against hope to find some magical treatment that would prove her doctors wrong and save her from another major surgery. But she was skeptical. "I have to be honest with you," she said in the no-nonsense voice she used to quiet her fourth-grade class, "I don't believe in this kind of stuff—herbs, acupuncture, New Age mumbo-jumbo. But I'm scared, I'm tired of feeling out of control, and I don't want to lose any more body parts. What can you do for me?"

A forty-seven-year-old ball of fire with naturally curly red hair just beginning to go gray at the temples, Alice didn't appear to be afraid of anything. Always direct and straightforward, she refused to censor her thoughts in deference to my feelings. More than once, she told me that my images and stories were nice but on the fuzzy side. She wasn't interested, she insisted, in metaphorical explanations.

"I don't believe that illness has meaning," she told me in that first session. "It just is what it is, and I hate it. Can you shrink these growths or not?"

"I have techniques that can help, but I can't promise you a perfect ending," I said.

"I don't believe in perfection," Alice countered.

"Have you ever heard the story? . . ." I began, and told her one of my favorites.

> *Mulla Nasrudin was quietly sipping his tea when a friend approached him and with great excitement announced his intention to be married.*
>
> *"Mulla, have you never thought of marriage yourself?" his friend asked.*
>
> *"When I was young all I could think about was finding the perfect wife," Nasrudin admitted. "I traveled far and wide searching for her. In Damascus I met a beautiful, tender-hearted, profoundly spiritual woman, but she had no knowledge of the world. So I kept on looking. In Isphahah, I met a woman who was beautiful in every way, spiritually and physically; but for some reason, we were not able to communicate with each other. So I kept on looking. After much effort, I found the perfect woman in Cairo. She was deeply spiritual, filled with grace and beauty, at home in both the physical world and the spiritual realm. At last I knew I had found the perfect wife."*

"Why did you not marry her, Mulla?" asked his friend.
"Alas," said Nasrudin as he took another sip of tea, "she was also
waiting for the perfect husband."

Alice gave me the gift of a deep belly laugh, and with the ice broken, we were able to get down to work. The color that immediately called out was red—Alice's hair was red, her complexion was ruddy, and whenever she became excited (which was often), a natural rosy flush deepened to crimson. Her pulses were tight and a bit wiry, particularly in the Liver position. I noted the thinness of the Liver and Heart pulses, each of which felt like a flimsy guitar string hitting my finger with a tight *ping*, but without much force behind it. This pulse quality indicated that the energy used to support her underlying imbalances and deficiencies was beginning to drain her vital organs of their essential constitutional energy.

Alice's tongue was red, almost purple, with bumps on the bottom of the tongue, a characteristic commonly seen in women with fibroids. The sides and tip of the tongue were a darker, deeper red, indicating heat in the Liver and possibly in the Heart, the result of a serious yin deficiency. Bright red splotches on the tip of her tongue confirmed this condition of heat in the Heart, which is typically expressed as symptoms of insomnia, memory problems, breathlessness, anxiety, and/or heart palpitations.

The existence of fibroids suggests that the Liver is overworked and thus cannot fulfill its function of keeping the energy flowing freely through its channels, resulting in a condition the Chinese call "constrained Liver *chi*." As the *chi* energy is gradually depleted, the blood slows down and thickens, creating "congealed blood," which results in chronic pain, migraine headaches, and physical masses such as fibroids and tumors. The standard treatment involves dispersing the congealed blood through the techniques of acupuncture and herbal therapy, which over a period of several weeks or months will help the energy and blood flow freely once again.

I selected eight acupoints to stimulate. Conception Vessel 4 (Gate at the Source), located on the midline of the body about halfway between the navel and the pubic bone, taps into our source or root energies—the pilot light for the entire body. Conception Vessel 6 (Sea of Chi), located one and a half inches below the navel on the midline, supports Kidney *chi* and yang. I chose to stimulate Alice's yang energy because the yang tends to be slightly more invigorating than the yin, thus creating more energetic movement toward the pelvic region.

Spleen 6 (Three Yin Meeting) works together with Spleen 8 (Earth's

Crux) and Spleen 10 (Sea of Blood) to invigorate the entire system and move the blood through the stuckness. Liver 3 (Great Rushing), located between the big toe and second toe, moves the *chi* to break up blockages, and Heart 7 (Gate of Spirit), located on the inner wrist crease, supports the Heart fires, stabilizing and calming the spirit and helping Alice to relax and find a peaceful center. Pericardium 6 (Inner Frontier Gate) has similar actions to Heart 7, calming and pacifying the spirit and also serving to protect the Heart from noxious invasion.

For herbs, I suggested a combination of chasteberry, a wonderful, balancing herb that supports the functions of the corpus luteum (thus promoting progesterone and helping to combat the effects of estrogen, which stimulates the growth of fibroids); sage, which the Chinese value as a blood mover, helping to relieve congestion and stagnation; dandelion root to nourish the Liver and promote its functions of keeping the energy, blood, and emotions flowing; red clover, a blood cleanser and mover that appears to inhibit the spread of cancers (particularly breast and ovarian); and valerian root, a nervous system tonic and mild sedative that would help Alice relax. I also recommended the Chinese ready-made formula Hsiao Yao Wan (Free and Easy Wanderer Pills), which includes the herbs Bupleurum and *Dong Quai* and in China is considered the archetypical formula to relax a constrained Liver and instigate movement of *chi* and blood.

For her diet, I recommended that Alice avoid meat, poultry, and dairy products because these foods are loaded with artificial estrogens (and fibroids are estrogen dependent, or fed by estrogen) and follow a fiber-rich diet with lots of fresh vegetables, whole grains, and soy products (tofu, soy sauce, tempeh). Soya products contain plant estrogens, or phyto-estrogens, that bind to the estrogen receptor sites in the body, thus preventing the more harmful synthetic estrogens from entering the system. For supplements I recommended Vitamin B_6 (100 mg/day) and gamma linoleic acid (GLA; available in oil of evening primrose, 1,000 mg/day), in addition to a good multivitamin.

Alice faithfully followed the prescribed regimen of biweekly acupuncture sessions, daily herbal treatments, regular exercise, and good nutrition. During the acupuncture sessions, I continued to talk about the "meaning" of her fibroid, hoping to help her understand that this mass was not just a piece of tissue stuck to the wall of her uterus, but a part of her, even an important and meaningful part. What was the meaning of the "blocked energy" in her pelvis? What could she learn from her fibroids about her relationship to her body, her creativity, and her emotions?

FIBROIDS

WESTERN INTERPRETATION AND TREATMENT

Fibroids are benign tumors made of fibrous tissue growing in or on the uterus; there is no known cause for these growths. Although the tumor itself is not considered dangerous, fibroids can cause problems such as profuse bleeding or, by pressing against other organs, urinary urgency, incontinence, and pain due to nerve pressure. Over 50 percent of women over the age of forty have fibroids, which are responsible for one-third of all gynecological hospital admissions.

If the fibroid is not causing symptoms, most doctors take a "wait and see" attitude, since the tumors often disappear during menopause. Drugs to induce premature menopause (Lupron or Synarol) are sometimes prescribed for short time spans, usually to shrink fibroids in preparation for surgery. Progesterone therapy is prescribed if bleeding is a problem. Myomectomy (surgical excision of the fibroid tumor) is sometimes recommended, and hysterectomy is frequently advised (30 percent of all hysterectomies are performed for fibroids).

CHINESE INTERPRETATION

The Chinese offer two interpretations for fibroids: (1) Liver *chi* builds up and stagnates in the Lower Heater (pelvic region) leading to congealed blood; if not corrected, the congealed blood is transformed into a mass (fibroid). (2) A deficiency of Liver or Spleen *chi* can also lead to a condition of congealed blood in the Lower Heater, for the deficient *chi* is unable to keep the blood moving, which leads to stagnation.

COMPLEMENTARY TREATMENTS

SUPPLEMENTS

- **B-complex vitamin** (use the high-potency B-100 formula*)
- **Vitamin E** (alpha tocopherol, 400–800 mg/day)
- **Magnesium** (1,000–1,500 mg/day)

*The B-100 designation indicates that the product contains 100 mg each of the B vitamins. Recommended dosage is one tablet per day, or as directed.

TOPICAL TREATMENT

Castor oil packs, applied over the lower belly, stimulate circulation to the uterus and may help to reduce fibroid size. Kits can be ordered from the Woman to Woman Center, One Pleasant Street, Yarmouth, Maine 04096; (207) 846–6163.

EXERCISE

Because stagnation is involved, daily exercise is considered vitally important; acupuncture, chiropractic, or body work may help to free the energy in the pelvic area.

DIET

Increase natural phyto (plant) estrogens (found in soya products, brown rice, yams). Avoid synthetic estrogenic foods (meats, poultry, dairy products, eggs), refined carbohydrate products (sugars, white flour products), alcohol, caffeine, nicotine, and oral contraceptives.

HERBAL ALLIES

These herbs can be combined to make an effective tonic. A balanced formula would be 40 percent chasteberry and 20 percent each sage, false unicorn root, and dandelion root.

- **Chasteberry**, to support progesterone production
- **Common garden sage**, to move the blood and support the circulation
- **False unicorn root**, to balance hormones
- **Dandelion root**, to help the Liver eliminate excess estrogen

CHINESE PATENT REMEDIES

- **Hsiao Yao Wan** (Relaxed Wanderer Pills) to support the Liver and encourage free movement of blood and *chi*

ACUPOINTS

Liver 3, Spleen 6, Spleen 10, and Liver 14

MIND/BODY/SPIRIT CONNECTION

The symptoms might be expressing these questions:

- "What is the purpose of the fibroid—what is it telling me about how I might have blocked my energy or creativity?"
- "Where do I feel stuck in my life?"
- "How can I free up my energy and live life more fully?"

Alice listened politely to my ramblings but kept her opinions to herself.

Six months after Alice first began treatments, she was lying down on the table, her eyes closed, when she announced that she had some news. In a businesslike tone, she told me that her gynecologist had informed her that the fibroid was only half its original size.

"That's wonderful!" I said. "How does that make you feel?" I expected to hear something along the lines of "It's about what I expected," but instead Alice put both hands on her lower abdomen, and the tension in her face and body relaxed for the first time since I had known her.

"I know this will sound strange coming from me," she said, "but I feel as if this fibroid is a baby. It's me as a baby, the person I never allowed myself to be. You see, I was always the rebel, the upstart, the obnoxious kid doing something to get into trouble, hoping to be noticed, while my parents were always obsessed with appearances, telling me to stick my stomach in, hold my chin up, and keep my thoughts and feelings to myself. I'll never forget my mother 'comforting' me by telling me to keep a stiff upper lip and to stop feeling sorry for myself, because there were so many people worse off in the world than me. And now I see that this growth was asking me to mother it, to take care of it, even to love it. I've become attached to it, as it is to me. I feel as if it's the 'me' that never got to grow up and express her feelings."

Alice was talking about the meaning of her fibroid—what it meant to her, and what she believed it was trying to tell her. She was asking for advice from within, turning to her body and using its wisdom to learn more about her heart and soul.

"I never realized how much it means to me to be a woman until I was faced with the thought of losing my uterus," she continued. "I remember thinking—how can I live with a hole at the center of my being? And I wondered what would take the place of that hole—would it fill up with fluids, would tissues from my bladder and other pelvic organs encroach, or would I just have a void at my center for the rest of my life?

"And I realized then that I didn't want to lose this vital organ," Alice concluded. "I never had the opportunity to have children, I never really wanted to have a child—but my uterus is part of me. I didn't want to continue on into the next part of my life without it. Now it looks like I won't have to. I feel intact, complete, healed. For the first time in many, many years, I feel as if I'm whole again."

The journey to wholeness is an ongoing process of give and take, catch and release, expand and contract. To become whole, we must let something die in order that something else might live. "Everything that comes alive seems to be in trade for something that dies, cell for cell," wrote Lewis Thomas in *The Lives of a Cell*. This continuous process of taking in and letting go distinguishes life from beginning to end, but women feel it most acutely during menopause, for this is the time when they must confront the death of their reproductive cells. As a woman grieves for the loss, she can begin to turn her attention to the gain: What will come alive now? What changes will take place? How will my life complete itself? *The I Ching* lovingly describes the give and take of life:

> When the sun goes, the moon comes; when the moon goes, the sun comes. Sun and moon alternate; thus light comes into existence. When cold goes, heat comes; when heat goes, cold comes. Cold and heat alternate, and thus the year completes itself. The past contracts. The future expands. Contraction and expansion act upon each other; hereby arises that which furthers.

In the autumn of her life, a woman takes these lessons deep within her, where they take root and grow. She has seen the beginning and the end of both spring and summer, and she feels the chill of approaching winter. Having lived this long, she understands the unrelenting nature of change, and rather than fight it, she learns to welcome the coming and going, the alteration and expansion, the ebb and flow, for in these continuous, predictable changes, she sees the cycle completing itself and then beginning over again.

When Thoreau was forty-three years old, just two years before his death, he stood in an open meadow by a brook and released the seeds from a milkweed pod. Enraptured, he watched the seeds soar, and his spirit seemed to lift off with them.

> When I release some seeds, the fine silky threads fly apart at once, opening with a spring—and then ray their relics out into a hemispherical form, each thread freeing itself from its neighbor, and all reflecting prismatic tints. These seeds are besides furnished with broad, thin margins or wings, which plainly keep them steady and prevent their whirling round. I let one go, and it rises slowly and uncertainly at first, now driven this way, then that, by invisible currents, and I fear it will make shipwreck against the neighboring wood. But no; as it approaches it, it surely rises above it, and then feeling the strong north wind, it is borne off rapidly in the opposite direction . . . ever rising higher and higher.

At this point in his musings, Thoreau shifts focus from the individual seed cases to the ongoing, never-ending cycle of the seasons. Generation after generation, the seeds sail off, each following its own separate path but all united in their need to take wing and fly off to new uncharted territories.

> Think of the great variety of balloons which at this season are buoyed up by similar means! How many myriads go sailing away thus, high over hill and meadow and river, on various tacks until the wind lulls, to plant their race in new localities. . . . And for this end these silken streamers have been perfecting themselves all summer, snugly packed in this light chest, a perfect adaptation to this end—a prophecy not only of the fall, but of future springs. Who could believe in prophecies . . . that the world would end this summer, while one milkweed with faith matured its seeds?

And so in the autumn of our lives, we learn to follow the milkweed's example, broadening our wings to keep steady, freeing ourselves from our neighbors, rising above, bounding across, buoyed and borne off by the winds, settling down only to rise again. With such deep faith in our own capabilities do we mature the seeds of heart and soul, creating ourselves anew from the inside out, over and over again. Perfectly poised between beginning and end, we see what we have never seen before, and the radiance of our vision lights the pathway before us.

> *The story is told that soon after his enlightenment the Buddha was walking down a country road. A passerby stopped him, awed by the radiant glow of peace and serenity that emanated from the Buddha's physical being.*
>
> *"What are you, my friend?" the man asked. "Are you a god or a messenger from the heavens?"*
>
> *"No," responded the Buddha.*
>
> *"Then you must be a sorcerer of some kind," said the man.*
>
> *"No," said the Buddha.*
>
> *"Are you just a human being?"*
>
> *"No."*
>
> *"Then what on earth could you be?"*
>
> *"I am awake," replied the Buddha.*

CHAPTER 16

WINTER: FROM BODY TO SOUL

If you stay in the center
and embrace death with your whole heart
you will endure forever.

—Tao te Ching

Our Native people rightly say that the responsibility of the nurturing and renewing of life is an enormous one, and thus requires an especially strong person to carry it off. They say the Moon pause women *are* especially strong because they retain the precious blood of life within them, and thus have extra energy available since there is no longer a need to make a place in the womb for a child every month. . . . This Moon pause grandmother . . . will be a very wise and visionary woman, because she will have retreated to Moon quest every Moon—thirteen times a year— for all the years of her menses, often thirty to forty years. *This depth of spirit and developed ability to call vision means she has powerful tools to use in her guidance of the people.*

—Brooke Medicine Eagle

As a woman enters into the winter season of life, her physical being may weaken, but her inner life—her soul—gains in strength and resilience. In the contracted and congealed world of winter, the pulse of life beats steady and strong. The seeds sleep in their bristly coffins, skidding along the frozen ponds and lakes or buried under soft blankets of snow. Beneath earth's surface, warm springs and underground currents nourish the roots with life-giving moisture. Water circulates in the deeper channels, pooling and conserving energy, patiently awaiting the resurgence of life that arises in spring.

Winter is the time for concentration and penetration, for going deep and turning inward, and Water is its element. From Water, women learn how to adapt and adjust, channeling their energies into creative pathways, sinking into the depths, settling, resting, reflecting, gathering energy. Following Water's example, a woman flows along the path of least resistance, learning to live within limitations and still retain her essential character. Seeking the lowest level where everything courses to her, she fills up, renewing herself, until she overflows with vital energy, and the cycle of life continues on uninterrupted.

In nature, Water changes shape and form, endlessly cycling through its solid, liquid, and vaporous phases. Surging rivers freeze solid, blocks of ice melt, puddles evaporate into mist and settle again as dew, moisture condenses into clouds and falls back to earth as rain or snow. Under all conditions, Water adapts and yields, pausing but never resting, bending but never breaking. Change defines its essential nature, for in a heartbeat, the river rushing by is entirely different, molecule for molecule, from the waters that flowed by just a moment before.

"You can't step twice into the same river," noted the Greek philosopher Heraclitus. The person you are today is not the one you were a day or even an hour earlier. Like the flowing river, human beings constantly recycle and renew themselves. In and around and through the body's 50 trillion cells, 6 trillion chemical reactions take place *each second*, making change the very nature of the human being. "If you could see your body as it really is, you would never see it the same way twice," writes endocrinologist Deepak Chopra in his book *Quantum Healing*.

> Ninety-eight percent of the atoms in your body were not there a year ago. The skeleton that seems so solid was not there

three months ago. The configuration of the bone cells remains somewhat constant, but atoms of all kinds pass freely back and forth through the cell walls, and by that means you acquire a new skeleton every three months.

The skin is new every month. You have a new stomach lining every four days, with the actual surface cells that contact food being renewed every five minutes. The cells in the liver turn over very slowly, but new atoms still flow through them, like water in a river course, making a new liver every six weeks. Even within the brain, whose cells are not replaced once they die, the content of carbon, nitrogen, oxygen, and so on is totally different today from a year ago.

It is as if you lived in a building whose bricks were systematically taken out and replaced every year. If you keep the same blueprint, then it will still look like the same building. But it won't be the same in actuality.

The essential nature of life is change, a scientific observation that confirms the three-thousand-year-old teachings of the Chinese philosophers. All life is characterized by and subject to change, and it is change itself—the constant, natural tension between yin and yang, creativity and receptivity, dark and light, day and night, the firm and the yielding, the sun and the moon—that generates and sustains life. Without the capacity to change, life would cease to exist, for it would have no means to express itself. In *The I Ching*, the nature of change is described as a natural process, synonymous with life itself:

> The changes are thought of here as natural processes, practically identical with life. Life depends on the polarity between activity and receptivity. This maintains tension, every adjustment of which manifests itself as a change, a process in life. If this state of tension, this potential, were to cease, there would no longer be a criterion for life—life could no longer express itself. On the other hand, these polar oppositions, these tensions, are constantly being generated anew by the changes inherent in life. If life should cease to express itself, these oppositions would be obliterated by progressive entropy, and the death of the world would ensue.

The Chinese believe that the same basic elements—Wood, Fire, Earth, Metal, and Water—govern organic and inorganic life; the ongoing, ever-changing interaction between these elements determines the unique nature and destiny of the organism. The body is thought to consist of five separate stratums, each of which is governed by one of the Five Transforming Powers. The skin, which is the outermost layer, is ruled by Metal. Just beneath the skin is the flesh, which is controlled by Earth. The third layer is comprised of the blood vessels, over which Fire maintains control. Next come the tendons and muscles, which are commanded by Wood. And at the deepest level are the bones, which are the domain of Water. Coursing through the marrow, rinsing, renewing, and enlivening, Water feeds and nourishes the bones, ensuring the flexibility and adaptability of the skeleton itself. Forming the foundation on which all the organs and tissues rest, the bones symbolize the indestructible nature of life.

In the process of aging, the skin, flesh, blood vessels, tendons, and muscles gradually lose shape and elasticity, but the bones maintain their essential character. Break a bone, and it will mend. Shatter a bone, and the fragments will persist in the fossil record for millions of years. Incinerate the bones, and bits and pieces of life linger on. Bones are the permanent, undying part of the human being. They speak of life; they defy even death.

In many cultures, certain wise elders are considered so powerful that they can bring the dead back to life. Ancient and decrepit, often toothless, always solitary, they are called the Bone People, and they wait in their hideouts by rivers or seas, in caves or dark forests, keeping watch until a wounded soul, lost and despairing of life, wanders into their territory. Then their work begins.

The following story about an encounter with the Bone People is adapted from *Rainbow Medicine*, by Wolf Moondance:

> "Why have you come?" the woman asked the skeleton.
> "To remind you of the way," the skeleton responded. "To remind you that nothing stays the same. . . . I call you to the bone people. I ask you to be a hollow bone. I ask that you watch, always, the movement of wisdom."

The Bone People remind us that change is the nature of life; they ask us to hollow ourselves out so that we can begin filling ourselves back up again. In her novel *The Bone People*, Keri Hulme weaves a strange but compelling tale about the people of the bones, also known as the beginning people or the people who make another people. One of the Bone People offers assistance to Kerewin, a lost soul who has returned to her ancestral home, preparing to die. "I am decaying piece by piece," Kerewin despairs. "I feel cold to my very bones."

Rising up from the ashes in the fireplace, the specter appears before her. Thin and wiry, browned and weathered, with silver hair, liquid eyes, and crooked teeth, the Bone Woman offers Kerewin a vile-tasting brew and whispers soothing words, assuring her that she is too full of life for death. She returns many times in the days and nights that follow, nourishing Kerewin's body with food and inflaming her soul with a fierce passion for life.

Late one night Kerewin walks to the ancestral burial site and calls out to the Bone Woman, hoping to learn why she has been saved and what is expected of her. In the stillness, she waits for an answer.

> Sea distant on the beach; birds in the night; her breath coming and going. Nothing else.
> I ask what it wants me to do, and there's silence.
> Nothing else.
> She sighs. . . . As she turns away, a great warmth flows into her. Up from the earth under her feet into the pit of her belly, coursing up like benevolent fire through her breast to the crown of her head.
> She feels her hair literally start to move.
> Shaking with laughter, shaking with tears, shook to the core by joy.

The Bone People cannot provide the answers to our questions; they can only affirm by their presence the reality of death and the gift of life. *"I have faced Death,"* Kerewin writes in her journal as she prepares to return home. *"I have been caught in the wild weed tangles of her hair, seen the gleam of her jade eyes. I will go when it is time—no choice!—but now I want life."*

In the winter of our lives, our wisdom sends its roots deep into the darkest rivers and shadowed pools of the inner self, and there in the reflective stillness we discover how to bend without breaking, to yield without succumbing, to age without decaying, to die and go on living. The Bone People transform us with their wisdom, dissolving our tired old bones and then breathing new life into the skeletal remains; they are at work within each of us from the moment we are born until the moment we die, adding marrow to the bones of the soul, fleshing out the person we are yet to become even as we die into ourselves, even as we bring back to life that which is dead and lifeless.

Breathing life into the bones is solitary work, reserved for those who have lived long, loved much, and suffered deeply, for the experiences of life teach us how to draw life's breath from the deepest, most truthful part of the self. In the waning years of life, when the outer layers of the physical body begin to lose shape and substance, the time comes to go searching for the bones. As the body ages, the soul ripens, for whatever is lost in strength or flexibility in the skin, flesh, blood vessels, muscles, and tendons is tacked onto the weight of the soul. Because the body is willing to make the sacrifice, the soul learns how to fill in the hollows at the deepest level of human being: the bones.

EMMA

Tiny, frail Emma greeted me with a firm handshake. Remnants of her beauty clung to her, for even after seventy-eight years of life, her features revealed a deep inner strength. Laugh lines radiated from her eyes, her sculpted jaw line spoke of a stubborn independent streak, and her soulful eyes were the color of a tropical sea just beyond the shallows, where turquoise makes the shift to a cooler, deeper blue. Although large boned with strong, square shoulders, a graceful neck, and the perfectly sculpted hands of an artist's model, Emma was painfully thin. Time, it seemed, had eaten away at her body; in her youth, she stood five feet seven inches tall and weighed 115 to 120 pounds, but now at the end of her seventh decade, she was barely five feet three inches tall and weighed no more than 100 pounds. When her niece made the appointment, she told me that her aunt was "wasting away" from pain.

"Tell me about the pain," I said.

"It's exquisite," Emma responded in a strong, resonant voice. "That's a term I heard from a doctor a long, long time ago. *Exquisite pain.* I've never forgotten it."

As Emma talked about her past, it was clear that "enduring the pain" had become her primary challenge in life, for life, she insisted, was synonymous with pain. When she was twenty-two years old, she broke her back.

Pregnant with her second child, holding her first child in her arms, she lost her footing, slid down an entire flight of uncarpeted stairs, and shattered two vertebrae at the base of her spine. For fifteen years, she lived with the pain, but when she could barely get out of bed in the morning to help her five children get ready for school, she agreed to have surgery to repair the shattered discs. After the operation, Emma experienced some relief from the pain, but as the years passed, and her children grew up and left home, she became increasingly sedentary, arthritis inflamed her joints, and the exquisite pain returned.

Emma related the details of her accident and its aftermath quickly and with little elaboration. A few minutes after she began her story, she sat with her hands folded in her lap, her blue eyes regarding me as if to say, "See, it's not so bad. I have nothing to complain about."

I often see this sense of resignation in the elderly, who seem to believe that degeneration and dementia are to be expected and accept these assaults as a natural part of aging. Becoming an invalid, in their minds, invalidates them as human beings who have a right to expect more from life. Giving into the pain, they give up any illusion or expectation of feeling better. But in Chinese thought the natural process of aging should proceed without significant pain or disability; where there is pain, there is blockage or obstruction, and much careful thought and skillful therapeutic intervention is focused on uncovering the root of the problem.

I asked Emma a number of specific questions, hoping to understand the source of her pain. *Where does it hurt the most? At what time of day are you most affected by the pain? What activities intensify or exacerbate the pain? What do you do to make your back feel better—do baths, massages, rest, or sleep help? Does the weather affect the pain? Is the pain dull, sharp, stationary, or variable? Are you ever without pain?* As she answered these questions, Emma began to reveal the extent of her pain and how deeply it had infiltrated her body, mind, and spirit.

Because it hurt to move, Emma had stopped moving. An avid golfer and bowler for much of her life, she could no longer pick up a bowling ball or swing a golf club without debilitating pain. She couldn't even walk around the block without stopping to rest every few minutes. As the pain gradually intensified, she became its prisoner, rarely venturing out of her home. An almost phobic fear ruled her life. She was afraid of falling down the stairs, afraid to drive long distances, afraid to walk on the uneven sidewalks of her neighborhood.

Painfully shy even in her youth, she had lived for years content in her husband's shadow, for he was a gregarious, extroverted, well-loved man with a wide circle of friends. When her husband was alive, his schedule kept her busy and active. But after his death when she was seventy-three, Emma became increasingly isolated from others. A natural affinity to solitude and reflection became a virtual imprisonment. All day, every day, Emma sat on her couch in front of the television, working on a needlepoint project or solving a complex crossword puzzle. The routine rarely varied.

Her kitchen cabinets were well stocked with canned foods, and her freezer was filled with frozen vegetables, chicken pot pies, and TV dinners. Her only exercise was to walk up and down the stairs in her apartment; before she negotiated the steps each morning, she checked to make sure that she had everything she needed so that she wouldn't have to go back up again until she was ready for bed. With little or no exercise, a diet consisting almost entirely of canned or frozen foods, and five to six cups of coffee every day, Emma's circulation was poor, arthritis had invaded virtually every joint of her body, she was chronically constipated, and urinary incontinence was becoming a problem.

Emma's strong bone structure, pale coloring, dry skin, and impatience with small talk revealed a strong affinity to Metal; her active, curious mind, and her penchant for solitude and reflective activities indicated that Water also exerted an important influence. Her face was very pale, almost without color, and a yellow-green tinge around her mouth confirmed her complaints of digestive problems. When I first put my finger to her pulses, I detected a strong, hammering quality, but when I pushed in and pressed down, the hammering disappeared. This "soft hammer" pulse indicates that the internal organs, particularly the Kidneys, are deficient in energy and fluids.

As the body's generator or pilot light, the Kidneys support and nourish all the other organs with *jing* and *chi*; when the Kidney energy is low, the yin (fluid) energy typically flickers out first, and the body has to rely on the yang (fire) energy to keep the blood and *chi* moving. Like an old but reliable engine that is pushed too hard and rarely tuned up, the gears begin to grind, the oil thickens and congeals, and spurts of smoke or blue flame warn of overheating. These "false yang" signs show up in the human body as a hammering pulse, heart palpitations, muscle aches and spasms, pounding headaches, night sweats, and insomnia.

Emma's tongue was bright red, which confirmed a deficient yin condition, and it was covered with numerous small cracks and fissures, indicating that her *chi* energy was being steadily consumed and near exhaustion.

Small brush fires were blazing here and there throughout Emma's system, and her body's water supply was so deficient that it could no longer contain the sparks. Although she was not in any immediate danger, her condition could be classified as semicritical; if her severely depleted reserves were not replenished, her entire system would be in jeopardy.

Emma's treatment involved two related but diverse strategies. Because her most serious presenting symptom was the chronic pain, the first strategy was to clear the surface by reinstigating the flow of energy and blood through the tendino-muscular channels, meridians that follow the same course as the organ meridians but travel much more superficially through the muscles and tendons themselves. These channels are said to carry *wei chi*, which is roughly analogous to immune energy. If we imagine that the periphery of the body is guarded by the tendino-muscular channels, the *wei chi* energy functions like a line of sentries guarding the borders of the kingdom. When an invasion (a cold or the flu, for example) is imminent, reinforcements are called up, and the battle begins in the tendons and muscles, creating the familar aches and pains associated with cold or flu symptoms.

Energy often gets trapped in these channels, causing pain and discomfort; the pain itself is a symptom of blockage, alerting the acupuncturist to treat the problem at the tendon and muscular level before it affects the organ meridians. When needling the tendino-muscular meridian, the acupuncturist uses a more aggressive technique called dispersing. First, the areas of blockage are located by pressing certain trigger points in the areas of pain called *ashi* or "ouch" points. (Emma, to my delight, began to refer to these as the "oh shit" points.) Once the specific points of energy blockage are located, the needles are inserted just under the surface of the skin and then gently twisted around to disperse the stagnant or occluded energy.

An ancient Chinese acupuncture technique known as *gua sya* involves covering the affected meridians with an ointment (salves like Tiger Balm and Vicks Vaporub work well) and then scraping the area with a special blunt instrument. The skin often becomes mottled and dark purple, revealing the trapped or congealed blood beneath the surface. Cupping, another pain-relieving technique, also helps to drain blocked energy and blood. Thick glass cups are placed over the trigger points, suction is created, and the stagnant energy is drawn to the surface where it can be dispersed. (The Chinese cupping technique is almost identical to the Jewish *bonkas* that my grandmother used during my childhood illnesses.) While these techniques may seem rather bizarre to the Western mind, they are extremely effective in relieving pain and discomfort and have been used with great success by skilled practitioners for thousands of years.

Emma mentioned that she had problems with insomnia, experiencing difficulty falling asleep and often waking up several times during the night. For years she had been bothered by "restless leg syndrome," an annoying and sometimes painful condition of twitching muscles and nervous tension; the Chinese interpret this syndrome as an "internal wind" condition, indicating a deficiency in Liver energy and a disturbance in the free flow of energy and blood throughout the body. The more superficial acupuncture techniques, which concentrated on the *ashi* points and used scraping and cupping to drain the blockage and relieve the pain, had an immediate and noticeable effect on Emma's twitching nerves and the radiating pains in her legs.

The second tier of Emma's treatment involved supporting her organ functions. Because Emma had a clear affinity to Metal and Water, and her symptoms indicated a depletion of Kidney and Liver energy, I decided to needle six acupoints. Kidney 3 (Great Stream), located just behind the inner ankle bone in the depression between the bone and the Achilles tendon, supports the Kidney as its source point, the point at which the energy in the meridian is the deepest and penetrates directly to the organ itself. Spleen 6 (Three Yin Meeting), located on the inner leg above the ankle bone, is an essential point for enriching the yin and regulating the various energies throughout the body. Conception Vessel 3 (Central Pole) and Conception Vessel 4 (Gate at the Source), located approximately an inch apart on the midline of the belly, strongly support the Kidney yin and *chi*. Lung 9 (Great Abyss) supports the circulation and integrity of the blood vessels; as the source point of the Lung channel, this point sustains the basic energy of Metal and, in Emma's case, would help her deal with her grief over her husband's death. As the authors of the acupuncture text *Grasping the Wind* phrase it, "the *chi* here is plentiful and deep like an abyss."

When I inserted the needle in Lung 3 (Heavenly Palace), approximately three inches below the armpit in the bicep muscle, I asked Emma to think about the meaning of this point, which I use only for psychological or spiritual matters. The Lung is concerned with receptivity and refinement, and this point helps us reconnect to this essential function, for it allows a sense of the spirit to radiate from the inside out. "Imagine that you are walking up the stairs to a dirty, dusty attic filled with windows covered with cobwebs," I suggested. "Think of this point as accessing the energy needed to wash the windows, sweep away the dust and dirt, and allow the sunlight to shine through and fill the space with streams of light."

To fortify the blood, nourish the Kidneys and Liver, and support the tendons and muscles, I recommended the herbal beverage Shou Wu Chih, which contains as its main ingredient polygonum, a Kidney *jing* supporter that is said to allow one "to age gracefully." Also included in this formula are the herbs *Dong Quai*, the archetypical female tonic, used to help support the blood, and rehmania, a strong Kidney yin tonic. A very tasty concoction, Shou Wu Chih is commonly used in China for the typical problems associated with aging, and many elderly Chinese women (and men) take several tablespoons every day as a daily supplement. I also recommended devil's claw, an anti-inflammatory herb; sage, which moves the blood and helps relieve stasis; and licorice, a harmonizing, yin-nourishing herb. (Licorice should not be used by people with high blood pressure as there is some evidence that it can raise the blood pressure.)

For Emma's diet, I strongly suggested cutting back on caffeine and refined carbohydrates, while adding more whole grains, fiber (bran cereal, psyllium, etc.), and fresh fruits and vegetables. Vitamin supplements included a multivitamin and magnesium (1,000 mg/day); deficiencies in magnesium have been associated with muscle cramping, irritability, and restless leg syndrome.

Exercise was vital to prevent stasis and stagnation, but this was a sticking point for Emma because any kind of movement that involved putting weight on her legs or stretching or bending her backbone caused severe pain. I explained the Chinese philosophy of pain, which states that if there is pain, there is obstruction; likewise, if there is no pain, we can assume that there is no obstruction. Pain is considered a sign of energy interference, and the acupuncturist's job is to locate the obstruction and use the needles to unblock it.

Acupuncture is famous for pain relief, and the herbal remedies would assist in moving the blood and energy, but Emma also needed to take responsibility for managing her pain. Because of the extent of her back injury, the buildup of scar tissue, the deeper blockages and resultant lack of flexibility and pressure on her nerves and muscles, Emma would never be completely free of pain. But the goal of treatment was to help her manage the pain so that she was in control rather than feeling that her life had to be lived in deference to the pain. After discussing a number of alternatives, Emma agreed to take a water aerobics class for seniors at the local YMCA and try some simple yoga stretching exercises.

OSTEOPOROSIS

WESTERN INTERPRETATION AND TREATMENT

Osteoporosis is a potentially serious condition involving a decrease in bone mass and an increase in bone brittleness; it is most common in postmenopausal women. The causes are multifactorial and include genetic predisposition, estrogen depletion, lack of exercise, unhealthy eating habits, smoking, and alcohol consumption. Bone scans are used to determine bone density and porosity.

Most physicians view osteoporosis as a symptom of hormonal deficiency, with estrogen depletion as the primary culprit. Estrogen replacement therapy, or ERT, has traditionally been the treatment of choice; however, due to the significantly increased risk of estrogen-related cancers, synthetic progesterones are now added and the treatment is labeled hormone replacement therapy, or HRT. HRT prevents osteoporosis, but once a woman stops taking the drugs, the bone loss continues and often escalates. Therefore, HRT is considered a lifetime commitment. Calcium supplements and exercise are also recommended to improve bone density and elasticity.

CHINESE INTERPRETATION

In Chinese thought, the Kidneys rule the bones, and osteoporosis is thought to reflect diminished Kidney function, especially the yin (fluid) energy. Kidney decline is viewed as a natural part of aging, and some loss of bone density is expected and considered normal. Only when the bone loss is excessive or interferes with aging gracefully are aggressive treatments suggested. As always in Traditional Chinese Medicine, prevention is emphasized.

COMPLEMENTARY TREATMENTS

SUPPLEMENTS

- **Calcium citrate**, either in calcium-fortified orange juice or calcium citrate, gluconate, or lactate capsules (500–1,000 mg/day. Avoid dolomite, bonemeal, and oyster shell, which contain lead and other harmful minerals; also avoid antacids, which are difficult to absorb and assimilate and can cause kidney stones or build up in joints, aggravating arthritic conditions.)

- **Magnesium**, to assist in the absorption of calcium into the bones (Take twice as much magnesium as calcium, 500–1,000 mg/day calcium and 1,000–2,000 mg/day magnesium.)
- **Vitamin D** to increase absorption of calcium (400 iu/day) (Sunlight is critically important to the body's ability to assimilate vitamin D; try to spend fifteen to twenty minutes every day in direct sunlight.)
- **Zinc** to support the bones, the immune system, and Kidney energies (30–50 mg/day)
- **Natural progesterone cream** prevents and reverses osteoporosis by helping to build new bone. (Estrogen retards the breakdown of old bone cells, but many complementary practitioners believe that estrogen can actually contribute to harder, less flexible bones. Since natural progesterone is a precursor to estrogen, progesterone cream may be sufficient for prevention and treatment of osteoporosis.)

EXERCISE

Since inactivity or lack of proper exercise can lead to bone loss, weight-bearing exercises—such as running or brisk walking while carrying light weights, bicycling, aerobics, and stair-stepping—are strongly advised. Incorporate weight-bearing exercises into your lifestyle by parking your car a distance away from the store and carrying your groceries or packages.

DIET

Add calcium- and magnesium-rich vegetables (spinach, kale, broccoli, seaweeds); also add seeds, nuts, legumes, whole grains, nonfat yogurt, and seafood. Avoid the following foods, beverages, or drugs, which contribute to calcium loss or interfere with calcium absorption: caffeine, alcohol, nicotine, sugar and refined carbohydrates, excess protein (meats, dairy, poultry), and phosphates (colas and root beer).

HERBAL ALLIES

The following herbs may be used alone or combined in equal parts to make a wonderful tonic:

- **Nettles**, a rich, nourishing herb full of minerals and nutrients
- **Horsetail** (*Equisetum arvense*), a plant rich in silica, which is essential to healthy bones

CHINESE PATENT REMEDIES

- **Liu Wei Di Huang Wan** (Six Flavor Rehmania Pill) for deficient Kidney yin, *or*
- **Shou Wu Chih**, a wine-type beverage containing *shou wu* (*polygonum multiflorum*), *Dong Quai*, and ginseng (one tablespoon twice daily) to support the Kidney *jing* and help you age gracefully

ACUPOINTS

Kidney 3, Kidney 10, and Spleen 6

MIND/BODY/SPIRIT CONNECTION

The symptoms might be expressing these questions:

- "How am I lacking support?"
- "How can I sustain my energies and, when I need support, ask for assistance from others?"
- "What is my foundation—how can I make it stronger?"
- "Where have I become hard, brittle, or rigid? What can I do to become more flexible and adaptable?"

"How about a weekly massage?" I asked Emma.

"No, I couldn't do that," she said, flushing bright red. I appealed to her sense of adventure, reminding her that if she were willing to have pins stuck in her body, what harm could a backrub do?

"It's a luxury I don't deserve," she finally confessed.

"Okay, I have a joke for you," I said. "How many Jewish grandmothers does it take to change a light bulb?" When Emma shook her head, I put on my best Jewish accent. "None. *Don't worry about me, darling, I'll just sit here in the dark.*"

Emma laughed until she cried. "All right, all right, I'll get a massage," she said.

Over the next six months Emma reported gradual but steady progress. The pain was diminished, and she could walk up and down the stairs without having to stop and rest. Changes in her diet, regular exercise, and daily doses of natural fiber (psyllium powder) regulated her bowel movements, while daily Kegel exercises (tightening the band of muscles that encircle the vagina in order to strengthen the pelvic floor) dramatically improved her bladder control. The yoga exercises, swim classes, and massages reduced her muscular tension and increased her flexibility.

During the acupuncture sessions, Emma began to talk about death and her ever-present grief. If pain was Emma's theme song, grief was its recurring melody. Whenever I mentioned her husband, her eyes flooded with tears. In our first sessions, she would dab at her tears with a tissue, take a deep breath, and quickly change the subject. As time went on, however, she began to talk more openly about her grief. At times, she would discuss the tragic situation of her older sister, who was confined to a nursing home and spent every moment of every day complaining about the emptiness of her life. Knowing that I was a collector of stories, she shared with me a story she had read in James Hillman's book *A Blue Fire*. Hillman, a Jungian analyst, was watching an elderly woman being interviewed by a psychiatrist:

> She sat in a wheelchair because she was elderly and feeble. She said that she was dead for she had lost her heart. The psychiatrist asked her to place her hand over her breast to feel her heart beating: it must still be there if she could feel its beat. "That," she said, "is not my real heart." She and the psychiatrist looked at each other. There was nothing more to say. Like the primitive who has lost his soul, she had lost the loving courageous connection to life—and that is the real heart, not the ticker which can as well pulsate isolated in a glass bottle.

"My sister's heart is still beating," Emma said as we talked about the meaning of the story, "but like that elderly lady, she has lost the deeper connection to life."

One day Emma talked about a decision she was having trouble making. Her three daughters lived within a hundred miles of each other on the

West Coast and wanted her to move into a retirement complex a few miles from the youngest daughter's home. "Nine of my fourteen grandchildren live out west," she said. "My two sons live on the East Coast, but they are both busy with their own lives, and I don't get to see them very often. So it would make sense to move, but I worry about giving up my independence. I don't want to become a burden. It seems that it might be better for everyone if I stayed put."

"But what a gift you would be giving your grandchildren!" I said. "For the rest of their lives, they would cherish their memories with you."

"I never thought of it that way," Emma said thoughtfully. Suddenly her eyes filled with tears. "But I can't leave Jim. Who would look after his grave, who would bring him flowers?" The grief that Emma had held inside for so long suddenly overflowed. A Hindu story about death seemed to comfort her.

> *Ramana Maharshi lay on his deathbed, troubled by the griefstricken cries of his followers. Reaching out to one of his attendants, he pulled him close and whispered, "Why are they so sorrowful?"*
> *"Because you are leaving them, master."*
> *Ramana looked bewildered. "But where do they think I could go?"*

A few weeks later Emma brought in the book *Ageless Body, Timeless Mind*, by Deepak Chopra. "Did you know that a honeybee can grow old and then become young again?" she asked me, her eyes bright with excitement. "Listen to this," she said, and began reading from the book:

> The common honeybee . . . can change its age at will. Every beehive needs young workers whose job is to stay indoors to feed and care for newly hatching larvae. After three weeks, these workers grow up and move on to become mature foragers, the bees who fly from the hive to collect pollen from flowers.
>
> At any given period, however, there may be too many young workers or too many old foragers. In the spring so many new larvae may be hatching that the hive lacks mature foragers and needs more very quickly. When that happens, some of the young workers age into foragers in one week instead of the usual three and fly off seeking food. On the other hand, if a swarm of bees splits off to form a new colony, it is likely to be composed mostly of old forager bees. Sensing a shortage of young workers, some of these old foragers will reverse their ages and become

young again—they regenerate the hormones of youthful workers and even regrow the withered glands needed to produce food for the hatching larvae.

"Imagine being able to do that," Emma marveled.

"Honeybees aren't the only creatures who have the ability to grow young as they age," I said. I told Emma about Mexico's Tarahumara Indians, who live in the mountains in northern Sonora and run twenty-five to fifty miles a day. The runners honored as the strongest and most physically fit are those in their sixties. When physiologists measured the lung capacity, cardiovascular fitness, and endurance of these marathon runners, they discovered that the elderly runners were indeed in the best physical shape.

"The Tarahumaras believe that the elders of the tribe are the strongest in body, mind, and spirit, and the aging runners live up to their tribe's expectations," I said. "In our culture, on the other hand, we succumb to what Harvard psychologist Ellen Langer has termed 'premature cognitive commitments,' assuming that as we grow older, we necessarily become more frail and feeble. This is the same mind-set that changed the destinies of a group of houseflies who were confined in a small jar for several days. The flies became committed to the belief that the inside of the jar was their entire world; when the lid was removed and they were free to take off, they kept flying in the same familiar circles, never venturing out of the previously restricted space. Their world literally was reduced to the limits of their imagination."

Emma shuddered involuntarily. "I'd rather be a honeybee, one of those old matrons who looks around, realizes the swarm needs her, and instantly becomes young again—what a wonderful image, buzzing around in this old body with the mind and spirit of a twenty-year-old!" She put her finger to her cheek and winked at me. "But now let me see—the twenties were rather tumultuous with all the childbearing, cooking, and cleaning. Maybe I'd rather be thirty or forty—those were both wonderful decades. My fifties and sixties were pretty darn good, too, and my seventies aren't turning out so bad. So maybe I'll just fly back and forth a bit, moving around from one decade to the next. What do you think?"

"I think you're wonderful," I said.

A few months later, Emma decided to move to California to live near her daughters and her grandchildren. I haven't seen her for several years, but every Christmas she sends me a card and relates the recent changes in her life. She continues to take a weekly water aerobics class and recently signed up for a hatha yoga class. When her restless leg syndrome started to bother her again, interfering with her "beauty sleep," as she put it, she found a qualified acupuncturist and herbalist whom she sees once a month for "maintenance work." Her grandchildren's soccer games and dance recitals keep her busy, and she has taken up photography, enrolling in several classes to perfect her darkroom techniques.

Twice a year, on her husband's birthday and their anniversary, Emma travels back east to visit her two sons and put fresh flowers on her husband's grave.

> *Dew evaporates*
> *and all our world*
> *is dew . . . so dear,*
> *so refreshing, so fleeting*
> —**Issa**
> (1763–1827),
> on the death of his child

Life is limited by death, but it is precisely the restriction imposed by that unyielding boundary that forces us to confront the meaning and purpose of our existence. "When it is accepted that there are clearly defined limits to life, then life will be seen to have a symmetry as well," writes Sherwin B. Nuland in *How We Die*. In death we discover the necessary counterweight to life, for death teaches us about the need for balance and equilibrium, for planting our feet squarely in the present moment and living so fully that if life were to end right now, it would be complete and whole. "Death is the only wise advisor that we have," Don Juan, a Yaqui Indian medicine man, instructed his disciple, Carlos Castaneda. "Turn to your death . . . nothing really matters outside its touch."

Turning to your death is not a matter for youth or inexperience. When we are young and full of ourselves, death seems far away, a frightening specter that threatens everyone else's life but our own. By purposely keeping death on the periphery of our vision, we can avoid looking it in the eye. But as the years pass, death moves from the threshold into the center of the room and assumes its importance as both teacher and healer. In a sense, death pushes us out of the center, for we begin to understand that life is not about me or you or them; its meaning is discovered in the ongoing, ever-changing connections between all living things. If at each moment we understand that death could present itself, then each moment becomes an opportunity to celebrate the wonder of being alive.

> *The old woman sat by the fire, looking into the flames and remembering the faces of all who had come and gone before her. When she heard the knock on the door, she was prepared.*
>
> *"I have traveled a long way," Death said, standing on the portal, "and I am weary."*
>
> *"I know, for I have seen you many times on my own journey," said the old woman, welcoming the traveler into her home. They sat down by the fire, and after a moment the old woman began to talk.*
>
> *"You were there when my house flooded," she began. "And you were there when our business was thriving. You appeared when the blizzards covered our door with snow. And when no rain came to bring green in the spring, I felt you nearby. You were in the room with me when I was ill. As friends came and went, you stayed close. When my children were sick, you kept me company. When I lost my beauty, you stood by me. When I was lonely, you comforted me. Just last year you wrapped my husband in your arms and eased his pain.*
>
> *"I meet with you in each breath I take, in each day that passes, in the ending and beginning of each season, in the dying leaves of autumn, and in the green shoots poking through the winter snow. You have taught me the difference between fear and readiness."*
>
> *The old woman had talked for a long time. She took one last deep breath, smiled, and reached for Death's hand. "Let's walk together, my friend, for by now the path is familiar, and I know the way."*

Death doesn't wait for us somewhere distant and far removed; death is here now, with you and with me, in the inhalation and exhalation of our breath, in the setting of the sun and the rising of the moon, in the flowers that bloom and the seeds that wither before they take root, in the leaf that greens and in full color dies. Each passing moment prepares us for our own death, for each moment can be seen as a complete cycle, the birth and the death of an instant. When each moment is greeted as perfect and whole, then we understand that death is not in front of us or even behind us, but in and of us at all times, a constant reminder of the evanescent nature of life.

In one of his shortest poems, Robert Frost wrote, "We dance round in

a ring and suppose, / But the Secret sits in the middle and knows."
Growing older and wiser, we enter the circle and confront the Secret.
What is it that the Secret knows?

Many wise women and men suggest that "the Secret" resides in the
simple act of living fully in the moment. Living in the moment is an art;
one might truthfully say that it is the art of life. "No thought, no action,
no movement, total stillness; only then can one manifest the true nature
and law of things from within and unconsciously and at last become one
with heaven and earth," wrote Lao-tzu thousands of years ago. A similar
sentiment is expressed by modern writer Iris Murdoch.

There is no beyond,
there is only here,
the infinitely small,
infinitely great and utterly
demanding present.

In the present, we are centered and balanced, which means paradoxically
that we remove ourselves from the center—the center of attention, the
central character, the focal point—and turn our attention outward toward
the larger world that encircles and enfolds all living things. Our sense of
the universe shifts, so that we no longer imagine that everyone else is
looking in at us, constantly assessing and judging, but that we are looking
out at the world, always striving not to judge or censure others.

Looking with the eyes of the soul rather than the eyes of the ego, "thee"
and "thine" become more important than "me" and "mine." Many wisdom
gatherers have attempted to describe this near-mystical experience of
centeredness and balance, but Black Elk of the Oglala Sioux, who died
at the ripe old age of eighty-seven, captures the experience:

Then I was standing on the highest mountain of them all,
and around about beneath me was the whole hoop of the
world. And while I stood there I saw more than I can tell
and I understood more than I saw; for I was seeing in a sacred
manner the shapes of all things in the spirit, and the shape
of all shapes as they must live together like one being. And
I saw the sacred hoop of my people was one of the many
hoops that made one circle, wide as daylight and as starlight,
and in the center grew one mighty flowering tree to shelter

all the children of one mother and one father. And I saw that
it was holy. . . .

But anywhere is the center of the world.

The center is everywhere, an expanding series of circles like ripples on
a pond, in which each successive ring expands the circles but does not
alter the central truth. A story is told about Copper Woman, a wise old
crone who instructed the women in her tribe about the power of the
blood. When it was time for her to leave her body behind, she whispered
the undying truths and prepared to greet her death knowing, as Ohiyesa
of the Santee Sioux knew, that "each soul must meet the morning sun,
the new sweet earth, and the Great Silence alone."

> *Copper Woman told {her daughter} Hai Nai Yu (whose name*
> *means The Wise One or The One Who Knows) that the wisdom must*
> *always be passed on to women, and reminded her that whatever the*
> *colour of the skin, all people come from the same blood and the blood*
> *is sacred. She said a time would come when the wisdom would nearly*
> *disappear, but it would never perish, and whenever it was needed, a*
> *way would be found to present it to the women, and they could then*
> *decide if they wanted to learn it or not. And Hai Nai Yu promised*
> *that when it came Time for her, she would be sure there was someone*
> *to replace her as the guardian of the wisdom.*
>
> *Copper Woman warned Hai Nai Yu that the world would change*
> *and times might come when Knowing would not be the same as Doing.*
> *And she told her that Trying would always be very important.*
>
> *Then she left the waiting house for the last time, and she ate a last*
> *meal with her family. She held them all and kissed them all, and*
> *reassured them she would always be there if there was Need.*
>
> *Then she walked to the beach and sat by herself and waited until*
> *the sun was gone and the moon was high in the sky, painting the*
> *waves with silver. She stood then, and said the words, sang the songs,*
> *danced the dances and prayed the prayers.*
>
> *Then she left her meat in her bag of skin, and took her bones with*
> *her, and became a spirit. She became Old Woman. She turned her bones*
> *into a broom and a loom.*
>
> **—The Daughters of Copper Woman** *(1981)*

The bones contain the undying spirit of the human being; from one
generation to the next, the spirit remains the same. From her bones,

Copper Woman created a broom, which would help her descendants clear the space necessary for meditation and reflection, and a loom, which would be used to weave together the strands of body, mind, and spirit, each essential to the woven whole, each forming an arc on the larger circle of life.

Copper Woman is the female spirit who seeks out the cycles, spheres, and spirals of life, weaving, spinning, braiding, and plaiting. With her broom and her loom, she creates a vast tapestry of life, which absorbs the golden sunlight and radiates the silver moonlight, changing in shape and texture from one moment to the next, reflecting the radiant spirit of the natural world. She is the essence of change, the bones of meaning, the heart that never stops beating, the gift we give to our children and they to theirs and on and on through the generations. The Apaches call her Changing Woman.

> *When Changing Woman gets to be a certain old age, she goes walking toward the east. After a while she sees herself in the distance looking like a young girl walking toward her. They both walk until they come together and after that there is only one. She is like a young girl again.*

The old woman journeys backward in time and space to discover her younger self, the child moves forward, and they meet in the center where "there is only one." The ending and the beginning are joined, the two halves are united, the broken parts are healed, life and death embrace. The circle is complete.

APPENDIXES

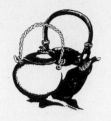

APPENDIX I

INVOKING THE GODDESS: A DIRECTORY OF HERBS

In this directory, we describe the spirit, personality, and common uses of twenty-one herbs renowned for their beneficial gynecological effects. Several of these cherished herbal allies have more general effects as immune enhancers, Heart strengtheners, Liver or Kidney tonics, but the focus here is on concerns specific to women. In general, these herbs (which represent Native American, European, Mediterranean, and Asian cultures and traditions) tend to favor the yin qualities, helping to subdue Fire, supporting the body's fluids (*chi*, blood, and water), and promoting a harmonious flow of energy throughout the body, mind, and spirit.

When I recommend a certain herb or combination of herbs to my patients, I emphasize that taking the herbs is a healing ritual in and of itself. The power of the Great Goddess lives on in the spirit and personality of the herb, and when we ask for the herb's help in promoting healing and wholeness, we can imagine the goddess working her magic within, strengthening, restoring, and renewing us with these simple gifts provided in abundance by Mother Earth.

If you would like to know more about how to use these essential female allies or investigate the healing properties of other remarkable herbs, we recommend the following sources:

General Herbology

Healing Herbal Remedies by Jason Elias and Shelagh Ryan Masline (New York: Dell, 1995).

The Healing Power of Herbs by Michael T. Murray (Roseville, CA: Prima Publishing, 1992).

The New Age Herbalist by Richard Mabey (New York: Collier Books, Macmillan, 1988).

The New Holistic Herbal by David Hoffman (Rockport, MA: Element Books, 1991).

Out of the Earth: The Essential Book of Herbal Medicine by Simon Mills (London, New York: Viking Arkana, 1991).

The Way of Herbs by Michael Tierra (New York: Pocket Books, 1980).

Herbals for Women

Breast Cancer? Breast Health! The Wise Woman Way by Susun Weed (Woodstock, NY: Ash Tree Publishing, 1995).

Herbal Healing for Women by Rosemary Gladstar (New York: Simon & Schuster, 1993).

Herbal Therapy for Women by Elisabeth Brooke, (San Francisco: Thorsons London, 1993).

Hygieia: A Woman's Herbal by Jeannine Parvati (Monroe, UT: Freestone Collective, 1978).

Menopausal Years: The Wise Woman Way by Susun Weed (Woodstock, NY: Ash Tree Publishing, 1992).

Wise Woman Herbal for the Childbearing Year by Susun Weed (Woodstock, NY: Ash Tree Publishing [P.O. Box 64, Woodstock, NY 12498], 1986).

Goddesses

For more information on the goddesses of the ancient world, we recommend the following sources:

Ancient Mirrors of Womanhood by Merlin Stone (Boston, MA: Beacon Press, 1979, 1984).

The Chalice and the Blade by Riane Eisler (New York: Harper/San Francisco, 1987).

The Goddesses and Gods of Old Europe by Marija Gimbutas (Berkeley and Los Angeles: University of California Press, 1982).

Goddesses in Everywoman by Jean Shinoda Bolen (New York: Harper & Row, 1984).

Gods in Everyman by Jean Shinoda Bolen (New York: Harper & Row, 1989).

The Language of the Goddess by Marija Gimbutas (New York: Harper & Row, 1989).

The Once and Future Goddess by Elinor Gadon (New York: Harper & Row, 1984).

When God Was a Woman by Merlin Stone (New York: Harcourt Brace Jovanovich, 1976).

The Woman's Encyclopedia of Myths and Secrets by Barbara Walker (New York: Harper & Row, 1983).

Women of Classical Mythology: A Biographical Dictionary by Robert E. Bell (New York: Oxford University Press, 1991).

INDEX OF HERBS

Black cohosh *(Cimicifuga racemosa)*
Black haw *(Viburnum prunifolium)*
Chasteberry *(Vitex agnus-castus)*
Dandelion root *(Taraxacum officinalis)*
Dong Quai *(Angelica sinensis)*
Echinacea *(Echinacea angustifolia)*
False unicorn root *(Chamaelirium luteum)*
Garlic *(Allium sativum)*
Ginger *(Zingiber officinale)*
Ginseng *(Panax ginseng, Panax quinquefolium, Eleutherococcus senticosus)*
Hawthorn berries *(Crataegus oxyacantha)*
Lady's mantle *(Alchemilla vulgaris)*
Milk thistle *(Carduus marianis, Silybum marianum)*

Motherwort *(Leonurus cardiaca)*
Nettles *(Urtica dioica)*
Raspberry leaf *(Rubus idaeus)*
Sage *(Salvia officinalis)*
St. John's wort *(Hypericum perforatum)*
Uva ursi *(Arctostaphylos uva ursi)*
Valeriana *(Valerian officinalis)*
Vervain *(Verbena officinalis)*

BLACK COHOSH
(Cimicifuga racemosa)

For thousands of years, Africans and Indians have chewed the root of this plant to calm their nerves and lift their spirits, and shamans have mixed the herb with water and sprinkled it around a room to ward off evil spirits. Gynecological uses of this herb are numerous and diverse. Traditionally used to spur on delayed menses and gently induce labor, black cohosh also possesses antispasmodic qualities that help to soothe nervous tension and lower the blood pressure. It also relieves numerous menopausal complaints, including hot flashes, headaches, joint pain, water retention, and fatigue. (Indeed, in clinical studies black cohosh proved to be as effective in relieving these symptoms as hormone replacement therapy.)

This herb invokes the North African goddess Lamia—Snake Woman— whose heart beats slow and sure, whose body remains ever flexible and adaptable, and whose spirit is renewed whenever she sheds her skin. Lamia is one of many goddesses intimately associated with the snake, "whose presence was a guarantee that nature's enigmatic cycle would be maintained and its life-giving powers not diminish," in archaeologist Marija Gimbutas's words.

Common Uses

- Helps to bring on delayed menstrual cycles
- Relieves tension and cramping associated with PMS
- Induces labor in a gentle, relaxing way (especially effective when used with blue cohosh, for these herbs seem to act synergistically to bring on contractions while relaxing and supporting the mother)
- Reduces breast soreness or tenderness

- Reduces or eliminates menopausal complaints, including hot flashes, arthritic degeneration, headaches, and fatigue
- Used in Europe primarily to relieve neuralgias (nerve pains), muscle cramps, or any inflammatory condition associated with spasm or tension

BLACK HAW
(Viburnum prunifolium)

The Native American herb black haw has been used for centuries to prevent miscarriage, stem heavy menstrual flow, and ease menstrual cramps. Like its brother herb cramp bark, black haw relaxes the smooth muscles of the body, with a particularly calming effect on the uterus. Gentle and maternal, this herb soothes the restless spirit and supports the embryo in utero, protecting the developing fetus from harm.

The spirit of Ops, the Roman goddess of plenty and fertility, lives on in this comforting herb. A nurturing, loving goddess, Ops governs the fertile powers of earth, offering food and shelter to those in need, while tenderly watching over pregnant women and newborns.

Common Uses

- Eases uterine cramping and dysmennorhea (painful periods)
- Prevents miscarriage (particularly effective when used with false unicorn root)
- Relieves tension and stress (particularly effective when used with valerian root)
- Suppresses excessive menstrual flow (particularly effective when used with lady's mantle)
- Reduces blood pressure

CHASTEBERRY
(Vitex agnus-castus)

Chasteberry, also known as monk's pepper, is a "wise mother" herb, nourishing and supporting the mind/body/spirit and gently restoring balance and harmony to the entire system. Chasteberry is my most cherished ally for women suffering from PMS or women who have difficulty negotiating the transition from summer to late autumn—the menopausal years—and it is also useful for a wide range of other gynecological conditions. The herb's effects are generally felt only after two or three months of faithful use; one to two years of regular use may be necessary for long-term improvement.

Chasteberry evokes Demeter, the kindly, nurturing Greek goddess whose powers govern the harvest months and who is considered the caretaker of women and children. Also known as the goddess of the waning moon, Demeter ensures an abundance of fruits and grains and guarantees the continuation of life in the enfolding mystery of the seed.

Common Uses

- Relieves symptoms of PMS, including irritability, depression, headaches, bloating, and cramping
- Relieves menopausal symptoms such as hot flashes, night sweats, depression, anxiety attacks, and flooding, or heavy periods
- Balances and regulates the menstrual flow
- Reduces uterine fibroids
- Helps resolve endometriosis
- Clears up hormonally related acne and other skin problems
- Protects against osteoporosis and reproductive cancers (especially breast and endometrial cancers)
- Induces emotional calm

DANDELION
(Taraxacum officinalis)

A story is told about a man who tried everything within his power to rid his garden of dandelions. Having exhausted all known possibilities, he appealed to an expert gardener, who gave him this advice: "I suggest you learn to love them." Once you learn about the astonishing healing powers of this simple weed, you will find it easier to cherish its ubiquitous presence.

One of the richest of all plants in nutritive value and a cornerstone of traditional herbal treatments, dandelion is the archetypical Liver tonic, helping this vital organ system detoxify and cleanse the blood. Dandelion is also highly valued as a nourishing kidney tonic; the French word for dandelion, *pissenlit*, literally means "piss in bed," a literary testament to dandelion's dramatic diuretic effects. Dandelion also has numerous gynecological benefits and is particularly helpful for relieving bloating and digestive disturbances associated with PMS or menopause, with the beneficial side effects of increasing energy, supporting digestion, and improving metabolism.

Dandelion invokes Yemaya, the powerful Nigerian Sea Mother. Surging and flowing through all of life without interruption, Yemaya washes away impurities, heals wounds of body, mind, and spirit, protects, comforts, and endures.

Common Uses

- Traditionally used for any condition involving the liver and gallbladder, including food sensitivities, hepatitis, and cirrhosis of the liver; also used to prevent gallstones and infections of the gallbladder
- Supports digestion and improves metabolism, allowing proper assimilation of food and drink
- Reduces bloating and/or water retention (extremely effective for premenstrual water retention)
- Gently cleanses the blood to help resolve acne, itchy or sensitive skin, and other skin conditions
- Regulates blood-sugar levels and resolves hormonally induced blood-sugar fluctuations
- Provides a rich source of usable iron, making it an invaluable ally for women who bleed heavily

DONG QUAI
(Angelica sinensis)

One of the most beloved and oft-prescribed of Chinese tonic herbs, *Dong Quai* is considered the archetypical female herb, used to promote fertility, support and stabilize pregnancy, and balance the menstrual cycles. It is an excellent menopausal tonic, used to ensure a healthy and problem-free menopause. The Chinese believe that *Dong Quai* enhances receptivity in the form of increasing fertility and opening the mind and spirit to revelatory visions.

Relaxing and nourishing, *Dong Quai* evokes the Chinese goddess Chang-O, who guards the power and mystery of menstrual blood, ruling over the never-ending cycle of life, death, and rebirth.

Common Uses

- Balances the menstrual flow and promotes fertility (In China, patients are warned to avoid this herb if they do *not* wish to conceive.)
- Relieves painful periods and cramping
- Relieves the symptoms of PMS
- Soothes the hot flashes, irritability, dry skin, and dry vaginal membranes associated with menopause
- Stabilizes cardiac function and lowers blood-cholesterol levels, preventing heart disease and reducing menopausal palpitations (racing heart)
- Clears a cluttered mind and soothes a troubled spirit

Caution: Due to its vasodilatory and blood-promoting action, *Dong Quai* should not be used if you are experiencing heavy menstrual periods. Although considered safe to use during pregnancy, use only under professional supervision. Occasionally, *Dong Quai* can cause loose bowels or diarrhea; discontinue use if these symptoms occur.

ECHINACEA
(*Echinacea angustifolia*)

The Native American herb echinacea (the purple coneflower) was used by natives and white settlers to treat a myriad of afflictions, including snakebites, burns, wounds, fevers, infections, toothaches, and sore throats. When used for preventative purposes, echinacea gears up the immune system to fight off threatening germs and diseases; after disease has taken hold, the herb valiantly battles the invading pathogens to restore health and wholeness.

This gentle but powerful herb invokes Athena, the ancient goddess of wisdom, whose chalice represented love of peace and harmony. In Greek mythology, Athena was recast as a protective warrior goddess, complete with helmet, spear, and shield. Both manifestations of the goddess—the wise, peace-loving matron and the mighty heroine who offered security and refuge to the besieged—can be found in echinacea, an herb imbued with both the wisdom of prevention and the power of healing.

Common Uses

- Enhances immune system functioning to prevent colds and flus and increase resistance to disease
- Acts as a diaphoretic (sweat inducer) to break a fever
- Treats and prevents yeast infections both systemically (taken internally) and vaginally (taken as a suppository or douche)
- Treats and prevents cystitis (urinary tract infections), pelvic inflammatory disease (PID), herpes, and other viral, fungal, and bacterial infections
- Used traditionally as an alterative (generally a remedy with detoxifying, cleansing, and eliminative actions) to treat skin diseases or disturbances, including eczema, psoriasis, allergic dermatitis, boils, and acne

FALSE UNICORN ROOT
(Chamaelirium luteum)

This Native American herb has been used for centuries for all manner of gynecological problems, ranging from weak or heavy periods to miscarriage and morning sickness, but its most treasured quality is its ability to promote fertility in both women and men. False unicorn root, also known as helonias root, is an adaptogenic herb, automatically adjusting its actions to the specific needs of the individual.

The ancient Irish earth goddess, Danu, lives on in this gentle herb. From her breasts and the river of blood that flowed from the cave between her legs, Danu created all life on earth. She gave birth to the moon by removing her cervix and gently placing it in the sky, and from that time on, women were blessed with the power to bleed in rhythm with the moon's cycles.

Common Uses

- Promotes fertility
- Prevents miscarriage (especially effective when used with black haw)
- Reestablishes menstrual regularity when natural rhythm has been lost
- Relieves chronic pelvic inflammation (especially effective when used with echinacea)
- Relieves symptoms of morning sickness
- Helps establish balance with erratic and heavy periods during the premenopausal and menopausal years

Caution: As with most herbs taken during pregnancy, false unicorn root should be used only with professional guidance.

GARLIC
(Allium sativum)

Garlic, a common household and culinary herb, has been used from time immemorial for a vast multitude of functions. Sanskrit records dating back more than five thousand years detail its astonishing healing capabilities; the Chinese have used the herb medicinally for more than three thousand years; and the Egyptians and Greeks used garlic for such diverse disorders as hypertension, earaches, infections, diarrhea, dysentery, and vaginitis. During the Middle Ages, wreathes of garlic were strung outside the house to guard against the plague, while bulbs were placed underneath children's pillows to protect them from evil during the night. Ancient Roman armies used the herb as an antiseptic and to treat lung diseases, and during World War I, the tradition continued as garlic was used to sterilize wounds and prevent gangrene, saving thousands of lives. Garlic's two main functions— its antimicrobial (antifungal, antibacterial, antiviral) actions and its supportive cardiovascular effects—have been extensively studied and validated scientifically.

The ancient goddess Gaea, who personified the earth itself, resides in this powerful but humble herb. All-producing and all-nourishing, Gaea is the Divine Mother who symbolizes the feminine power to nurture, protect, comfort, and heal.

Common Uses

- Prevents and provides relief from common colds and flus
- Heals intestinal and stomach infections or inflammations, from dysentery to irritable bowel syndrome
- Works gently and effectively as a urinary antibiotic for cystitis and various kidney disorders
- Treats causes and symptoms of pelvic inflammatory disease (PID) and various types of vaginal infections
- Used for any infection or inflammation of the respiratory system, including chronic sinusitis, bronchitis, and pneumonia
- Reduces blood pressure
- Reduces blood-cholesterol levels (reduces harmful LDL levels, while increasing the beneficial HDL levels)
- Reduces tumorous growths (considered to have anticancer actions)
- Balances sugar (glucose) levels in the body and can be used to treat hypoglycemia and diabetes

GINGER
(Zingiber Officinale)

A common culinary herb, ginger has enjoyed a worldwide reputation as a spice capable of warming the body, mind, and spirit. Shamans, wise women, and medicine men from all cultures and traditions have used ginger in love potions to create the heat necessary to kindle the fires of passion. In modern times, ginger is used for more strictly medicinal purposes—as a digestive tonic to relieve nausea and vomiting, as a powerful circulatory stimulant, and for fast and effective symptom relief from colds and flus. Gynecologically, ginger is valued for its ability to improve circulation to the entire pelvic cavity, reducing the symptoms of dysmenorrhea (cramping before or during menstruation) and stimulating menstrual flow.

Ginger evokes the Greek goddess Hestia, a grandmotherly divinity who rules over the hearth and home life, tending the eternal flame of domestic tranquillity to promote congeniality, devotion, intimacy, and affection.

Common Uses

- Eases menstrual cramps
- Promotes menstrual flow
- Relieves the symptoms of morning sickness (see Caution below)
- Relieves nausea and indigestion, calms an upset stomach, often used to prevent sea or motion sickness (a safe, natural alternative to Dramamine and various prescription drugs)
- Stimulates circulation, particularly for cold hands and feet
- Reduces blood-cholesterol levels
- Treats and/or prevents colds, flus, and respiratory problems

Caution: Large quantities of ginger should be avoided in pregnancy. For morning sickness, it is best to sip on a cup of mild ginger tea or place a drop of ginger tincture on your tongue; sometimes a small glass of ginger ale is all that is needed to settle the stomach.

GINSENG
(Panax ginseng, Panax quinquefolium, Eleutherococcus senticosus)

Ginseng has been used for thousands of years as a digestive aid, lung tonic, immune enhancer, energy tonic (to promote longevity and sexual prowess), and general aid to increase clarity of vision and thought. Ginseng comes in many varieties, all relatively interchangeable although with subtle variations in effect. American ginseng (*Panax quinquefolium*) is gentler and not quite as stimulating as the Asian varieties, and therefore more nourishing to the yin (Water) qualities; Korean and Chinese Ginseng (*Panax ginseng*) and Siberian ginseng (*Eleutherococcus senticosus*) tend to be warmer and more stimulating (supporting the yang or Fire qualities).

Although generally considered a male (yang) tonic, ginseng is rich in micronutrients specifically supportive of hormonal balance; in women, the herb exerts distinctively estrogenic effects, increasing vaginal moisture and elasticity, enhancing libido, and relieving numerous menopausal symptoms. The Chinese believe that ginseng allows both women and men to "age gracefully," but perhaps its most important function is its adaptogenic (individualized) effects on the adrenal glands, making it a superior tonic for the stresses of modern life.

In the realm of goddesses, ginseng evokes *Cerridwen*, the ancient Celtic goddess of intelligence, knowledge, and inspiration. Cerridwen possessed a magic cauldron in which she cooked precious herbs, and whoever drank from her Cauldron of the Deep was instantly filled with power and wisdom. Merlin, the magician of Arthurian legend, allegedly received all his magical powers from Cerridwen's cauldron.

Common Uses

- Relieves stress and dispels tension
- Eases depression and anxiety
- Builds strength and endurance
- Reduces or eliminates hot flashes
- Eases menopausal headaches
- Keeps the vaginal lining elastic and moist
- Reduces menstrual flooding
- Reinstates a normal rhythm to the menstrual cycle
- Reduces blood-cholesterol levels
- Regulates blood pressure
- Improves digestion
- Lowers blood-sugar levels

Caution: Ginseng can have a stimulating effect, especially when combined with caffeine; therefore avoid other stimulants if you regularly use ginseng. If you have high blood pressure, use only under professional supervision. If your menstrual cycle is extremely erratic, it is best to avoid using ginseng.

HAWTHORN BERRIES
(Crataegus oxyacantha)

Sometimes called ginseng for the heart, hawthorn has been used traditionally as a heart stabilizer to mitigate arrhythmias, such as palpitations (heart flutters) and tachycardia (very rapid hearbeats), and as a circulatory agent, stimulating blood flow through the vessels and improving circulation throughout the body. Slow-acting but reliable, hawthorn is a supreme menopausal ally, strengthening the heart muscle, improving circulation to the pelvic area, and supporting peripheral circulation. For use at any age, hawthorn is a soothing, supportive, balancing herb for high-strung, emotional individuals (the Fire or Heart type in Traditional Chinese Medicine).

Hawthorn invokes the gentle but powerful Sumerian goddess Inanna, Lady of the Morning and Evening Stars. Inanna rules over her vast empire with great compassion, healing the sick and wounded, providing for the hungry, protecting lost souls, and consoling the grief-stricken.

Common Uses

- Increases the blood supply to the heart, toning and strengthening the heart and blood vessels
- Stabilizes the heartbeat (particularly useful for arrhythmias or palpitations)
- Reduces hypertension
- Relieves hot flashes
- Calms the emotions
- Relieves insomnia (without the sedative effects of many sleeping medications)
- Increases the blood flow to the pelvic cavity and is thus useful for treating pelvic inflammatory disease (PID) and endometriosis
- Controls diarrhea, colic, and other intestinal spasms
- Provides digestive relief, helping to break up stagnant food and allow food and fluids to move more freely (traditionally used in China as a digestive aid)

LADY'S MANTLE
(Alchemilla vulgaris)

Lady's mantle has a long history as a sacred, magical herb; in ancient times alchemists would gather the dew that collected on the plant's foliage and use it to enhance the potency of their formulas. The principal quality of this herb is its astringency, which makes it the perfect antidote to heavy menstrual flow, breakthrough bleeding, or heavy discharges (leukorrhea). Lady's mantle also increases the blood supply to the reproductive organs, stimulating menstruation and supporting a balanced menstrual flow. Its proven anti-inflammatory properties confirm its historical role as an effective healing agent for wounds.

Lady's mantle invokes the Northern European goddess Freya, Mother of All—goddess of love, goddess of the plow—who is worshiped for her astonishing fertility. Freya embodies beauty, sensuality, compassion, and productivity; her magical number is thirteen, which represents the Sacred Thirteen Moons of the menstrual cycle.

Common Uses

- Controls heavy menstrual bleeding, flooding, or discharges (especially effective when combined with agrimony)
- Regulates menstrual cycles
- Promotes fertility
- Tones and strengthens the uterus and ovaries
- Promotes menstruation
- Acts as a powerful mouthwash for oral ulcers and cold sores and as an effective gargle for laryngitis

MILK THISTLE
(Carduus marianus, Silybum marianum)

As its common name implies, milk thistle has been used for thousands of years to promote milk production in lactating mothers; in Europe, wet nurses regularly ingested this plant to ensure an abundant flow of milk. In the Middle Ages, herbalists discovered milk thistle's value as a liver tonic and cleanser; numerous modern-day studies confirm its wide range of clinical uses for liver and gallbladder disorders. As the liver is arguably the most overworked of all our vital organs due to the stress and tension of modern life and the ubiquitous presence of environmental toxins, I regularly recommend milk thistle as a general support for vital liver functions and a specific aid in times of extreme stress or fatigue.

Milk thistle invokes the Central American mother goddess Mayahuel—the Woman with Four Hundred Breasts. Also known as the Mother Pot of the World and the Endlessly Milking One, Mayahuel nourishes, sustains, and transforms the world, giving freely of herself in order that others might live and thrive. Timeless and eternal, Mayahuel is said to sing the song that never ends.

Common Uses

- Supports liver and gallbladder function and helps these organs to renew and regenerate dead or dying cells
- Acts as a liver cleanser, reducing or eliminating toxins from the liver
- Stimulates the flow and production of milk in lactating mothers
- Clears the mind of depression
- Eases the physiological effects of stress, fatigue, and overexertion

MOTHERWORT
(Leonurus cardiaca)

An excellent all-purpose herb, motherwort is particularly effective for menopausal complaints and the tension and discomfort associated with premenstrual syndrome. Its calming (but nonsedating) effects extend to the mind and the spirit, helping to restore emotional balance by relieving tension, anxiety, confusion, and irritability.

Motherwort's botanical name means "lionhearted," and this herb can be imagined as the noble and courageous Egyptian goddess Isis, Mother of All. When her husband, Osiris, was murdered, the loyal Isis breathed life back into his body, sparking his spirit. In ancient Egypt, Isis represented the symbol of royal power, and the pharaohs would sit on her throne as a child sits on her mother's lap.

Common Uses

- Relieves and reduces hot flashes
- Reduces cramping with periods (PMS or otherwise)
- Helps to stimulate menstrual flow and reinstate regular periods
- Reduces pain and discomfort associated with menstruation
- Thickens and moistens vaginal walls
- Relieves anxiety and irritability
- Promotes a good night's sleep

- Tones and strengthens heart muscles and blood vessels
- Eases heart palpitations, calms a rapidly beating heart (tachycardia), and reinstates a steady heartbeat

Caution: Because motherwort can induce uterine contractions, avoid during pregnancy.

NETTLES
(Urtica dioica)

Nettles, also called stinging nettles, have a strong spiritual heritage and were used traditionally to remove curses or spells, directing them back to the sender (thus the sting). An extremely powerful and invasive plant, nettles extract high concentrations of nutrients from the soil and are especially rich in iron, vitamin C, calcium, and chlorophyll; these and other nutrients in the plant have powerful and diverse effects on the human body. Nettles have been used with great success to treat arthritic diseases and inflammations, to support kidney and bladder functions, and to control hemorrhaging. The Native Americans used nettles primarily as a gynecological herb and general womb tonic to increase fertility, support pregnancy, control bleeding during childbirth, and ease the transition through menopause.

Artemis, the Greek goddess of the moon and protectress of children, resides in this herb. Although loving and nurturing (particularly to women and children), Artemis could sting like nettle and was swift to punish when she was displeased. Complex and multifaceted, Artemis enjoyed almost limitless power in the ancient world.

Common Uses

- Promotes fertility
- Stimulates milk in nursing mothers
- Acts as a superfood to ensure good nutrition and health during pregnancy
- Establishes regular menstrual cycles
- Stems heavy bleeding or hemorrhages from the womb (also used for nosebleeds, coughing up of blood, and other hemorrhages)

- Nourishes the kidneys and adrenal glands (excellent for arthritis and gout, helping to excrete uric acid and other toxic metabolites)
- Creates strong, flexible bones
- Strengthens nervous system, increasing stamina and energy without stessing nerves
- Relieves menopausal symptoms such as anxiety, depression, fatigue, irritability, mood swings, and exhaustion
- Thickens and nourishes vaginal tissues
- Reduces vaginal itch and burning associated with yeast infections

RASPBERRY LEAF
(Rubus idaeus)

One of the few herbs universally considered safe to take during all stages of pregnancy, raspberry promotes fertility, enhances and strengthens the womb for pregnancy, and helps to prevent miscarriage. When taken during pregnancy, raspberry provides gentle relief of morning sickness and gastro-intestinal distress. During labor, the herb helps to reduce pain, allows the uterine contractions to work more effectively (although it does *not* strengthen contractions), and prevents excessive blood loss. When taken after childbirth, the plant works to replenish uterine tissues, toning and strengthening the muscles.

A mild yet strongly supportive plant, raspberry invokes the great mother goddess Huitaca, worshiped by the Chibcha of Colombia. Queen of Love and Pleasure, Huitaca oversees the ongoing cycle of renewal and creation, ensuring fertility and the safe delivery of healthy babies. It is said that the spirit of this playful peasant goddess lives under the skin of those who know her, reminding them to attend to the simple pleasures of life—eating, drinking, dancing, and lovemaking.

Common Uses

- Increases fertility (particularly effective when combined with false unicorn root)
- Supports and strengthens the uterus, preventing miscarriages and contributing to problem-free pregnancies
- Alleviates symptoms of morning sickness and gastrointestinal distress
- Helps nursing mothers produce an abundant supply of milk

- Tones and strengthens the uterus after childbirth
- Dries up abnormal uterine discharges

SAGE
(Salvia officinalis)

"Where sage doth grow well and vigorous, therein rules a strong woman," goes the old wives' saying. A common garden and culinary herb, sage is among the most sacred and cherished of medicinal plants. Native Americans used a sage smudge to purify the air to prepare the way for the Great Spirit. In Europe, sage was placed over the doorway to absorb any evil spirits that might seek entry. And in China, sage is considered a preeminent blood mover, helping to move *chi* and blood through physical and emotional obstructions to resolve stuckness.

Sage invokes the Indian goddess of mystery, Maya, who represents the untiring life force that manifests itself in the never-ending cycles of growth, decay, and renewal. Maya is never still or static, but always moving, changing shape, and transforming energy from one state into another. In the emptiness that flows into the fullness that flows into the emptiness of Maya, it is said, one can find enlightenment.

Common Uses

- Reduces or eliminates hot flashes, night sweats, and cold sweats associated with menopause
- Balances the female reproductive cycle
- Reduces or eliminates headaches, especially those associated with menopausal changes
- Resolves psychological feelings of being blocked or stuck
- Eases irritation, lifts depression, evens out mood swings
- Relieves menstrual cramps
- Helps nursing mothers dry up their breast milk
- Acts as an effective mouthwash for cold sores and mouth ulcers and as a gargle for sore throats and laryngitis

Caution: Discontinue use if the mouth or vagina is excessively dry. Avoid using large amounts of this herb over long periods of time.

ST. JOHN'S WORT
(Hypericum perforatum)

In medieval times, St. John's wort was burned in the fireplace to create a protective energy around the home and its inhabitants. A powerful restorative and soothing herb, St. John's wort has been used with great success for relieving symptoms of nervous tension including insomnia, menstrual cramps, intestinal colic, irritable bowel, and general anxiety. In addition to its ability to relax tension and muscle spasms, St. John's wort acts to calm and soothe the nervous system, resolving anxiety and irritability, alleviating depression, and assuaging pain. The gentle balancing actions of this herb—its ability to strengthen the nerves, increase energy and resilience, restore the spirit, and relieve muscle spasms and cramps—combine to make it a valuable ally for women experiencing difficulty with the transition from summer to autumn (the menopausal years).

This gentle but powerful herb can be imagined as Hecate, the Turkish goddess of the crossroads. Old as the earth itself, Hecate appears in the dark of the moon, offering comfort and protection to travelers who have lost their way or those who need assistance in making life's difficult decisions.

Common Uses

- Relieves irritability and depression
- Increases energy and stamina
- Deepens sleep, preventing insomnia
- Soothes and strengthens nerves
- Relieves muscle spasms and cramps (useful for intestinal colic and irritable bowel syndrome)
- Reduces pain and intensity of menstrual cramps
- Relieves menopausal symptoms, including hot flashes, night sweats, fluid retention, fatigue, anxiety, and mental confusion
- Provides effective treatment for wounds, burns, and skin problems, including eczema, psoriasis, and cold sores, and quick relief for stiff or painful joints and muscles (Such treatments use the oil extracted from the leaves and flowers of the plant.)

Uva Ursi
(*Arctostaphylos uva ursi*)

Native Americans considered uva ursi, also known as bearberry or mountain cranberry, a visionary plant and frequently smoked the leaves during sacred pipe rituals. In both European and Native American traditions, this herb traditionally has been used as a general tonic for the urinary system. Uva ursi has antiseptic (antibacterial) and astringent (drying) effects, making it an invaluable ally in the treatment of urinary tract infections, intestinal irritations, and vaginal or uterine discharges.

The Zulu goddess Mbaba Mwana Waresa, the Great Rain Mother of All, reigns in this sacred herb. Mbaba Mwana Waresa cleanses, cools, and nourishes all of life with her hallowed waters; the rainbow, it is said, is her smile. (This is a wonderful image, reinforcing the goddess's strong connection to Mother Earth—for if the rainbow is her smile, her head must be buried in the earth!)

Common Uses

- Helps prevent and treat cystitis, urethritis, and prostatitis (see Caution below)
- Soothes and strengthens the tissues of the urinary tract
- Acts as a strong diuretic (see Caution below), reducing the bloating associated with PMS
- Helps to control diarrhea
- Soothes intestinal irritations

Caution: Avoid large doses and prolonged usage. Discontinue if kidney symptoms (pain or discomfort in the kidney area of the back) occur. Because uva ursi has strong diuretic qualities, use only with professional guidance during pregnancy.

Valerian
(*Valeriana officinalis*)

Traditionally used as a heal-all for numerous physical, emotional, and spiritual problems, valerian is primarily used today as a calming and tranquilizing agent to ease anxiety and relieve tension. Although valerian is sometimes referred to as a plant sedative, it does not create drowsiness and in fact has a well-deserved reputation as a nervous system restorative, even acting as a gentle stimulant in cases of extreme fatigue.

The Chinese Mother of Mercy, Kuan Yin, resides in this herb. Kuan (earth) Yin (the spiritual energy that ebbs and flows) fills us with the force of her gentle healing powers, easing our pain and loneliness, soothing hurt feelings, promoting reconciliation, and strengthening feelings of love and devotion.

Common Uses

- Induces a state of tranquility and calm
- Reduces anxiety
- Eases symptoms associated with PMS (cramps, tension, irritability, mental confusion, fatigue, depression, anxiety)
- Relieves menopausal symptoms such as depression, irritability, insomnia, and racing heart (tachycardia)
- Relieves migraine headaches

VERVAIN
(Verbena officinalis)

In ancient times, vervain was considered a sacred herb with magical powers capable of warding off evil spirits, creating a spirit of peace and harmony, ensuring fidelity, and promoting marital bliss. In the Native American Moon Lodge, vervain was used to promote menstruation, ease cramps, reduce flooding, and increase libido.

This soothing, harmonizing herb can be imagined as Juno Lucina, the Italian Queen of Celestial Light, who rules over marriages and family matters and whose steady hand and gentle wisdom guide us through the dark phases of our lives, leading us ever so surely into the light. Every lunar month, as the story is told, Juno Lucina places her crescent pendant in the heavens; when the sliver of moon catches the silver light reflected from her face, it glows.

Common Uses

- Dispels depression
- Reduces chronic anxiety and restlessness
- Relieves insomnia and deepens sleep
- Eases headaches, especially those caused by nervous tension (migraines, for example)
- Increases the flow of mother's milk
- Brings on delayed menses

Caution: Although vervain is often used for anxiety during pregnancy, it should be taken only in minimal doses and always under a professional's guidance.

APPENDIX 2

THE POETRY OF THE POINTS: A DIRECTORY OF ACUPUNCTURE POINTS

While many books on Traditional Chinese Medicine discuss the locations and general functions of specific acupuncture points, in this appendix we offer a detailed look at the spiritual nature of the points. Each of the 365 acupuncture points in the human body has a unique energy or essence evoked by its name and its actions in the body/mind/spirit. When a specific point is needled or pressed, meditating on the "poetry of the point" often helps to accelerate the healing process. In acupuncture and herbal medicine, the mind, body, and spirit are considered inseparable; when they are permitted to communicate freely with each other, balance and harmony are soon restored.

Our directory includes twenty acupuncture points, all of which have a strong history of traditional use in the treatment of problems or symptoms associated with puberty, pregnancy, childbirth, menopause, and postmenopause. (They have many other general uses as well.) The choice of the points is somewhat idiosyncratic, as every acupuncturist has favorite points that he or she relies on as one would trust a devoted friend in time of need or crisis. It is that close, personal relationship with the points that we try to capture in this appendix.

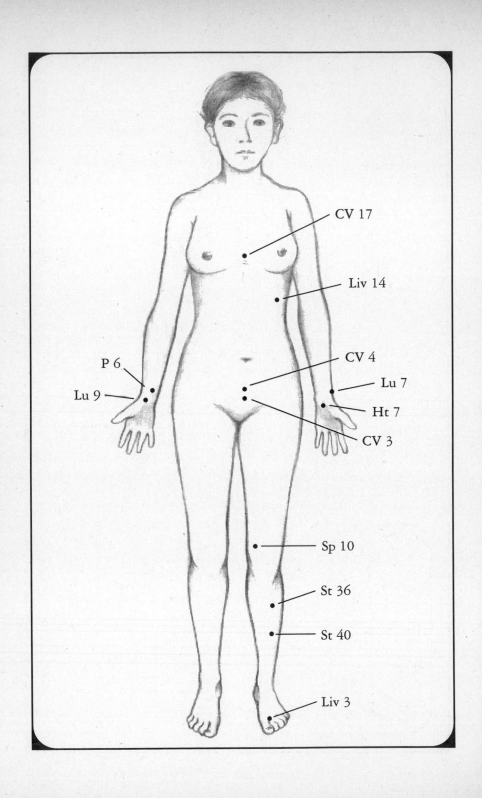

CV 17

Liv 14

P 6

Lu 9

CV 4

Lu 7

Ht 7

CV 3

Sp 10

St 36

St 40

Liv 3

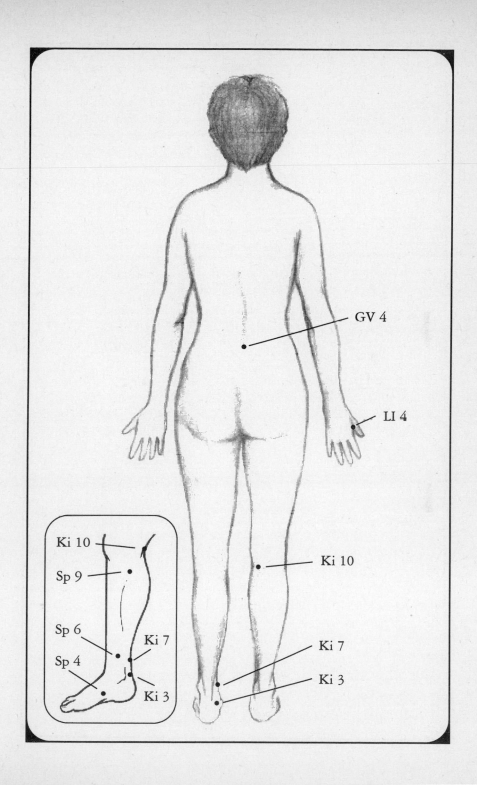

GV 4

LI 4

Ki 10

Ki 10

Sp 9

Sp 6

Ki 7

Sp 4

Ki 3

Ki 7

Ki 3

In selecting the points, we have included only those that are relatively easy to locate and stimulate yourself by pressing directly on the point (the technique known as acupressure). To find the point, read the general description of its location and then let the point guide you to it by sliding your fingers along the general area until they stop in a natural depression or hollow, which tends to be slightly more sensitive to the touch than the surrounding area. When an imbalance or disharmony of energies exists, the acupoint is often extremely sensitive, even painful to the touch.

If your interest in the technique or practice of acupuncture extends beyond this brief appendix, we recommend the following books:

Acupuncture for the Beginner

Between Heaven and Earth: A Guide to Chinese Medicine by Harriet Beinfield and Efrem Korngold (New York: Ballantine Books, 1991).

Plain Talk about Acupuncture by Ellinor R. Mitchell (New York: Whalehall, Inc., 1987).

Traditional Acupuncture: The Law of the Five Elements by Dianne M. Connelly (Columbia, MD: Center for Traditional Acupuncture, 1979).

The Web That Has No Weaver by Ted Kaptchuk (New York: Congdon and Weed, 1983).

Acupuncture: Metaphor and Meaning

Character and Health: The Relationship of Acupuncture and Psychology by Yves Requena (Brookline, MA: Paradigm Publications, 1989).

Dragon Rises, Red Bird Flies: Psychotherapy and Chinese Medicine by Leon Hammer (Barrytown, NY: Station Hill Press, 1990).

The Joy of Feeling: Bodymind Acupressure by Iona Marsaa Teeguarden (New York: Japan Publications, 1984).

INDEX OF ACUPUNCTURE POINTS (pages 330–331)

Conception Vessel 3 (CV 3),   *Zhong Ji* or *Ren 3* (Central Pole)
Conception Vessel 4 (CV 4),   *Guan Yuan* (Gate at the Source)

Conception Vessel 17 (CV 17),   *Dan Zhong* (Central Altar, Sea of the Chest Chi)

Governing Vessel 4 (GV 4),   *Ming Men* (Vital Gate, Life Gate Fire)

Heart 7 (Ht 7),   *Shen Men* (Spirit Gate)

Kidney 3 (Ki 3),   *Tai Xi* (Great Stream)

Kidney 7 (Ki 7),   *Fu Liu* (Recover Flow)

Kidney 10 (Ki 10),   *Yin Gu* (Yin Valley)

Large Intestine 4 (LI 4),   *He Gu* (Union of the Valleys, Great Eliminator)

Liver 3 (Liv 3),   *Tai Chong* (Great Rushing)

Liver 14 (Liv 14),   *Qi Men* (Gate of Hope)

Lung 7 (Lu 7),   *Lie Que* (Broken Sequence)

Lung 9 (Lu 9),   *Tai Yuan* (Great Abyss)

Pericardium 6 (P 6),   *Nei Guan* (Inner Frontier Gate, Inner Gate)

Spleen 4 (Sp 4),   *Gong Sun* (Ancestor and Descendant)

Spleen 6 (Sp 6),   *San Yin Jiao* (Three Yin Meeting)

Spleen 9 (Sp 9),   *Yin Ling Quan* (Yin Mound Spring)

Spleen 10 (Sp 10),   *Xue Hai* (Sea of Blood)

Stomach 36 (St 36),   *Zu San Li* (Walks Three Miles)

Stomach 40 (St 40),   *Feng Long* (Abundant Splendor, Bountiful Bulge)

CONCEPTION VESSEL 3, *ZHONG JI* OR *REN 3*
(Central Pole)

Conception Vessel 3 is the point where the three yin channels—the Spleen, Kidney, and Liver—join their forces and merge with the archetypical yin channel, the Conception Vessel. This point, like Spleen 6 (page 346), is a very strong supporter of the yin (fluid or water energy) and is traditionally used for almost all gynecological problems. Located directly over the womb, it guides the energies to the lower pelvic area, influencing the uterus and ovaries.

When I stimulate this point, I ask the patient to imagine a strong, flexible pole extending downward from her belly to penetrate deep into the earth. When the pole reaches the underground source of water and life energy, the fluid light can be drawn back up the Central Pole to nourish the body/mind/spirit with yin essence.

Common Uses

• Supports Kidney function, particularly the yin aspect of the Kidney

(The Kidney is considered the root of both yin and yang and plays a vital role in sexual function; thus this point is used to resolve vaginal dryness, restore interest in sex, "cool" hot flashes, and mitigate anxiety and general irritability.)

- Supports and nourishes the uterus, balancing the menstrual cycle; used for numerous menstrual disturbances including pelvic inflammatory disease (PID), fibroids, irregular menses, PMS, and amenorrhea
- Promotes urination and is often used for cystitis and incontinence (known as the *mu* [supportive] point for the Urinary Bladder)

Location: Conception Vessel 3 is located on the midline of the lower belly, about one thumb-width (a term that is used interchangeably with inch) below the midpoint between the umbilicus and the top of the pubic bone (approximately one inch beneath Conception Vessel 4).

CONCEPTION VESSEL 4, *GUAN YUAN*
(Gate at the Source)

Conception Vessel 4 is also known as the *tantien* (center) point, signifying the center of gravity or place of total balance. This acupoint, which connects directly to the Kidney and the Uterus, is used to access hidden reservoirs of *yuan chi* (original *chi*), sparking all the vital functions. When a patient feels scattered or lost, I ask her to place her hands over her *tantien* and imagine that she is able to use her *chi* and yang energies as a kind of welding torch to mend the broken pipes leading to the deep reservoirs of energy. Breathing deep, she can then pull the energy up to her center, from which it is dispersed throughout the body/mind/spirit.

Common Uses

- Tones and strengthens the Kidneys and Uterus
- Supports *chi* and is used for any form of depletion, including fatigue, lethargy, lack of self-interest, and lack of motivation
- Warms the uterus and lower pelvic area and is used to regulate the menstrual flow, assisting in the treatment of such problems as amenorrhea (lack of periods), irregular periods, scanty flow, PMS, infertility, and menopausal lethargy and/or depression

- Resolves digestive and intestinal problems
- Assists the Small Intestine in its role of separating the pure from the impure, eliminating toxic substances from the mind and the body

Location: Conception Vessel 4 is located on the midline of the body, halfway between the pubic bone and the belly button (approximately one hand-width below the belly button).

CONCEPTION VESSEL 17, *DAN ZHONG*
(Central Altar, Sea of the Chest Chi)

The Central Altar helps to regulate the physiological activities of the chest organs—the Lungs, Heart, and Pericardium. As these organs also govern spiritual issues, this point is commonly used for disharmonies involving *shen*, such as thought disturbances, sleep problems, manic behaviors, or depression. When emotional tensions build, we can often feel the energy getting stuck in this area; the symptoms of this stagnation of *chi* include difficulty breathing, tightness in the chest, heart palpitations, and other arrhythmias. When you stimulate this point, imagine that you are sending out a strong current of energy that radiates throughout the chest area to scatter and diffuse the tension, allowing the light and vital energy to penetrate the darkness.

Common Uses

- Protects and supports the Heart and Pericardium and calms the spirit; useful for any emotional disturbance including insomnia, anxiety, and restlessness
- Supports the Lung energy and can be used for any disturbance of the Lungs, including colds, flus, tightness in the chest, difficulty breathing, asthma, and bronchitis
- Facilitates and supports lactation; used for numerous breast disorders, including distention, pain or soreness of the breasts, cystic breasts, lactation problems, and mastitis

Location: Conception Vessel 17 is located on the midline of the breastbone, directly between the nipples.

GOVERNING VESSEL 4, *MING MEN*
(Vital Gate, Life Gate Fire)

Considered the "pilot light" of the entire body/mind/spirit, Life Gate Fire is located on the Governing Vessel, a major pathway that runs up the center of the spinal cord, along the top of the head to the face, where it joins up with the Conception Vessel. If you could draw a line straight from the umbilicus through the body to the spine, you would touch this point; as the umbilicus connects us to the mother, Life Gate Fire is said to connect to the root (essential, or primary) source of life energy. The main yang (Fire) point in the body, Life Gate Fire invigorates the entire system, bringing the spark back into life. Imagine it as the match that ignites the Fire (located in the Kidneys) that generates and sustains life.

Common Uses

- Fortifies Kidney energy and Kidney yang
- Supports the lower back and allows you to stand up for yourself
- Regulates the menstrual cycle
- Creates the Fire needed to dry up vaginal discharges
- Supports sexual vitality in both women and men

Location: Life Gate Fire is located on the spine in the small of the back at the central point between the Kidneys (approximately one hand-width above the tailbone).

HEART 7, *SHEN MEN*
(Spirit Gate)

This point settles the spirit. The Heart is said to store spirit, or *shen*, which the Chinese believe is reflected in and through the eyes. When the eyes sparkle and shine, the *shen* is considered strong and indicates good health; when the eyes appear dull or hazy, the *shen* is weak, indicating serious underlying problems in the body/mind/spirit. Spirit Gate can be imagined as the doorway to the palace where *shen* is stored; when this point is stimulated, a troubled or anxious spirit is soothed and the Heart is permitted to relax and settle into a steady rhythm.

Common Uses

- Calms and pacifies the spirit *(shen)*, thus relieving disorders of *shen*, including generalized anxiety, nervousness, mania, obsessive-compulsive behaviors, agitation, memory problems, and sleep disturbances
- Regulates and stabilizes the Heart *chi* and is useful for many heart problems including palpitations and arrythmias
- Supports the yin qualities of the Heart, clearing the heat; helps to relieve menopausal symptoms such as night sweats and hot flashes
- Lowers blood pressure

Location: Heart 7 is located on the inner crease of the wrist in a depression located approximately half an inch in from the pinky side of wrist.

KIDNEY 3, *TAI XI*
(Great Stream)

The source point on the Kidney channel, Kidney 3 tones and supports every aspect of Kidney function including the yin, yang, *chi*, and *jing*. As the generator and root of both yin and yang energies, the Kidney requires support for many conditions of depleted energy. Stimulating this point allows us to replenish our body, mind, and spirit in the great stream of life's energy. When you press this point, imagine taking a dip in an ice-cold mountain stream; feel the invigorating waters penetrate deep into your being—deeper than the skin, tendons, and muscles, deeper even than the tissues and organs, filtering into your bones to renew and regenerate life at the core.

Common Uses

- Supports and nourishes the Kidneys
- Relieves Kidney conditions characterized by depletion of energy, including low back and/or knee pain, urinary incontinence or retention, lack of sexual vigor and/or interest; also useful for depleted emotional conditions such as lethargy or lack of drive and motivation
- Nourishes the Kidney yin and indirectly supports the Liver yin. Commonly used for depleted conditions where heat symptoms are

prevalent, such as agitation, hot flashes, night sweats, insomnia, restless sleep, or hot (itchy or irritated) eyes

Location: Kidney 3 is located in the depression between the inside ankle bone and the Achilles tendon; use your fingers to poke around in the valley until you feel the tender spot.

KIDNEY 7, *FU LIU*
(Recover Flow)

Traditionally used to support and fortify Kidney energy in all of its forms, especially *chi* and yang, this is an important point for numerous gynecological problems, particularly those connected with the urinary system. Kidney 7 provides a jump start to help you rekindle vital energy that may have been depleted from stress, a long illness, or generalized states of exhaustion. When I stimulate this point, I like to think that I am tapping into a potent source of electrical energy that can then be used to "recover the flow" essential to life itself.

Common Uses

- Strengthens vital energy throughout the body, mind, and spirit
- Adjusts and regulates the menstrual cycles
- Supports the immune system, helping to build and balance the protective *wei chi* energy (the Chinese equivalent of the immune system)
- Promotes perspiration when the body needs to expel toxins and pathogens (such as those related to colds, flus, etc.), but helps to prevent excessive sweating and the loss of vital *chi* when a deficiency exists

Location: Located two inches above Kidney 3, Kidney 7 lies between the Achilles tendon and the inner ankle bone.

KIDNEY 10, *YIN GU*
(Yin Valley)

The Water point on the Kidney channel (a Water orb), Kidney 10 is known as the Master Point, providing essential support for yin energies.

When stimulating this point, imagine a beautiful valley that has filled up with water; underground springs gently diffuse and disperse the water throughout the surrounding forests and farmlands, naturally irrigating the earth and providing abundant sources of liquid nourishment. If you are suffering from a heat condition such as vaginitis or cystitis with burning urination, imagine the Water being channeled into the lower (pelvic) regions, where it disperses the heat and the Fire.

Common Uses

- Assists the Kidney, particularly with its yin functions
- Clears heat from the lower burner (the organs located below the umbilicus)
- Removes heat from the blood and helps relieve such symptoms as acne, boils, and other inflammations of the skin, including eczema or psoriasis

Location: Kidney 10 is located at the innermost aspect of the crease of the knee, between the two large tendons.

LARGE INTESTINE 4, *HE GU*
(*Union of the Valleys, Great Eliminator*)

This sensitive point is often used for draining or dispersing stuck energy in the upper part of the body, especially the head and neck areas, relieving headaches of all varieties, congestion in the sinus cavities, stuffy nose, sore throat, swollen glands, eye problems, and neck or shoulder tightness with pain and spasm. Liver 3 (located in the webbing between the big toe and the second toe) performs a similar function for the lower body, moving and unblocking energy that is stuck below the shoulders; when used together, these points are called the Four Gates, and are said to "clean the house." Thus, the Great Eliminator can be imagined as a powerful internal vacuum cleaner that sucks the negative energy out of the upper body, relieving congestion and allowing us to breathe freely and see clearly.

Common Uses

- Supports the Lung, helping to eliminate pathogens; excellent for relieving sinus infections, headaches, and the heavy, "filled with cotton" sensations that accompany many head colds
- Clears the lungs and helps to resolve heat conditions such as sore throats and swollen lymph glands
- Promotes menstruation, expedites labor, and assists in delivery of the afterbirth (Though extremely useful during labor and childbirth, this point is contraindicated in pregnancy.)
- Regulates the intestines and traditionally used for intestinal problems such as diarrhea, irritable bowel, and constipation
- Helps to brighten the eyes and is used in conjunction with any eye condition, including itchy, irritated eyes, conjunctivitis, or swollen eyes

Location: Located on the top of the hand in the webbing between the thumb and index finger.

LIVER 3, *TAI CHONG*
(Great Rushing)

The source point for the Liver meridian, Liver 3 is often used when the Liver energy is constrained or deficient. The Chinese Liver rules "flowing and spreading" and is responsible for the circulation and distribution of blood and *chi* throughout the body. Like the Western liver, the Chinese Liver filters, purifies, and detoxifies every substance we take into our bodies, but in Chinese thought, the Liver is also thought to detoxify the spirit. One of the branches of the Liver meridian opens into the eyes; thus the Chinese believe that the Liver rules internal and external problems with vision.

Great Rushing can be imagined as a physical, emotional, and spiritual Roto-Rooter, breaking up blockages and obstructions and allowing energy and blood to flow through the system unimpeded. A stream that finds its source high atop a mountain and runs freely and without interruption to the sea is considered healthy and full of life energy; if the water meets an obstruction and cannot move through it, illness and disease will occur.

Common Uses

- Supports the Liver, promoting the free flow of energy and blood
- Relieves gynecological symptoms such as cramping, irritability, anxiety, depression, heavy menstrual bleeding (especially with clots), headaches (especially migraines), and digestive problems associated with stress
- Expels "wind" conditions, which are thought to be caused by an imbalance in Liver *chi*, including tremors, muscle twitches, pain that tends to move around from joint to joint or muscle to muscle, dizziness, and headaches
- Effective for pain relief associated with wind conditions
- Brightens the eyes, helping to resolve physiological and psychological problems with vision.

Location: Liver 3 is located on the upper aspect of the foot in the depression in the webbing between the big toe and the second toe.

LIVER 14, *QI MEN*
(Gate of Hope)

The alarm point for the Liver orb, Liver 14 becomes extremely sensitive to the touch when the Liver is stressed or near exhaustion. Gate of Hope helps to resolve stagnation of energy, stimulating movement of energy, blood, and *chi* while rekindling a sense of hope and confidence in the future. When I stimulate this point, I ask the patient to imagine that she has been standing in one place, pulling and tugging on a door or gate that will not open no matter how hard she tries. Rather than continue to deplete her energies, I suggest that she look around at the other doors that are available to her, all of which have freely swinging gates and will allow her entry to wherever she needs or wants to go. By changing her perspective, I remind her, she can change her world.

Common Uses

- Supports Liver functions, stimulating the flow of *chi* and helping to resolve blockages; helps you to move through emotional stuckness and feelings of helplessness and hopelessness

- Rules flow and helps to reestablish a normal menstrual cycle; very effective for PMS, particularly for breast distention, bloating, cramping, and emotional upheavals
- Transforms "congealed blood" by activating the energy through the meridians and breaking up blockages; useful for such conditions as cystic breast disease, ovarian cysts, and uterine fibroids (In Chinese thought, all masses are thought to result from conditions of congealed blood.)
- Relieves the stabbing pain (another symptom of congealed blood) associated with endometriosis, migraine headaches, and stomach, chest, or genital distress
- Promotes digestion, relieving constipation and bloating

Location: Liver 14 is located two ribs directly below the nipples on the mammillary line, in the space between the ribs.

LUNG 7, *LIE QUE*
(Broken Sequence)

Lung 7 opens the Conception Vessel (*Renmo*), which is the major support of the yin qualities of the body/mind/spirit. This point is traditionally used as a powerful support for the Lungs, circulating and spreading Lung energies to resolve colds, respiratory infections, and asthmatic symptoms. Because it is connected to the Conception Vessel, Lung 7 also helps to balance hormonal levels, actively stimulating and propelling the yin energy throughout the body. When I stimulate this point, I like to think that I am opening up release valves on a dammed-up river, allowing the power and vitality of the waters to flood through the body, mind, and spirit, nourishing, moistening, and invigorating the vital organs.

Common Uses

- Supports and moves the energy of the Lung; useful for all congestive problems involving the Lung, including asthma, bronchitis, sinus infections, coughs, and excess phlegm (especially effective when used with Large Intestine 4)
- Supports the production of *wei chi*, the Chinese equivalent of the immune system

- Opens and closes the pores of the skin, helping to eliminate toxins through perspiration while retaining vital stores of *chi*
- Supports the yin-circulating functions of the Conception Vessel
- Helps to increase feelings of power and self-confidence when stimulated in conjunction with Conception Vessel 3 and 4, permitting us to feel more at home in ourselves

Location: Lung 7 is located two inches above the wrist crease on the inner forearm; run your fingers along the bone on the inner (thumb) side of the forearm, moving them over the bone until they stop in a depression.

LUNG 9, *TAI YUAN*
(Great Abyss)

As the source point on the Lung channel, Great Abyss offers a direct line to the Lung orb and is used to activate and energize the Lung *chi*. This *chi* can be imagined as a waterfall that plunges from high atop a mountain into the great abyss of the body's interior, where it surges and swells, an abundant source of powerful energy. Lung 9 is often used to support Metal energies when they are out of balance. (Metal is the power that governs the activities of the Lungs.)

Common Uses

- Supports and strengthens the Lung *chi*, helping to resolve problems associated with the Lung, including colds, bronchitis, asthma, and sinus infections
- Supports the *wei chi* (immune energy), which originates in the Lung
- Regulates the blood vessels and is often used to support and move the blood and to stop heavy bleeding
- Supports the yin, especially the chest yin, and is useful for anxiety, palpitations, and irritability; especially effective when used with Heart 7 and Pericardium 6

Location: Lung 9 is located on the crease on the palm side of the wrist in the depression at the base of the thumb (about half an inch in from the side of the wrist).

PERICARDIUM 6, *NEI GUAN*
(Inner Frontier Gate, Inner Gate)

Inner Gate offers a metaphor for the function of the Pericardium, the muscle that surrounds and protects the heart. When the gate swings freely, blood, energy, and nutrients are permitted into the body/mind/spirit, while stress, toxins, and disturbing thoughts are barred entrance. Disease occurs when the hinges to the inner gate are rusty, and the gate is stuck either open or closed; when this occurs, we can no longer keep careful guard over the entryway to our inner being. When this point is pressed or needled, I ask the patient to imagine that she is oiling and lubricating the hinges of her Heart. By stimulating this point, she can either permit or deny entrance into the inner sanctum of the Heart, protecting herself from physical and psychic harm, while allowing essential information and nutrients to enter.

Pericardium 6 is traditionally used for a wide variety of symptoms ranging from nausea, motion sickness, and morning sickness to tightness of the chest, anxiety attacks, and heart palpitations. This point is also used to unblock constrained Liver *chi*, thus promoting the free and unimpeded flow of energy and blood through the body/mind/spirit.

Common Uses

- Tones and supports Heart functions
- Corrects "Heart imbalances," a traditional Chinese medical diagnosis for symptoms such as palpitations, anxiety, disturbed sleep, and poor memory
- Calms "rebellious Stomach *chi*," a traditional diagnosis for symptoms such as nausea and heartburn (In Western medicine, these symptoms are often considered psychosomatic in origin.)
- Relaxes muscle constriction in the chest, relieving tension and shortness of breath
- Relieves symptoms of morning sickness (A combination of herbs and acupuncture is particularly effective for the nausea, heartburn, and bloating associated with early pregnancy. In Western herbalism, ginger is the herb of choice, while practitioners of Traditional Chinese Medicine tend to prefer tangerine peel.)

Location: Pericardium 6 is located on the inner part of the forearm, two thumb-widths above the crease of the wrist in the depression between the two tendons.

SPLEEN 4, *GONG SUN*
(Ancestor and Descendant)

Spleen 4 is the opening point on a special channel known as the *chong mo*, or penetration channel, which provides a direct route for nourishment to penetrate deep into our inner being. Chong mo is always associated with the access and use of the inherited energy known as *jing*, the gift passed down from ancestor to descendant (thus the name of this point). In opening the penetration channel, we acknowledge that we are worthy of nourishment—not just physical sustenance but emotional and spiritual support as well. Spleen 4 is a particularly important point for those who tend to mother their friends and family members but find it difficult to allow others to care for them.

Common Uses

- Regulates the manufacture and quality of the blood
- Breaks up stagnation of blood and is therefore useful for conditions of congealed blood, such as painful menstrual periods, fibroids, ovarian cysts, and heavy periods with clotting
- Normalizes the menstrual cycles
- Supports and regulates the functions of the Spleen and Stomach, allowing the proper assimilation of foods and fluids
- Resolves digestive problems by dissolving stagnation in the digestive system; effective for symptoms such as gastroenteritis, excessive gas and bloating, chronic nausea and vomiting

Location: Spleen 4 is located on the inside of the foot, along the arch ("where the red and the white skin meet"), in a hollow one and one-half inches behind the knuckle (bunyon bone) of the big toe.

SPLEEN 6, *SAN YIN JIAO*
(Three Yin Meeting)

The three yin meridians—the Liver, Kidney, and Spleen—meet at this
point, which is one of the most oft-used points in acupuncture for depleted
yin or disturbed yang. Considered a universal gynecological point, Three
Yin Meeting can be imagined as three mountain streams joining up to
create a powerful whitewater river. At the widest and deepest point of
the river, the energy of this point is generated and constantly renewed.
Like many of the herbs discussed in appendix I (specifically false unicorn
root and chasteberry), Spleen 6 has an adaptogenic effect and is capable
of altering its effects to meet the individual's specific needs.

Common Uses

- Nourishes the blood
- Helps to support and balance the menstrual cycle and is used for
  almost all gynecological complaints
- Nourishes and supports the yin, relieving deficient yin conditions
  such as dry or itchy skin, lack of vaginal moistness, insomnia, and
  constipation
- Subdues the yang, relieving hot flashes, night sweats, irritability,
  agitation, nervousness, flushing, and skin irritations
- Strengthens the Stomach and Spleen functions, supporting digestion
  and assimilation of nutrients

Location: Spleen 6 is located approximately three thumb-widths above
the interior ankle bone, in a depression just to the side of the tibia bone.

SPLEEN 9, *YIN LING QUAN*
(Yin Mound Spring)

When the heat and humidity rise in the summer months, isolated pools
of water fill up with bacteria and become stagnant over time. Yin Mound
Spring provides an abundant source of fresh, nutrient-rich water that can
be used to flush out and replace the polluted pools. It is said to clear the
body's waterways of "damp-heat conditions," which result when water
gets stuck and creates areas of swelling or inflammation. At a deeper

(organic) level, Spleen 9 can be used to support the functions of the Spleen and Stomach orbs and is a valued adjunct to any treatment for replenishing the yin energies and improving nourishment.

Common Uses

- Promotes urination and resolves edema (swelling due to water retention)
- Reduces swelling around the joints, relieving arthritic symptoms
- An excellent point for treating cystitis and urethritis (and prostatitis in men)
- Supports the function of the Spleen and Stomach and resolves digestive "dampness," which results in such symptoms as loose bowels, bloating, and gurgling stomach

Location: Spleen 9 is located in the depression on the inside of the lower leg, just below the knee. With your knee bent, slide your fingers along the bone on the inside border of the knee until they stop in a natural depression; this point is often extremely sensitive to the touch.

SPLEEN 10, *XUE HAI*
(Sea of Blood)

Spleen 10 nourishes and moves the blood and is considered the archetypical point for virtually any condition involving blood and menstruation, particularly when stagnation or depletion exists. (This point is contraindicated in cases of excessive menstrual bleeding or heavy breakthrough bleeding.) When needling or pressing this point, imagine within yourself a sea where blood is stored and continually replenished with flowing streams of vital energy and nutrients. Stimulating this point provides new outlets for the water to circulate throughout the body, flushing out the toxins while oxygenating and nourishing the cells.

Common Uses

- Moves stagnant blood and is useful for any gynecological condition

involving pain, including cramping, premenstrual tension, and
migraines
- Resolves congealed blood and is useful for such symptoms as fibroid
tumors, ovarian cysts, and other masses or growths anywhere in the
body
- Supports and nourishes the blood and helps to resolve "blood-deficient
conditions," such as irregular menstrual periods or missed periods
(amenorrhea)
- Aids in the treatment of skin problems, which the Chinese view as
symptoms of excess heat in the blood

Location: Sea of Blood is located on the inside of the knee in the fleshy
part of the bulge, approximately two and a half inches above the kneecap
(on the thigh).

STOMACH 36, *ZU SAN LI*
(Walks Three Miles)

Stomach 36 assists the Stomach and Spleen in their task of transforming
nutrients into usable energy. A powerfully energizing point, Stomach 36
supports the assimilation of food and fluids and actively converts nutrients
into *chi* and blood. One of the most frequently used acupoints (gynecological and otherwise), Walks Three Miles gets its name from ancient times,
when monks traveled long distances by foot to visit different monasteries.
When they felt exhausted and unable to continue, the monks would needle
or press this point and gain the energy needed to walk an additional three
miles.

Common Uses

- Energizes and strengthens the Spleen, Stomach, Small Intestine and
Large Intestine, helping to regulate digestive problems
- Builds *chi* by helping the Stomach and Spleen produce "acquired *chi*,"
and assists the Kidney in its job of protecting its stores of "inherited
chi"
- Restores health after debilitating disease or exhaustion (a powerful
point for building *chi* after pregnancy and childbirth)

- Supports "upright *chi*" and is used traditionally to prevent prolapses such as hemorrhoids, hernias, prolapsed uterus, and prolapsed bladder
- Rids the body of excess dampness, helping to resolve edema (water retention), vaginal discharges, and any other form of emotional or spiritual dampness such as heaviness of limbs, foggy thinking, and lethargy
- Assists with numerous gynecological functions: brings on menses, helps to establish regular periods, promotes lactation, and provides relief from menopausal symptoms

Location: Stomach 36 is located three inches below the dimple or depression on the outside (pinky) side of the knee; approximately an inch from the crest of the shinbone, Stomach 36 lies in a groove or natural depression in the muscle.

STOMACH 40, *FENG LONG*
(Abundant Splendor, Bountiful Bulge)

Stomach 40 is the archetypical point used to disperse excess dampness in the Stomach channel, helping to resolve such symptoms as lethargy, foggy thinking, heaviness of limbs, and aching joints. When I stimulate this point, I like to imagine that a strong wind of energy blows through the body, mind, and spirit, dispelling the fog and revealing the abundant splendor that existed all along. When the clouds lift, the body/mind/spirit is warmed and rejuvenated by the healing rays of the sun.

Common Uses

- Eliminates and transforms dampness and congealed fluids; useful for any condition of excess phlegm or edema, including digestive bloating, water retention, and chronic loose stools
- Regulates the functions of the Stomach and Spleen by supporting metabolism and eliminating *tan* (undigested fluids)
- Calms the spirit and helps to resolve what the Chinese call "Heart phlegm," which causes muddled thinking, dull affect, slurred speech, and depression

• Supports the lungs and helps to resolve excess mucous conditions such as chronic bronchitis, chronic sinusitis, and asthma

Location: Stomach 40 is located midway between the ankle and knee, on the outer side of the lower leg, two inches lateral (toward the side of the leg) from the shinbone, in a bulge on the calf muscle.

APPENDIX 3

RESOURCES

PRACTITIONERS

In selecting a practitioner from any tradition, it is important to do your homework. Ask around and get feedback on various practitioners in your area from their patients. Word of mouth is probably the most valuable resource you have. Ask your prospective practitioner many questions. How long have they been in practice? Which modalities, if any, do they use to complement their specialty? How do they feel their specialty can be of help to you? Remember that you are in control—you are hiring someone to work for you.

HOLISTIC WESTERN MEDICINE

American Holistic Medical Association
4101 Lake Boone Trail, Suite 201

Raleigh, NC 27607
(919) 787-5181

Can give references to M.D.s who subscribe to a holistic approach.

ACUPUNCTURE

American Association of Acupuncture and Oriental Medicine (AAAOM)
433 Front St.
Catasauqua, PA 18032–2506
(610) 433-2448

Both the AAAOM and NAAOM (address and phone number below) offer referrals to qualified practitioners in your area and can provide information on qualifications for licensure and certification for each state.

National Alliance of Acupuncture and Oriental Medicine (NAAOM)
638 Prospect Ave.
Hartford, CT 06105
(203) 586-7509

National Commission for the Certification of Acupuncturists (NCCA)
1424 16th St. NW, Suite 105
Washington, DC 20036
(202) 232-1404

Can give you a list of fully certified acupuncturists (those who have graduated from an accredited school, with a minimum of three years postcollege training, and passed the NCCA comprehensive exams) in your area.

National Council of Acupuncture Schools and Colleges (NCASC)
PO Box 954
Columbia, MD 21044
(301) 997-4888

If you're interested in pursuing an education and career in acupuncture, this resource will let you know which schools are certified, and prepare you for the national boards (a prerequisite for most state licensure).

HERBAL MEDICINE

Crane Enterprises
45 Samoset Ave.
RFD #1
Plymouth, MA 02360
(800) 227-4118

Offers a referral service and can recommend a trained practitioner of Chinese herbal medicine in your area.

National Commission for the Certification of Acupuncturists (NCCA)
1424 16th St. NW, Suite 105
Washington, DC 20036
(202) 232–1404

The NCCA department in Chinese herbal medicine requires that certain educational standards be met and a comprehensive exam passed. But this is a new department, and there are many competent herbal practitioners who are not yet board certified. It is best to ask practitioners where they received their training, how long they have been practicing, and whether or not they have access to supervision. Herbs can be potent medicine, and it is important for you to trust that your herbalist is well trained.

Note: There are many training programs in Western herbal medicine, but as of yet, no licensing in this country. Many of the best herbalists are carrying on, with great skill, the wise woman traditions of connectedness to the earth and its many gifts, and very often these wise individuals are also very learned about the scientific applications of herbal medicine.

The best way to find a good herbal practitioner is by word of mouth. Ask a holistically oriented physician or chiropractor to recommend an herbalist. Find out how they learned their art and with whom they studied, and ask for the names of some of their patients you could talk to.

NATUROPATHIC PHYSICIANS

Naturopathic physicians are well trained in vitamin, mineral, and herbal methods of healing, as well as Western medical physiology and pathology.

American Association of Naturopathic Physicians
2366 Eastlake Ave., East Suite 322
Seattle, WA 98102

Send a SASE to the above address and request a listing of certified naturopathic physicians in your area.

JOURNALS AND NEWSLETTERS

American Botanical Council and the Herb Research Foundation
PO Box 201660
Austin, TX 78720
(800) 748-2617
(800) 373-7105

Offers a wonderful journal on herbology called *HerbalGram*, and can give advice on how to find an herbalist. Most schools offering courses of study in herbal medicine advertise in this journal.

Medical Herbalism
PO Box 33080
Portland, OR 97233

Publishes an informative newsletter geared toward herbal practitioners.

Northeast Herbal Association
PO Box 146
Marshfield, VT 05658-0146

Publishes a newsletter and maintains a directory of practicing herbalists in the northest states.

BUYING HERBS BY MAIL

The following is a list of reputable dealers who grow and sell good-quality, usually organic, dried herbs, both in bulk or in capsules, tinctures, etc. Send for a catalog.

Avena Botanicals
PO Box 365
West Rockport, ME 04865

Frontier Cooperative Herbs
Rte. 1, Box 31
Norway, Iowa 52318

Gaia Herbs
62 Old Littleton Rd.
Harvard, MA 01451

Green Terrestrial
PO Box 41, Rte. 9W
Milton, NY 12547

Herbalist and Alchemist
PO Box 458
Bloomsbury, NJ 08804

The Herb Closet
104 Main St.
Montpelier, VT 05602

Herb Pharm
PO Box 116
Williams, OR 97544

Island Herbs
c/o Ryan Drum
Waldron Island, WA 98297

ITM Herb Products
2017 SE Hawthorne
Portland, OR 97214
(800) 544–7504

Carries a wide range of Chinese patent remedies in addition to their own
excellent products and formulas.

Meadowbrook Herbs
Whispering Pines Rd.
Wyoming, RI 02898

Sage Mountain Herb Products
PO Box 420
East Barre, VT 05649

WOMEN'S HEALTH

GENERAL INFORMATION

American College of Obstetricians and Gynecologists
409 12th St. SW
Washington, DC 20024–2188
(202) 638–5577

Provides information for patients on various gynecological issues but does not provide referrals. Let them know what topics you're interested in, and include a self-addressed stamped envelope.

Boston Women's Health Book Collective
240-A Elm St.
Somerville, MA 02144
(617) 625–0271

Offers an information line and provides a safe place to ask questions. Will send you information on topics of concern, and offers access to their extensive library devoted to women's health. Can also refer you to organizations in your area.

MENSTRUATION AND FERTILITY

American Society for Reproductive Medicine
1209 Montgomery Hwy.
Birmingham, AL 35216–2809
(205) 978–5000

Offers a list of physician referrals by state and provides information packets and resource lists on fertility issues.

Womankind: Life Cycles Curriculum
104 Petaluma Ave.
Sebastopol, CA 95472
(707) 829-2744

Dedicated to helping women reclaim their menstruating power and fertility. Organizes "coming of age" programs and offers referrals to practitioners or groups in your area.

PREGNANCY AND BIRTHING

International Childbirth Education Association
PO Box 20048
Minneapolis, MN 55420
(612) 854–8660

Offers a publications catalog that covers a wide variety of issues concerning childbirth, and provides referrals to childbirth education classes worldwide.

La Leche League International
1400 North Meacham Rd.
Schamburg, IL 60173
(708) 519–7730

Provides information and referrals on every aspect of breast-feeding.

ENDOMETRIOSIS

Endometriosis Alliance of Greater New York
Old Chelsea Station, Box 634
New York, NY 10113–0634
(212) 533–3636

Offers a phone menu that lists the services available. Will return phone calls (but only collect) to answer questions.

Endometriosis Association
8585 North 76th Pl.

Milwaukee, WI 53223
(800) 992–3636

Will send information packets on endometriosis.

HYSTERECTOMY

**HERS Foundation (Hysterectomy Education
    Resources and Services)**
422 Bryn Mawr Ave.
Bala-Cynwyd, PA 19004
(215) 667–7757

An excellent resource for information about hysterectomy. Information
packets available by mail.

CANCER

American Cancer Society
1599 Clifton Rd. NE
Atlanta, GA 30329
(800) ACS-2345

Provides information on available treatment programs (from a Western
perspective) for various types of cancer and can refer you to other organizations for services. Does not provide referrals to individual doctors.

MENOPAUSE

A Friend Indeed Publications, Inc.
PO Box 1710
Champlain, NY 12919–1710
and
Box 515
Place du Parc Station
Montreal, Canada H2W 2P1
(514) 843-5730

Puts out an excellent newsletter and offers info on menopause and midlife
issues.

Older Women's League (OWL)
666 Eleventh St. NW, Suite 700
Washington, DC 20001
(202) 783-6686

Offers information on the politics of women's health and health reform. Provides a list of publications and member organizations and offers a "model benefits package."

Natural Feminine Products

These companies offer natural cloth products, including menstrual pads, underwear, and panty liners. Write for their mail-order catalogs. New Cycle is more focused on natural menstrual care products, while Seventh Generation offers a wide range of natural care products for home and body care.

New Cycle Products
PO Box 3248
Santa Rosa, CA 95402
(707) 571-2036

Seventh Generation
Colschester, VT 05403
(800) 456-1177

Natural Pharmaceuticals

Madison Pharmacy Associates
429 Gammon Pl.
Madison, WI 53719
(800) 558-7046

Offers information on a wide variety of gynecological issues and makes excellent women's products, which are available both over the counter and by prescription.

Melaleuca, Inc.
3910 South Yellowstone Hwy.
Idaho Falls, Idaho 83402-6003

Melaleuca is the botanical name for the tea tree. Not only can you purchase tea tree oil, but they also offer a wide variety of environmentally friendly household products (many of which use melaleuca oil as their active ingredient).

Professional and Technical Services
333 Northeast Sandy Blvd.
Portland, OR 97232
(800) 648-8211

Makes excellent natural products, including ProGest cream, and offers advice on a variety of gynecological conditions, and information on where you can get their products (available only through health professionals).

Transitions for Health
621 SW Alder, Suite 900
Portland, OR 97205
(800) 888-6814

Offers information packets on a wide variety of issues, including PMS and menopause, a catalog of their products geared to the layperson, and a free newsletter.

Women's Health America
PO Box 9690
Madison, WI 53715
(608) 833-9102

An extension of Madison Pharmacy (see above). Offers books, videos, and over-the-counter pharmaceuticals for all sorts of women's health issues.

The Women's International Pharmacy
5708 Monona Drive
Madison, WI 53716
(800) 279-5708
fax: (800) 279-8011

They offer excellent quality natural pharmaceutical products for women, both prescription and nonprescription, and will supply information packets on various gynecological conditions.

NUTRITIONAL SUPPLEMENTS

Most of the companies listed below are widely represented in health food stores, but good vitamins are certainly not limited to the brands listed. Consult a professional about other brands.

Alacer Corporation—good products, especially vitamin C.

Kal-Healthway—good-quality vitamins easily found in stores.

McZand or Zand Herbal Products—high-quality Western and Chinese herbal products.

Michael's Naturopathic Formulas—excellent herbal and vitamin formulas for various syndromes and diseases.

Nature's Herbs—excellent herbal products, with assured potency and certifiably organic.

Nature's Way—high-quality herbal products.

New Chapter Vitamins—excellent herbal tonics and vitamin products.

Nutricology—specially prepared formulas for various syndromes and diseases.

The following companies produce good-quality, widely available vitamin and mineral supplements: **Nature's Plus, Richlife, Schiff Products, Solgar,** and **Twinlabs**.

ENDNOTES

(title) "The feminine nature . . .": Marija Gimbutas, *The Goddesses and Gods of Old Europe* (Berkeley and Los Angeles: University of California Press, 1982), 152.

ACKNOWLEDGMENTS

(vii) "All wisdom . . .": Hugh Kerr, "Preacher, Professor, Editor," *Theology Today* 45:1 (April 1988): 1.

PRELUDE

(xvi) "the thoughts of . . .": Richard Wilhelm and Cary F. Baynes, trans., *The I Ching*, 3rd ed. (Princeton: Princeton University Press, 1967), xxxv. All quotes from *The I Ching* are taken from this edition.

(xviii) "Nothing in the world . . .": Lao-tzu, *Tao te Ching*, trans. Stephen Mitchell (New York: HarperPerennial, 1991), 78.

(xx) "The more you know . . .": Ibid., 47.

(xxiii) "When male and female . . .": Ibid., 42.

CHAPTER 1, A SENSE OF BALANCE

(3) "What can we . . .": Thomas Merton, trans., *Wisdom of the Desert: Sayings from the Desert Fathers of the Fourth Century* (Boston and London: Shambhala, 1994), 16. (Hereafter referred to as *Wisdom of the Desert.*)

(3) "If you want . . .": Lao-tzu, *Tao te Ching*, trans. Stephen Mitchell (New York: HarperPerennial, 1991), 22.

(4) "the level of . . .": Joseph Campbell, *The Power of Myth* (New York: Doubleday, 1988), 174.

(4) Rachel Naomi Remen, M.D., discusses the story of the cancer patient in two of her four talks in her audiotaped series *Beyond Cure: Four Talks on Healing for Health Professionals* (Bolinas, Calif.: Institute for the Study of Health and Illness, 1992). Another version of this story, also told by Dr. Remen, appears in Christina Feldman and Jack Kornfield, *Stories of the Spirit, Stories of the Heart: Parables of the Spiritual Path From Around the World* (New York: HarperSanFrancisco, 1991), 78. (Hereafter referred to as *Stories of the Spirit.*)

Dr. Remen's insights into the healing process have been elucidated by many others. In *A Blue Fire* (New York: Harper & Row, 1989, 162) psychotherapist James Hillman explains that healing comes "not because one is whole, integrated, and all together, but from a consciousness breaking through dismemberment"; and Jungian analyst Marion Woodman identifies addiction as the "wound" that permits full consciousness of the human condition: "Addiction keeps a person in touch with the god. . . . At the very point of vulnerability is where the surrender takes place—that is where the god enters. The god comes through the wound" ("Worshipping Illusions," in *Parabola* 12:2, May 1987, 64).

(7) "A neighbor . . .": Noah benShea, *Jacob the Baker: Gentle Wisdom for a Complicated World* (New York: Ballantine, 1989), 32. (Hereafter referred to as *Jacob the Baker.*)

(7) "There ain't . . .": Gertrude Stein is quoted in Jon Winokur, comp. and ed., *Zen to Go* (New York: New American Library, 1989), 11.

(8) "There once was . . .": This traditional story is adapted from a retelling by Feldman and Kornfield, *Stories of the Spirit*, 345.

CHAPTER 2, THE WISDOM OF THE WHOLE

(9) "All know that . . .": Jon Winokur, comp. and ed., *Zen to Go* (New York: New American Library, 1989), 148.

(9) "Your vision will . . .": Carl Jung is quoted in Jess M. Brallier, ed., *Medical Wit and Wisdom* (Philadelphia: Running Press, 1993), 19.

(9) "In the point . . .": Dag Hammarskjöld, *Markings* (New York: Knopf, 1965), 174.

(10) "Many hundreds of years . . .": This story has been told and retold dozens of times. Our version is loosely based on a retelling in Idries Shah, *Tales of the Dervishes* (New York: Dutton, 1970), 25.

(12) "there is nothing . . .": René Descartes is quoted in Fritjof Capra, *The Turning Point: Science, Society, and the Rising Culture* (New York: Bantam, 1983), 62. (Hereafter referred to as *Turning Point.*)

(12) "Think of your body . . .": Quoted in Lynn Payer, *Medicine and Culture: Varieties of Treatment in the United States, England, West Germany, and France* (New York: Penguin Books, 1988), 148.

(13) "Would you . . .": Murray Haydon is quoted in Brallier, *Medical Wit and Wisdom*, 27.

(13) Mr. Hipp joke: Jeff Rovin, *Five Hundred Great Doctor Jokes* (New York: Signet, 1993), 28.

(14) "My physician provided . . .": Arthur Frank, *At the Will of the Body* (New York: Houghton-Mifflin, 1991), 10.

(14) "The help I want . . .": Ibid., 14.

(15) "Heard . . . if they only understood . . .": Ram Dass and Paul Gorman, *How Can I Help? Stories and Reflections on Service* (New York: Knopf, 1988), 112.

(16) "It can be . . .": Riane Eisler, *The Chalice and the Blade: Our History: Our Future* (New York: HarperSanFrancisco, 1987), 183.

(16) The story of Isis and Osiris is discussed in Joseph Campbell, *The Power of Myth* (New York: Doubleday, 1988), 177.

(18) "thinking is the most . . .": Oscar Wilde quoted in Brallier, *Medical Wit and Wisdom*, 107.

(18) "Every time they asked . . .": Capra, *Turning Point*, 76.

(18) "Can nature possibly . . .": Werner Heisenberg is quoted in Capra, *Turning Point*, 76.

(18) "As we penetrate . . .": Ibid., 81.

(19) "Today there is . . .": James Jeans is quoted in Capra, *Turning Point*, 86. Capra cites Jeans, *The Mysterious Universe* (New York: Macmillan, 1930).

(19) "A continuous dancing . . .": Capra, *Turning Point*, 88.

(19) "The world thus . . .": Werner Heisenberg is quoted in ibid., 81.

(20) "And I have felt . . .": From William Wordsworth, "Lines Composed a Few Miles above Tintern Abbey . . .", in John O. Hayden, ed., *William Wordsworth: The Poems*, vol. 1 (New Haven and London: Yale University Press, 1981), 360.

(20-22) Interviews with Thomas Delbanco, Candace Pert, and David Felten in Bill Moyers, *Healing and the Mind* (New York: Doubleday, 1993), 13, 188–189, 231.

(22) "The group therapy . . .": David Spiegel, M.D., *Living beyond Limits: New Hope and Help for Facing Life-Threatening Illness* (New York: Random House, 1993), xiii.

(23) "I had to sit . . .": Ibid., 78.

(23) "Something in the group . . .": Spiegel is quoted in Moyers, *Healing and the Mind*, 68.

(23) The rabbit study is discussed in Larry Dossey, *Space, Time, and Medicine* (Boston: Shambhala, 1982), 61–62; and in Deepok Chopra, M.D., *Quantum Healing: Exploring the Frontiers of Mind/Body Medicine* (New York: Bantam, 1989), 33.

(24) "Just as the physical . . .": David Felten is quoted in Moyers, *Healing and the Mind*, 234.

(25) "To know yet to think . . .": Lao-tzu, *Tao te Ching*, trans. D. C. Lau (Hong Kong: Chinese University Press, 1989), 105.

(25) "When you're green . . .": Ray Kroc is quoted in Jon Winokur, comp. and ed., *Zen to Go* (New York: New American Library, 1989), 125.

(25) "Mulla Nasrudin . . .": This story appears in many collections; our version is adapted from Anthony de Mello, *The Song of the Bird* (New York: Doubleday, 1982), 27.

(26) "When we must . . .": Carl Jung is quoted in Larry Dossey, *Meaning and Medicine: A Doctor's Tales of Breakthrough and Healing* (New York: Bantam, 1991), 201.

(26) "One of the devotees . . .": This story is adapted from Christina Feldman and Jack Kornfield, *Stories of the Spirit* (New York: HarperSanFrancisco, 1991), 214.

(27) "An old man . . .": Noah benShea, *Jacob the Baker* (New York: Ballantine, 1989), 50.

(28) "COME TO THE EDGE . . .": Guillaume Apollinaire is quoted in Bernie S. Siegel, M.D., *Love, Medicine, and Miracles* (New York: Harper & Row, 1986), 204.

CHAPTER 3, THE GODDESS AND THE WITCH

(29) "When you have . . .": Joseph Campbell, *The Power of Myth* (New York: Doubleday, 1988), 167.

(29) "This is a story . . .": Starhawk is quoted in the videotaped series *Women and Spirituality*, directed by Donna Read; coproduction of the National Film Board of Canada and the Great Atlantic and Pacific Film Company.

(31) Joseph Campbell, *The Masks of God*, 4 vols. (New York: Viking Penguin, 1991).

(31) "I am Nature . . .": The second-century Roman writer Apuleius, an African priest of Isis, left a fascinating account of the Great Goddess. See Robert Graves, trans., *The Golden Ass* (New York: Pocket Books, 1951), 36.

(32) "He shaped my loins . . .": Diane Wolkstein and Samuel N. Kramer, *Inanna: Queen of Heaven and Earth* (New York: Harper & Row, 1983), 4.

(33) "The male divinity . . .": Marija Gimbutas, *The Goddesses and Gods of Old Europe* (Berkeley and Los Angeles: University of California Press, 1974), 237.

(33) "The whole . . . ": Nicholas Platon, *Crete* (Geneva, Switzerland: Nagel, 1966), 148.

(34) "One of the better known . . .": Jeanne Achterberg, *Woman as Healer: A Panoramic Survey of the Healing Activities of Women from Prehistoric Times to the Present* (Boston: Shambhala, 1990), 32.

(35-37) We are indebted to Merlin Stone for her illuminating discussions of the laws, priestly pronouncements, and biblical edicts designed to destroy the power of women in ancient times. See Stone, *When God Was a Woman* (New York: Harcourt Brace Jovanovich, 1976), 189–192.

(37) "For as regards . . .": Heinrich Kramer and James Sprenger, *Malleus Maleficarum*, trans. Montague Summers (London: Pushkin Press, 1951), 45.

(39) "All witchcraft . . .": Ibid., 47.

(40) "When a woman . . .": Ibid., 43.

(40) "For other things . . .": Francesca Maria Guazzo, *Compendium Maleficarum (The Montague Summers Edition)*, trans. E. A. Ashwin (New York: Dover, 1988), 137.

(40) "Whose fervour is . . .": Ibid., 137.

(40) "Further, since women . . .": Ibid., 137.

(41) "Gilly Duncan . . .": Achterberg, *Woman as Healer*, 90.

(41) "At Dammartin . . .": Nicole Stephanie's story is told in Guazzo, *Compendium Maleficarum*, 126–128.

(43) The Scottish law of 1563 is discussed in Hans Peter Duerr, *Dreamtime: Concerning the Boundary between Wilderness and Civilization* (Oxford, U.K.: Basil Blackwell, 1987), 161, n. 60.

(43) "There is no . . .": Guazzo, *Compendium Maleficarum*, 125.

(43) "For this must . . .": An English witch-hunter is quoted in Barbara Ehrenreich and Deirdre English, *Witches, Midwives and Nurses: A History of Women Healers* (New York: Feminist Press, 1973), 12.

(44) "And what, then . . .": Kramer and Sprenger, *Malleus Maleficarum*, 121.

(45) "usually lascivious . . ." and "When you see . . .": Duerr, *Dreamtime*, 57. In a footnote, 266, Duerr notes that this quotation is from J. Michelet, *Die Hexe* (Munich: n.p., 1974), 133, and comments: "The quote seems somewhat unlikely to me, but if not true, it is well invented."

(46) "torture nature's . . .": Francis Bacon is quoted in Fritjof Capra, *Turning Point* (New York: Bantam, 1983), 56. Capra cites Carolyn Merchant, *The Death of Nature* (New York: Harper & Row, 1980), 169.

(46) "There was a man . . .": Noah benShea, *Jacob the Baker* (New York: Ballantine, 1989), 90.

(47) "The memory of . . .": Dominic Maruca, "A Reflection on Guilt," *Human Development* 3:1 (Spring 1982): 42.

(47) "How should one . . .": This story is adapted from Abraham Twerski, *Living Each Day* (New York: Mesorah, 1988), 342.

CHAPTER 4, SPEAK TO THE EARTH

(49) "Speak to the earth . . .": Job 12:8.

(49) "The purpose of . . .": Mad Bear is quoted in Dell Boyd, *Rolling Thunder* (New York: Dell, 1974), 244.

(50) The story of Albert Isaiah Coffin and the Seneca wise woman appears in Barbara Griggs, *The Green Pharmacy: The History and Evolution of Western Herbal Medicine* (Rochester, Vt.: Healing Arts Press, 1981), 199–200. (Hereafter referred to as *Green Pharmacy*.) We are indebted to Griggs for her pioneering work on the history of herbal medicine. In her brilliant discussion of heroic chemical

cures, Griggs discusses two "truths" about medical treatment that have held through the centuries (83–85): (1) "It is a curious and depressing truth, demonstrated again and again in medical history, that the desire of the average physician to administer powerful and active drugs is only equalled by the desire of the average patient to have powerful and active drugs administered to him." (2) "Once a powerful and potentially dangerous drug is accepted into practice on the grounds that extremely serious illness justifies its use, it tends to be increasingly prescribed for quite trivial ailments. (Modern antibiotics are an excellent example of this tendency.)"

(50) "Every person is . . .": Boyd, *Rolling Thunder*, 244.

(52) "The most basic . . .": Ibid., 199.

(53) The authors are indebted to Ernest Kurtz, Ph.D., coauthor of *The Spirituality of Imperfection* (New York: Bantam, 1992) for his insights into the concept of *dukkha* and William James's related notion of *torn-to-pieces-hood*.

(54) "I hate it . . .": Jeff Rovin, *Five Hundred Great Doctor Jokes* (New York: Signet, 1993), 45.

(55) "When she came out . . .": The story is told by Thomas Delbanco, M.D., in Bill Moyers, *Healing and the Mind* (New York: Doubleday, 1993), 10.

(55) "We once had . . .": The story is related by Ron Anderson, M.D., in ibid., 41.

(56) "Imagine you're outside . . .": The story is told by Anthony Robbins in his audiotaped workshop *Living Health: The Lifestyle of Vibrant Health and Energy* (Robbins Research International, 1991).

(57) "The Reason Why . . .": We discovered the Al-Razi letter and book titles in Ivan Illich, *Medical Nemesis: The Expropriation of Health* (New York: Random House, 1976), 27, n. 49.

(58) "a cure can . . .": Dr. Al-Razi's advice to avoid complex remedies appears in Griggs, *Green Pharmacy*, 24.

(59) The rich, who could afford the expensive mercury treatments, were the primary victims of this therapy. In Hermannus, *An Excellent Treatise teaching how to cure the French-Pocked* (London: n.p., 1590), this interesting comment appears: "The common people, perceiving so manie to be spoiled and killed with Quicksilver would not willinglie be cured therewith." See also Griggs, *Green Pharmacy*, 38.

(59) "He was getting . . .": Griggs, *Green Pharmacy*, 85.

(59) "pearls, hyacinths, corals . . .": Ibid., 79.

(60) "gnaw their bodies . . .": Dr. Culpepper is quoted in ibid., 94–98.

(60) The calomel saga is drawn from ibid., 155–159.

(60) Dr. Thomas Graham's contributions are drawn from ibid., 189–190.

(61) "a great-grandmother . . ." and "why our young men . . .": Florence Nightingale and Oliver Wendell Holmes are quoted in ibid., 237–238. Griggs cites Wendell Holmes, "Currents and Counter-Currents in Medical Science," in *Medical Essays 1842–1882* (Boston and New York: Houghton, Miflin, 1891), 199, 202, 294.

(61) Illich, *Medical Nemesis*, 1, 26.

(62) "Because the patient . . .": Eugene Robin, M.D., *Matters of Life and Death: Risks vs. Benefits of Medical Care* (Stanford, Calif.: Stanford Alumni Association, 1984), 58.

(62) The quotations relating to iatroepidemics appear in "The Harm That Medicine Does—Iatroepidemics," ibid., chap. 8.

(63) "Now we have . . .": Robert S. Mendelsohn, M.D., *Confessions of a Medical Heretic* (Chicago: Contemporary Books, 1990), 62.

(63) "Antibiotics: The End of Miracle Drugs?" *Newsweek*, 28 March, 1994, 46–51.

(64) John Shen is an "old master" acupuncturist and Chinese herbalist; this anecdote is taken from a lecture by Dr. Shen at the Tri-State Institute for Traditional Chinese Acupuncture.

(64) "The doctor took . . .": Rovin, *Five Hundred Great Doctor Jokes*, 20.

(65) Hippocrates, Galen, Paracelsus, and Voltaire are quoted in Jess. M. Brallier, *Medical Wit and Wisdom* (Philadelphia: Running Press, 1993), 62, 64, 65, 142.

(65) "al the vertue . . .": Conrad Gesner, *The Treasure of Euonymous* (Amsterdam and New York: Da Capo, 1969; orig. pub. England: n.p., 1559), 36. See also Griggs, *Green Pharmacy*, 68.

(65)   "A mountain of . . .": Griggs, *Green Pharmacy*, 330.

(65)   The Bio-Strath story appears in ibid., 304–308.

(66)   The material on comfrey is adapted from Rosemary Gladstar, *Herbal Healing for Women* (New York: Simon & Schuster, 1993), and Simon Y. Mills, *Out of the Earth: The Essential Book of Herbal Medicine* (New York: Viking Arkana, 1991).

(67)   "The logical inference . . .": Griggs, *Green Pharmacy*, 313.

(68)   "There exists . . .": Mark J. Plotkin, Ph.D., *Tales of a Shaman's Apprentice: An Ethnobotanist Searches for New Medicines in the Amazon Rain Forest* (New York: Viking, 1993), 7.

(70)   "humility is . . .": Dag Hammarskjöld, *Markings* (New York: Knopf, 1965), 174. Emphasis is his.

(70)   "Not all of the knowledge . . .": Boyd, *Rolling Thunder*, 260.

(71)   "As a youth . . .": This story is adapted from Frederick Franck, "The Mirrors of Mahayana," *Parabola* 11:2 (May 1986): 66.

(71)   "Teach your children . . .": Chief Seattle is quoted in Elizabeth Roberts and Elias Amidon, eds., *Earth Prayers from Around the World: 365 Prayers, Poems, and Invocations for Honoring the Earth* (New York: HarperSanFrancisco, 1991), 10.

CHAPTER 5, THE STREAM OF LIFE

(75)   "After a time . . .": Richard Wilhelm and Cary F. Baynes, trans., *The I Ching*, 3rd ed. (Princeton: Princeton University Press, 1967), 97.

(75)   "When we experience . . .": Charlene Spretnak, *States of Grace: The Recovery of Meaning in the Postmodern Age* (New York: HarperSanFrancisco, 1991), 24.

(75)   "The waters on the surface . . .": *The I Ching*, 35.

(76)   "There is no . . .": Jon Winokur, comp. and ed., *Zen to Go* (New York: New American Library, 1989), 102. Winokur cites Lao-tzu, *Tao te Ching*, trans. D. C. Lau (New York: Penguin, 1963).

(77)   "God created . . .": This story is a recollection of a discourse by Bhagwan Shree Rajneesh at his ashram in Poona, India.

(78)   "The Book of Changes . . .": *The I Ching*, lviii.

(78)   "There is nothing . . .": Ibid., 299.

(79)   "There was something . . .": Lao-tzu, *Tao te Ching*, trans. Stephen Mitchell (New York: HarperPerennial, 1991), 25.

(79)   "Everything on earth . . .": *The I Ching*, 50.

(79)   "Men are born . . .": Lao-tzu, *Tao te Ching*, trans. Mitchell, 76.

(80)   "A stream, from . . .": Idries Shah, *Tales of the Dervishes* (New York: Dutton, 1970), 23. We have taken the liberty of revising the stream's gender from male to female.

(82)   "the moon becomes . . .": *The I Ching*, 238.

(82)   "to undermine . . .": Ibid., 64.

(82)   "water washes . . .": Ibid., 155.

(82)   "We should not . . .": Ibid., 25.

(82)   "holy seriousness . . .": Ibid., 83.

(82)   "self-knowledge does not . . .": Ibid., 85.

(83)   "Many years ago . . .": This story is adapted from Abbot Zenkei Shibayama (Nanzenji Monastery, Kyoto, Japan), *A Flower Does Not Talk*, trans. Sumiko Kudo (Rutland, Vt.: Tuttle, 1970), 189.

(84)   "The secret of tao . . .": *The I Ching*, 300.

(84)   "allows the divine light . . .": Ibid., 387.

(84)   "The earth is still . . .": Ibid., 152.

(85)   "The gentlest thing . . .": Lao-tzu, *Tao te Ching*, trans. Mitchell, 43.

(85)   "The hard and stiff . . .": Ibid., 76.

Endnotes369

(86)"When the master ...": This story is adapted from Anthony de Mello, *One Minute Wisdom* (New York: Doubleday-Image, 1988), 137.

(86)"Two monks were ...": This story appears in many collections; our version is adapted from Paul Reps, comp., *Zen Flesh, Zen Bones: A Collection of Zen and Pre-Zen Writings* (New York: Anchor Books, 1961), 114 (hereafter cited as *Zen Flesh, Zen Bones*); and Jon Winokur, comp. and ed., *Zen to Go* (New York: New American Library, 1989), 51.

(87)"The sages did not ...": Ilza Veith, trans., *The Yellow Emperor's Classic of Internal Medicine* (Berkeley and Los Angeles: University of California Press, 1949), 105. All references to this work, hereafter referred to as *The Yellow Emperor's Classic*, are to this edition.

(89)"When the Five Phase Theory ...": Fritjof Capra, *Turning Point* (New York: Bantam, 1983), 313.

CHAPTER 6, AFFINITIES

Chapters 6 through 11 borrow from many important works, including Harriet Beinfield and Efrem Korngold, *Between Heaven and Earth: A Guide to Chinese Medicine* (New York: Ballantine, 1991); Diane Connelly, *Traditional Acupuncture: The Law of the Five Elements* (Columbia, Md.: The Center for Traditional Acupuncture, 1979); Leon Hammer, M.D., *Dragon Rises, Red Bird Flies* (Barrytown, N.Y.: Station Hill, 1990); Yves Requena, *Character and Health: The Relationship of Acupuncture and Psychology* (Brookline, Mass.: Paradigm, 1989); and Iona Marsaa Teeguarden, *The Joy of Feeling: Bodymind Acupressure* (New York: Japan Publications, 1987).

(91)"Things that accord ...": Confucius is quoted in Richard Wilhelm and Cary F. Baynes, trans., *The I Ching*, 3rd ed. (Princeton: Princeton University Press, 1967), 9.

(91)"The interaction of the Five Elements ...": Ilza Veith, trans., *The Yellow Emperor's Classic* (Berkeley and Los Angeles: University of California Press, 1949), 136.

(92)"The sages combined ...": Ibid., 149.

CHAPTER 7, WOOD: THE VISIONARY

(99)"The supernatural [powers] ...": Ilza Veith, trans., *The Yellow Emperor's Classic* (Berkeley and Los Angeles: University of California Press, 1949), 118.

(100)"A thunderstorm brings ...": Richard Wilhelm and Cary F. Baynes, trans., *The I Ching*, 3rd ed. (Princeton: Princeton University Press, 1967), 16.

(100)"A young female disciple ...": This story is adapted from Christina Feldman and Jack Kornfield, *Stories of the Spirit* (New York: HarperSanFrancisco, 1991), 297.

(101)"In springtime when ...": *The I Ching*, 101.

(101)"Beginning and creation ...": *The Yellow Emperor's Classic*, 147.

(102)"has the functions ...": Ibid., 133.

(102)"occupies the position ...": Ibid., 133.

(103)"The load is ...": *The I Ching*, 111.

(103)"She accepts no advice ...": Ibid., 113.

(104)"The master Bankei ...": This story appears in many collections; our version is adapted from Paul Reps, comp., *Zen Flesh, Zen Bones* (New York: Anchor Books, 1961), 8.

(105)"She who pushes ...": *The I Ching*, 181.

(106)"When adversity befalls ...": Ibid., 182.

(106)"butts her head ...": Ibid., 183.

(107)"Wood in the earth ...": Ibid., 179.

CHAPTER 8, FIRE: THE COMMUNICATOR

(109) "The supernatural [powers] . . .": Ilza Veith, trans., *The Yellow Emperor's Classic* (Berkeley and Los Angeles: University of California Press, 1949), 118.

(110) "Rumi knocked . . .": This story is adapted from Christina Feldman and Jack Kornfield, *Stories of the Spirit* (New York: HarperSanFrancisco, 1991), 357.

(111) "A quiet, wordless . . .": *The I Ching*, 225.

(111) "Fire clings to wood . . .": Ibid., 121.

(112) "the complexion of . . .": *The Yellow Emperor's Classic*, 119.

(112) "period of luxurious . . .": Ibid., 102.

(112) "the heart craves . . .": Ibid., 141.

(112) "The joyous mood . . .": *The I Ching*, 224.

(116) "If a woman is . . .": Ibid., 226.

(117) "What is dark . . .": Ibid., 119.

CHAPTER 9, EARTH: THE PEACEMAKER

(119) "The [mysterious] powers . . .": Ilza Veith, trans., *The Yellow Emperor's Classic* (Berkeley and Los Angeles: University of California Press, 1949), 119.

(120) "The symbol of heaven . . .": Richard Wilhelm and Cary F. Baynes, trans., *The I Ching*, 3rd ed. (Princeton: Princeton University Press, 1967), 14.

(120) "The wind blows . . .": Ibid., 235.

(120) "A bird should not . . .": Ibid., 240.

(121) "When a woman . . .": Ibid., 10.

(121) "Just as the earth . . .": Ibid., 80.

(121) "Two old men . . .": This story appears in many collections; our version is adapted from Thomas Merton, trans., *Wisdom of the Desert* (Boston and London: Shambhala, 1994), 116.

(122) "just stay at the center . . .": Lao-tzu, *Tao te Ching*, trans. Stephen Mitchell (New York: HarperPerennial, 1991), 19.

(122) "In a little hut . . .": This story is adapted from Abbot Zenkei Shibayama (Nanzenji Monastery, Kyoto, Japan), *A Flower Does Not Talk*, trans. Sumiko Kudo (Rutland, Vt.: Tuttle, 1970), 137.

(123) "Everything that is created . . .": *The Yellow Emperor's Classic*, 148.

(123) "that which is correct . . .": *The I Ching*, 131.

(126) "She who seeks . . .": Ibid., 109.

(128) "The earth in its . . .": Ibid., 13.

CHAPTER 10, METAL: THE ARTIST

(131) "The [mysterious] powers . . .": Ilza Veith, trans., *The Yellow Emperor's Classic* (Berkeley and Los Angeles: University of California, 1949), 119.

(131) "The mountain rests . . .": Richard Wilhelm and Cary F. Baynes, trans., *The I Ching*, 3rd ed. (Princeton: Princeton University Press, 1967), 94.

(132) "Here at the highest . . .": Ibid., 93.

(132) "tranquil beauty . . .": Ibid., 91.

(132) "When desire is . . .": Ibid., 91.

(133) "Which is the right way . . .": This story is adapted from Christina Feldman and Jack Kornfield, *Stories of the Spirit* (New York: HarperSanFrancisco, 1991), 273.

(133) "Precious metals and jade . . .": *The Yellow Emperor's Classic*, 147.

(134) Depiction of the lung as the "tender organ" is taken from Ted J. Kaptchuk, *The Web That Has No Weaver: Understanding Chinese Medicine* (New York: Congdon and Weed, 1983), 56.
(135) "The end is reached . . .": *The I Ching*, 126.
(137) "If you want . . .": Lao-tzu, *Tao te Ching*, trans. Stephen Mitchell (New York: HarperPerennial, 1991), 22.
(137) "On their way . . .": This story appears in many collections; our version is adapted from Anthony de Mello, *The Song of the Bird* (New York: Doubleday, 1982), 108.
(138) "like old Jell-O . . .": Harriet Beinfield and Efrem Korngold, *Between Heaven and Earth: A Guide to Chinese Medicine* (New York: Ballantine, 1991), 208.
(139) "We cannot lose . . .": *The I Ching*, 102.

CHAPTER 11, WATER: THE SAGE

(141) "The [mysterious] powers . . .": Ilza Veith, trans., *The Yellow Emperor's Classic* (Berkeley and Los Angeles: University of California Press, 1949), 120.
(141) "In order to find . . .": Richard Wilhelm and Cary F. Baynes, trans., *The I Ching*, 3rd ed. (Princeton: Princeton University Press, 1967), 17.
(142) "If a person . . .": Ibid.
(142) "Water on top . . .": Ibid., 581.
(142) "What is the truth path . . .": This story appears in many collections; our version is adapted from Christine Feldman and Jack Kornfield, *Stories of the Spirit* (New York: HarperSanFrancisco, 1991), 307.
(143) "They will say . . .": Antonio Porchia, *Voices*, trans. W. S. Merwin (Chicago: Big Table, 1969), 24.
(143) "A lake evaporates . . .": *The I Ching*, 224.
(144) "I am in the present . . .": Igor Stravinsky is quoted in Jon Winokur, comp. and ed., *Zen to Go* (New York: New American Library, 1989), 72.
(144) "A community leader . . .": Noah benShea, *Jacob the Baker* (New York: Ballantine, 1989), 22.
(145) "In winter . . .": *The I Ching*, 98.
(147) "When the kidneys . . .": *The Yellow Emperor's Classic*, 205.
(150) "Abbot Pastor . . .": This story is adapted from Thomas Merton, trans., *Wisdom of the Desert* (Boston and London: Shambhala, 1994), 72.
(151) "Water . . . flows . . .": *The I Ching*, 115.

CHAPTER 12, A CIRCLE WITH NO BEGINNING OR END

(155) "Like the day . . .": Richard Wilhelm and Cary F. Baynes, trans., *The I Ching*, 3rd ed. (Princeton: Princeton University Press, 1967), 271.
(157) "When Nasrudin . . .": This story appears in many collections; our version is adapted from Christina Feldman and Jack Kornfield, *Stories of the Spirit* (New York: HarperSanFrancisco, 1991), 212. See also Anthony de Mello, *The Song of the Bird* (New York: Doubleday, 1982), 153.

CHAPTER 13, SPRING: FROM CHILD TO WOMAN

(159) "Know the male . . .": Lao-tzu, *Tao te Ching*, trans. Stephen Mitchell (New York: HarperPerennial, 1991), 28.

(159) "It is said . . .": Brooke Medicine Eagle, *Buffalo Woman Comes Singing* (New York: Ballantine, 1991), 338.

(160) "The force that through the green fuse drives the flower" is the title of a Dylan Thomas poem; see Daniel Jones, ed., *The Poems of Dylan Thomas* (New York: New Directions, 1971), 77.

(161) "The goddess Chang-O . . .": This story is adapted from Luisa Francia, *Dragontime: Magic and Mystery of Menstruation* (Woodstock, N.Y.: Ash Tree, 1993), 38.

(162) "And if a woman . . .": Leviticus 15:19–30.

(162) "the monthly flux . . .": Pliny the Elder is quoted in Christiane Northrup, M.D., *Women's Bodies, Women's Wisdom: Creating Physical and Emotional Health and Healing* (New York: Bantam, 1994), 105. (Hereafter referred to as *Women's Bodies*). Northrup cites Dr. Ronald Norris's November 1982 lecture on PMS in Rockland, Maine. Pliny is also quoted in Claudia de Lys, *The Giant Book of Superstitions* (Secaucus, N.J.: Citadel, 1979), 46.

(162) "I first got . . .": Dena Taylor, *Red Flower: Rethinking Menstruation* (Freedom, Calif.: Crossing Press, 1988), 5.

(163) "I was 10 . . .": Ibid.

(163) "My period first came . . .": Lara Owen, *Her Blood Is Gold: Celebrating the Power of Menstruation* (New York: HarperSanFrancisco, 1993), 10. Owen also discusses the Jewish tradition of slapping the face (11–12).

(164) "When You're a Wife . . .": 1963 Tampax insert quoted in Northrup, *Women's Bodies*, 108.

(164) "A menstruating woman . . .": Thomas Buckley and Alma Gottlieb, eds., *Blood Magic: The Anthropology of Menstruation* (Berkeley and Los Angeles: University of California Press, 1988), 190.

(165) "Let me take you . . .": Medicine Eagle, *Buffalo Woman Comes Singing*, 327.

(172) "De chi le mei you . . .": This typical conversation between acupuncturist and patient is reported in David Eisenberg, M.D., with Thomas Lee Wright, *Encounters with Qi: Exploring Chinese Medicine* (New York: Penguin, 1985), 72.

(172) *The Essentials of Chinese Acupuncture*, comp. by Beijing College of Traditional Chinese Medicine, Shanghai College of Traditional Chinese Medicine, Nanjing College of Traditional Chinese Medicine, and the Acupuncture Institute of the Academy of Traditional Chinese Medicine (Beijing, China: Foreign Languages Press, 1980).

(178) The poem "Struggle" appeared in *Quote* magazine, Las Cruces, N. Mex.; reprinted with permission from editor Tom Kelley.

(179) "The Lady of the Wild Things" and "The epiphany . . .": Marija Gimbutas, *The Goddesses and Gods of Old Europe* (Berkeley and Los Angeles: University of California Press, 1974), 182.

(182) "My body is . . .": Max Sugar, M.D., ed., *Female Adolescent Development* (New York: Brunner/ Mazel, 1979), 236.

(182) "I remember when . . .": Lynda Madaras, *The What's Happening to My Body? Book for Girls* (New York: Newmarket, 1988), 30.

(182) Statistics about adolescent body image and dieting are borrowed from: Andrea Blum, Julie Harrison, Barbara Ess, and Gail Vachon, eds., *The Facts About Women* (New York: New Press, 1993), 20. Blum et al. cite Naomi Wolf, *The Beauty Myth* (New York: Morrow, 1991).

(183) "When I become . . .": Northrup, *Women's Bodies*, 114.

(185) "The word *ritual* . . .": Elinor Gadon, *The Once and Future Goddess* (New York: Harper & Row, 1989), 2.

(186) "The secret of beginning . . .": Christina Feldman and Jack Kornfield, *Stories of the Spirit* (New York: HarperSanFrancisco, 1991), 83.

(186) "ripping the lettuce . . .": Tom Robbins, *Another Roadside Attraction* (New York: Bantam, 1991), 177.

(188) "When our young people . . .": Dell Boyd, *Rolling Thunder* (New York: Dell, 1974), 12.

(190) "When I went . . .": Owen, *Her Blood Is Gold*, 60.

(190) "Something I found . . .": Medicine Eagle, *Buffalo Woman Comes Singing*, 332.

(190) "Getting my pads . . .": Owen, *Her Blood Is Gold*, 142.

(191) "They'd take you . . .": Anne Cameron, *The Daughters of Copper Woman* (Vancouver, B.C.: Press Gang, 1981), 102.

(192) "The women, who . . .": Penelope Shuttle and Peter Redgrove, *The Wise Wound* (New York: Grove Press, 1986), 173.

(192) "I love my daughter . . .": Amy Tan is quoted in Melissa Stein, comp., *The Wit and Wisdom of Women* (Philadelphia: Running Press, 1993), 103.

(192) "My mother is . . .": Marge Piercy is quoted in ibid., 102.

(195) "Innocence is . . .": Annie Dillard is quoted in ibid., 182.

(195) "The way to do . . .": Lao-tzu is quoted in Jon Winokur, comp. and ed., *Zen to Go* (New York: New American Library, 1989), 102.

(196) "The Zen teacher . . .": We are once again grateful to Dr. Ernest Kurtz for bringing this story to our attention; Dr. Kurtz discovered this story, which we have adapted, in an otherwise unidentified clipping from the periodical *The Utne Reader*, May–June 1989, which cited Shawn Gosieski, *New Cyclist*, Fall 1988.

CHAPTER 14, SUMMER: FROM LOVER TO MOTHER

(197) "The Tao is called . . .": Lao-tzu, *Tao te Ching*, trans. Stephen Mitchell (New York: HarperPerennial, 1991), 6.

(197) "American Indian women . . .": Paula Gunn Allen, *The Sacred Hoop: Recovering the Feminine in American Indian Traditions* (Boston: Beacon Press, 1992), 28.

(198) "'I love you,' . . .": William Goldman, *The Princess Bride: A Hot Fairy Tale* (New York: Ballantine, 1973), 47.

(199) The Skeleton Woman story is adapted from Clarissa Pinkola Estés, Ph.D., *Women Who Run with the Wolves* (New York: Ballantine, 1992). Estés's version of the story and her commentary appear in chap. 5, "Hunting: When the Heart Is a Lonely Hunter," 130.

(209) "The forecasters were . . .": This story was told to Jason Elias by a friend.

(213) "When a father's . . .": Bob Flaws, *Endometriosis, Infertility and Traditional Chinese Medicine: A Laywoman's Guide* (Boulder, Colo.: Blue Poppy Press, 1989), 80.

(218) The fertility awareness method is described in detail in Barbara Kass-Annese, R.N., and Hal Danzer, M.D., *The Fertility Awareness Handbook* (Alameda, Calif.: Hunter House, 1992). See also Evelyn L. Billings and Anne O'Donovan, *The Billings Method* (New York: Random House, 1980).

Special thanks to nurse practitioner Sil Reynolds for introducing us to the concept of conscious fertility, and to Serafina Corsello, M.D., for her theories on unopposed estrogens. Dr. Corsello is founder and director of the Corsello Centers for Nutritional and Complementary Medicine in New York City and on Long Island and hosts a radio talk show on complementary medicine called *Second Opinion* (WOR radio, New York City).

(220) We are indebted to Susun Weed for her pregnancy tonic formula, which Jason Elias uses regularly and with great success in his practice.

(224) "In ancient times . . .": This story is taken from an audiotaped discourse by Don Pachuta, M.D., at the Traditional Acupuncture Institute in Columbia, Md.

(226) "develop or give birth . . .": Christiane Northrup, M.D., *Women's Bodies* (New York: Bantam, 1994), 100.

(229) For more information on hormone replacement therapy, unopposed estrogens, and synthetic vs. natural progesterones, see John Lee, M.D., *Natural Progesterone: The Multiple Roles of a Remarkable Hormone* (Sebastopol, Calif.: BLL Publications, 1993); Dee Ito, *Without Estrogen* (New York: Random House, 1994); Betty Kamin, *Hormonal Replacement: Yes or No* (Novato, Calif.: Nutritional Encounter, 1993); and "The Estrogen Complex," *Newsweek*, 21 March 1994, 76.

(231) "oil the hormonal machinery . . .": This quotation is taken from an interview with Dr. Serafina Corsello.

(235) "One of the old men . . .": This story is adapted from Thomas Merton, trans., *Wisdom of the Desert* (Boston and London: Shambhala, 1994), 123.

(237) "Tem Eyos Ki . . .": Anne Cameron, *The Daughters of Copper Woman* (Vancouver, B.C.: Press Gang, 1981), 57.

CHAPTER 15, AUTUMN: FROM MATRIARCH TO WISE WOMAN

(239) "Whoever is soft . . .": Lao-tzu, *Tao te Ching*, trans. Stephen Mitchell (New York: HarperPerennial, 1991), 76.

(239) "The power of woman . . .": Paula Gunn Allen, *Grandmothers of the Light: A Medicine Woman's Source Book* (Boston: Beacon Press, 1991), 13.

(240) "Here, in the seed . . .": Richard Wilhelm and Cary F. Baynes, trans., *The I Ching*, 3rd ed. (Princeton: Princeton University Press, 1967), 271.

(240) "From such small . . .": Henry David Thoreau, *Faith in a Seed: The Dispersion of Seeds and Other Late Natural History Writings*, ed. Bradley P. Dean (Washington, D.C.: Island Press, 1993), 66.

(240) "We find ourselves . . .": Ibid., 101.

(240) "The very earth . . .": Ibid., 151.

(240) "That which seemed . . .": Ibid., 88.

(240) "The Wellingtonia gigantea . . .": Ibid., 178.

(241) The way of the gatherer is explored in Allen, *Grandmothers of the Light*, 12–14.

(241) "There are great obstacles . . .": *The I Ching*, 89.

(250) "Abbot Mark . . .": This story is adapted from Thomas Merton, trans., *Wisdom of the Desert* (Boston and London: Shambhala, 1994), 123.

(251) "passionate, idealistic . . .": Germaine Greer, *The Change: Women, Aging, and the Menopause* (New York: Knopf, 1992), 53.

(251-252) Gail Sheehy discusses her "introduction to the scandalous politics of menopause" in *The Silent Passage: Menopause* (New York: Random House, 1991), 15–23.

(253) "When a woman . . .": This story is adapted from Brooke Medicine Eagle's discussion of the Grandmother Lodge in her audiotape *Moon Time*, which can be ordered from Harmony Network, PO Box 2550, Guerneville, CA 95446; 707-869-0989.

(254) "The Kidney is . . .": Harriet Beinfield and Efrem Korngold, *Between Heaven and Earth: A Guide to Chinese Medicine* (New York: Ballantine, 1991), 125.

(258) For more information on hormone replacement therapy, see Saja Greenwood, M.D., *Menopause Naturally* (Volcano, Calif.: Volcano Press, 1989); Greer, *The Change*; Dee Ito, *Without Estrogen* (New York: Random House, 1994); Betty Kamin, *Hormonal Replacement: Yes or No* (Novato, Calif.: Nutritional Encounter, 1993); Linda Ojeda, *Menopause without Medicine* (Alameda, Calif.: Hunter House, 1992); Sheehy, *The Silent Passage*; and Sidney M. Wolfe, M.D., and the Public Citizen Health Research Group with Rhoda Donkin Jones, *Women's Health Alert: What Most Doctors Won't Tell You about Birth Control, C-Sections, Weight Control Products, Hormone Replacement Therapy, Osteoporosis, Breast Implants, Tranquilizers, Hysterectomies, and Other Medications, Procedures, and Conditions That Could Endanger Your Life* (Reading, Mass.: Addison-Wesley, 1991).

(259) The 1986 study is discussed in Wolfe et al., *Women's Health Alert*, 199.

(260) "Female reproductive hormones . . .": Ibid., 194.

(260) "the best way . . .": Christiane Northrup, M.D., *Women's Bodies* (New York: Bantam, 1994), 468.

(264) "A university professor . . .": This story appears in many collections; our version is adapted from Paul Reps, comp., *Zen Flesh, Zen Bones* (New York: Anchor Books, 1961), 5. See also Stephen

Levine, *Who Dies? An Investigation of Conscious Living and Conscious Dying* (New York: Anchor Books, 1982), 70.

(266) "Perhaps middle age . . .": Anne Morrow Lindbergh is quoted in Carol Spenard LaRusso, ed., *The Wisdom of Women* (San Rafael, Calif.: New World Library, 1992), 67.

(267) "Pragmatic Americans . . .": Luigi Barzini, *The Europeans* (London and New York: Penguin Books, 1984), 239.

(267) "After the last . . .": Ralph C. Wright, "Hysterectomy: Past, Present and Future," *Obstetrics and Gynecology* 35 (1969): 560.

(267) "Hysterectomy fits . . .": Dr. Eleanor B. Easley, "The Dilemma of Women in Our Culture: Gynecologic Repercussions, Part II," *American Journal of Obstetrics and Gynecology* 110 (1971): 858.

(267) "Menstruation is . . .": Editorial in *Lancet*, 15 August 1987, 376.

(269) "Most people begin . . .": Levine, *Who Dies?*, 34.

(269) "We could never . . .": Helen Keller is quoted in Melissa Stein, *The Wit and Wisdom of Women* (Philadelphia: Running Press, 1993), 122.

(270) "The brother had . . .": This story is adapted from Merton, *Wisdom of the Desert*, 48.

(271) "Mulla Nasrudin . . .": This story is adapted from Christina Feldman and Jack Kornfield, *Stories of the Spirit* (New York: HarperSanFrancisco, 1991), 241.

(276) The Chinese view of fibroids is shared by a growing number of mainstream medical practitioners; see Northrup, *Women's Bodies*, 84: "Whenever I see a woman with a uterine problem such as fibroid tumors—which are present in 40 percent of American women—I ask her to meditate upon her relationships, creativity, and sense of security. What is her fibroid telling her about these areas? Fibroids, endometriosis, diseases of the ovaries, and other pelvic disorders are manifestations of 'blocked energy' in the pelvis."

(277) "Everything that comes . . .": Lewis Thomas, *The Lives of a Cell: Notes of a Biology Watcher* (New York: Bantam, 1975), 116.

(277) "When the sun . . .": *The I Ching*, 338.

(278) "When I release . . .": Thoreau, *Faith in a Seed*, 432.

(278) "Think of the great . . .": Ibid., 93.

(279) "The story is told . . .": This story is adapted from Feldman and Kornfield, *Stories of the Spirit*, 392.

CHAPTER 16, WINTER: FROM BODY TO SOUL

(281) "If you stay . . .": Lao-tzu, *Tao te Ching*, trans. Stephen Mitchell (New York: HarperPerennial, 1991), 33.

(281) "Our Native people . . .": Brooke Medicine Eagle, *Buffalo Woman Comes Singing* (New York: Ballantine, 1991), 339. Emphasis in original.

(282) "You can't step . . .": Heraclitus is quoted in Stephen Mitchell, ed., *The Enlightened Mind: An Anthology of Sacred Prose* (New York: HarperPerennial, 1991), 8.

(282) "Ninety-eight percent . . .": Deepak Chopra, M.D., *Quantum Healing: Exploring the Frontiers of Mind/Body Medicine* (New York: Bantam, 1989), 48.

(283) "The changes are . . .": Richard Wilhelm and Cary F. Baynes, trans., *The I Ching*, 3rd ed. (Princeton: Princeton University Press, 1967), 323.

(284) "Why have you come? . . .": This story is adapted from Wolf Moondance, *Rainbow Medicine* (New York: Sterling, 1994), 147.

(285) "I am decaying . . .": Keri Hulme, *The Bone People* (New York: Penguin Books, 1986), 420.

(285) "I feel cold . . .": Ibid., 423.

(285) "Sea distant on the beach . . .": Ibid., 430.

(285) "I have faced Death . . .": Ibid., 436.

(295) "She sat in a wheelchair . . .": James Hillman, *A Blue Fire: Selected Writings by James Hillman* (New York: HarperCollins, 1991), 18.

(296) "Ramana Maharshi . . .": This story is adapted from Christina Feldman and Jack Kornfield, *Stories of the Heart* (New York: HarperSanFrancisco, 1991), 344.

(296) "The common honeybee . . .": Deepak Chopra, M.D., *Ageless Body, Timeless Mind: The Quantum Alternative to Growing Old* (New York: Harmony Books, 1993), 308.

(297) Chopra discusses the Tarahumara Indians in *Quantum Healing*, 220–221, 232.

(297) The flies experiment is discussed in the audiotaped series *The Quantum Healing Workshop with Deepak Chopra* (New York: Mystic Fire Audio, 1990).

(298) "Dew evaporates . . .": Issa, in *Japanese Haiku: Three Hundred and Thirty Examples of Seventeen-Syllable Poems* by Basho, Buson, Issa, Shiki, Sokan, Kikaku, Ransetsu, Joso, Yaha, Boncho, and others, in new translation (Mount Vernon, N.Y.: Peter Pauper, 1956).

(298) "When it is accepted . . .": Sherwin B. Nuland, *How We Die* (New York: Knopf, 1994), 87.

(298) "Death is the only . . .": Carlos Castaneda, *Journey to Ixtlan: The Lessons of San Juan* (New York: Simon & Schuster, 1972), 55.

(299) "The old woman . . .": This story was mentioned in Clarissa Pinkola Estés, Ph.D., *Women Who Run with the Wolves* (New York: Ballantine, 1992), 162.

(299) "We dance round . . .": Robert Frost, "The Secret Sits," in *Complete Poems of Robert Frost* (New York: Holt, Rinehart and Winston, 1962), 495.

(300) "No thought . . .": Lao-tzu is quoted in Jon Winokur, comp. and ed., *Zen to Go* (New York: New American Library, 1989), 110.

(300) "There is no beyond . . .": Iris Murdoch is quoted in Melissa Stein, *The Wit and Wisdom of Women* (Philadelphia: Running Press, 1993), 112.

(300) "Then I was . . .": Black Elk is quoted in Cousineau, *The Soul of the World*, who cites John G. Neihardt, *Black Elk Speaks* (New York: Washington Square Books, 1959).

(301) "each soul must . . .": Charles Alexander Eastman (Ohiyesa of the Santee Sioux) is quoted in Kent Nerburn and Louise Mengelkoch, *Native American Wisdom* (San Rafael, Calif.: New World Library, 1991), 57.

(301) "Copper Woman . . .": Anne Cameron, *The Daughters of Copper Woman* (Vancouver, B.C.: Press Gang, 1981), 53.

(302) "When Changing Woman . . .": Carolyn Niethammer, *Daughters of the Earth: The Lives and Legends of American Indian Women* (New York: Macmillan, 1977), 47. See also Carolyn McVickar Edwards, *The Storyteller's Goddess* (New York: HarperSanFrancisco, 1991), 60. Edwards attributes this story to the Navajos.

APPENDIX 2

We relied on several scholarly sources in our discussions of the different acupuncture points and their interpretations: Arnie Lade, *Acupuncture Points, Images and Functions* (Seattle: Eastland Press, 1989); Malvin Finkelstein, *The Energetic Function of Points* (Eugene, Ore.: Eugene Center for Acupuncture and Acupressure, 1984); and Andrew Ellis, Nigel Wiseman, and Ken Boss, *Grasping the Wind: An Exploration Into the Meaning of Chinese Acupuncture Point Names* (Brookline, Mass.: Paradigm, 1989).

INDEX

Calcium citrate, 292–93
Calendula, 208
Calomel, 60–61
Cameron, Anne, 191
Campbell, Joseph, 4, 16, 29, 31, 32
Camphorwood Gate acupoint, 250
Cancer, 4–5, 22–23, 259–60, 268, 273
Candida albicans, 202
Capra, Fritjof, 18–19, 89
Castaneda, Carlos, 298
Catholicism, 43–44
Centeredness, 300–301
Centering, 52–53, 57
Central Altar acupoint, 335
Central Pole acupoint, 172, 206, 217, 244–45,
    264, 290
  described, 333–34
Cerridwen, 316–17
Cervical dysplasia, 189
Cervical mucus, 180, 219
Cervix, 218–19
Chai Pai Di Huang Wan, 223
Chalice and the Blade, The (Eisler), 16
Change, cycle of, 79–84, 123, 282–84
Change, The (Greer), 251
Chang Huang, 213
Changing Woman, 302
Chang-O, 161, 312
Channels, 170–71, 289
Chasteberry, 175, 231, 233, 262, 263, 265,
    273, 275
  described, 309–10
Chemical medicines, 58–61, 69
Chest cold, 58
Chi, 85–88, 170–71, 205, 206, 217, 231
  aging process and, 254, 288
  ching, 134, 146
  constrained Liver, 272
  de, 172
  manipulating the energy of, 88
  reckless bleeding and, 243–44
  source, 245
  upright, 127
  wei, 134, 289
  yuan, 146
Childbearing, 35–36, 44
Children, 213–17, 235
Chlamydia, 202
Chlorine, 229
Cholera, 58
Cholesterol, 259, 268
Chong mo, 250
Chopra, Deepak, 282–83, 296–97
Christianity, witchcraft and, 38–45
Chronic yeast infections, 202–12
  acupuncture for, 206–207, 209, 212
  antibiotics and, 203
  Chinese interpretation, 210

Chinese patent remedies, 212
  diet for, 207, 211
  douche for, 208
  exercise and, 207
  Five Transforming Powers and, 203–206
  herbal allies for, 207–208, 211
  mind/body/spirit connection, 212
  pH level and, 202, 208
  stress and, 204
  supplements for, 207, 210–11
  topical strategies for, 211
  Western interpretation and treatment,
    210
Church, Catholic, and human dissection, 12
Cinnamon, 195
Circle of life, 4, 10, 133
Circulation Sex, 112, 113, 114
Cleavers, 233
Clement, Saint, 37
Clomid, 213
Codeine, 67
Coffin, Albert Isaiah, 50
Colic, 59
Columbus, Christopher, 58
Comfrey, 66
Communication, 14–15, 22
  breakdown in, 13–14, 55
Communicator, the, *see* Fire
Compassion, 4, 5
Compendium Maleficarum, 40, 41, 43
Conception Vessel 2 acupoint, 205
Conception Vessel 3 acupoint, 172, 205, 218,
    244–45, 264, 290
  described, 333–34
Conception Vessel 4 acupoint, 218, 245, 272,
    290
  described, 334–35
Conception Vessel 6 acupoint, 272
Conception Vessel 17 acupoint, 335
Confessions of a Medical Heretic (Mendelsohn),
    63
Confucius, 91
Congealed blood, 272
Connelly, Dianne, 114
Conscious fertility, 219
Contemplation, 82, 132
Control Cycle, 94
  Generation Cycle combined with, 95
Copernicus, 45
Copper Woman (Cameron), 191, 301–302
Core Issues, 132
Coronary artery disease, 63
Corpus luteum, 181, 228, 273
Corsello, Dr. Serafina, 219, 231
Cosmology, 45
Cramping, 183, 184–85
  acupoints for, 185
  body/mind/spirit connection for, 185